Smart Medical Data Sensing and IoT Systems Design in Healthcare

Chinmay Chakraborty
Birla Institute of Technology, India

A volume in the Advances in Healthcare Information Systems and Administration (AHISA) Book Series

IGI Global
DISSEMINATOR OF KNOWLEDGE

Published in the United States of America by
IGI Global
Medical Information Science Reference (an imprint of IGI Global)
701 E. Chocolate Avenue
Hershey PA, USA 17033
Tel: 717-533-8845
Fax: 717-533-8661
E-mail: cust@igi-global.com
Web site: http://www.igi-global.com

Library of Congress Cataloging-in-Publication Data

Names: Chakraborty, Chinmay, 1984- editor.
Title: Smart medical data sensing and IoT systems design in healthcare / Chinmay Chakraborty, editor.
Description: Hershey PA : Medical Information Science Reference, [2020] | Includes bibliographical references.
Identifiers: LCCN 2019019595| ISBN 9781799802617 (hardcover) | ISBN 9781799802624 (ebook)
Subjects: | MESH: Internet | Delivery of Health Care | Medical Informatics | Telemedicine | Smartphone
Classification: LCC R858 | NLM W 26.55.C7 | DDC 610.285--dc23 LC record available at https://lccn.loc.gov/2019019595

This book is published in the IGI Global book series Advances in Healthcare Information Systems and Administration (AHISA) (ISSN: 2328-1243; eISSN: 2328-126X)

British Cataloguing in Publication Data
A Cataloguing in Publication record for this book is available from the British Library.

All work contributed to this book is new, previously-unpublished material. The views expressed in this book are those of the authors, but not necessarily of the publisher.

For electronic access to this publication, please contact: eresources@igi-global.com.

Advances in Healthcare Information Systems and Administration (AHISA) Book Series

Anastasius Moumtzoglou
Hellenic Society for Quality & Safety in Healthcare and P. & A. Kyriakou Children's Hospital, Greece

ISSN:2328-1243
EISSN:2328-126X

Mission

The **Advances in Healthcare Information Systems and Administration (AHISA) Book Series** aims to provide a channel for international researchers to progress the field of study on technology and its implications on healthcare and health information systems. With the growing focus on healthcare and the importance of enhancing this industry to tend to the expanding population, the book series seeks to accelerate the awareness of technological advancements of health information systems and expand awareness and implementation.

Driven by advancing technologies and their clinical applications, the emerging field of health information systems and informatics is still searching for coherent directing frameworks to advance health care and clinical practices and research. Conducting research in these areas is both promising and challenging due to a host of factors, including rapidly evolving technologies and their application complexity. At the same time, organizational issues, including technology adoption, diffusion and acceptance as well as cost benefits and cost effectiveness of advancing health information systems and informatics applications as innovative forms of investment in healthcare are gaining attention as well. **AHISA** addresses these concepts and critical issues.

Coverage

- Decision Support Systems
- Virtual health technologies
- Role of informatics specialists
- Medical Informatics
- Rehabilitative Technologies
- E-Health and M-Health
- IT security and privacy issues
- Clinical Decision Support Design, Development and Implementation
- Measurements and Impact of HISA on Public and Social Policy
- IT Applications in Physical Therapeutic Treatments

IGI Global is currently accepting manuscripts for publication within this series. To submit a proposal for a volume in this series, please contact our Acquisition Editors at Acquisitions@igi-global.com or visit: http://www.igi-global.com/publish/.

The Advances in Healthcare Information Systems and Administration (AHISA) Book Series (ISSN 2328-1243) is published by IGI Global, 701 E. Chocolate Avenue, Hershey, PA 17033-1240, USA, www.igi-global.com. This series is composed of titles available for purchase individually; each title is edited to be contextually exclusive from any other title within the series. For pricing and ordering information please visit http://www.igi-global.com/book-series/advances-healthcare-information-systems-administration/37156. Postmaster: Send all address changes to above address.

Titles in this Series

For a list of additional titles in this series, please visit: www.igi-global.com/book-series

Emerging Trends and Innovations in Privacy and Health Information Management
Cristina Albuquerque (University of Coimbra, ortugal)
Medical Information Science Reference • ©2019 • 376pp • H/C (ISBN: 9781522584704) • US $275.00

Mobile Health Applications for Quality Healthcare Delivery
Anastasius Moumtzoglou (P&A Kyriakou Children's Hospital, Greece)
Medical Information Science Reference • ©2019 • 327pp • H/C (ISBN: 9781522580218) • US $265.00

Intelligent Systems for Healthcare Management and Delivery
Nardjes Bouchemal (University Center of Mila, Algeria)
Medical Information Science Reference • ©2019 • 377pp • H/C (ISBN: 9781522570714) • US $245.00

Human Rights, Public Values, and Leadership in Healthcare Policy
Augustine Nduka Eneanya (University of Lagos, Nigeria)
Medical Information Science Reference • ©2019 • 311pp • H/C (ISBN: 9781522561330) • US $225.00

Contemporary Applications of Mobile Computing in Healthcare Settings
R. Rajkumar (VIT University, India)
Medical Information Science Reference • ©2018 • 259pp • H/C (ISBN: 9781522550365) • US $205.00

Handbook of Research on Emerging Perspectives on Healthcare Information Systems and Informatics
Joseph Tan (McMaster University, Canada)
Medical Information Science Reference • ©2018 • 641pp • H/C (ISBN: 9781522554608) • US $355.00

Big Data Analytics in HIV/AIDS Research
Ali Al Mazari (Alfaisal University, Saudi Arabia)
Medical Information Science Reference • ©2018 • 294pp • H/C (ISBN: 9781522532033) • US $215.00

Advanced Systems for Improved Public Healthcare and Disease Prevention Emerging Research and Opportunities
Thierry Oscar Edoh (Technical University of Munich, Germany)
Medical Information Science Reference • ©2018 • 262pp • H/C (ISBN: 9781522555285) • US $185.00

Global Perspectives on Health Communication in the Age of Social Media
Seif Sekalala (Kean University, USA) and Brandon C. Niezgoda (Drexel University, USA)
Medical Information Science Reference • ©2018 • 348pp • H/C (ISBN: 9781522537168) • US $225.00

IGI Global
DISSEMINATOR OF KNOWLEDGE

701 East Chocolate Avenue, Hershey, PA 17033, USA
Tel: 717-533-8845 x100 • Fax: 717-533-8661
E-Mail: cust@igi-global.com • www.igi-global.com

Table of Contents

Detailed Table of Contents

Mobile health (mHealth), the application of mobile technologies for healthcare services, has been the driving force in healthcare in the last few decades; from healthcare service delivery to low-cost tools for effective disease diagnosis, prediction, monitoring, and management. The main purpose of this chapter was to identify the scope and range of studies on mHealth used as low-cost tools for effective disease diagnosis, prediction, monitoring, and management. The authors identified 55 papers that met the inclusion and exclusion criteria after searching different academic databases. The findings revealed that low-cost mHealth approaches such as text messaging and mobile applications developed using artificial intelligence algorithms have been used for disease diagnosis, prediction, monitoring, and management. The findings of this scoping review present information regarding different mHealth approaches that can be used by researchers and practitioners interested in the application of low-cost mHealth solutions in low-resource settings.

Security is the primary issue nowadays because cybercrimes are increasing. The organizations can store and maintain their data on their own, but it is not cost effective, so for convenience they are choosing cloud. Due to its popularity, the healthcare organizations are storing their sensitive data to cloud-based storage systems, that is, electronic health records (EHR). One of the most feasible methods for maintaining privacy is homomorphism encryption (HE). HE can combine different services without losing security or displaying sensitive data. HE is nothing but computations performed on encrypted data. According to the type of operations and limited number of operations performed on encrypted data, it is categorized into three types: partially homomorphic encryption (PHE), somewhat homomorphic encryption (SWHE), fully homomorphic encryption (FHE). HE method is very suitable for the EHR, which requires data privacy and security.

Nearest neighbor algorithms like kNN and Parzen Window are generative algorithms that are used extensively for medical diagnosis and classification of diseases. The data generated or collected in healthcare is high dimensional and cannot be assumed to follow a particular distribution. The conventional approaches fail due to computational complexity, curse of dimensionality, and varying distributions. Hence, this chapter deals with a blending technique for evaluation of nearest neighbor algorithms based on various parameters such as the size of data, dimensions of data, window size, and number of nearest neighbors to make it suitable for massive datasets. Dimensionality reduction and clustering are combined with nearest neighbor classifier such as kNN and Parzen Window to observe the performance of the blended models on various types of datasets. Experimental results on 15 real datasets with various models reveal the efficacy of the proposed blends.

Telemedicine is defined as the means of providing healthcare for people from a distance by the use of telecommunication and information technology. This technology is mainly useful in overcoming the obstacles of distance and provide enhancement in the access of medical services that would not be easily available in different rural areas. Telemedicine security includes issues such as confidentiality, integrity, and authentication that are also present in other systems involving information and data. Maintaining integrity of data stored and used is a huge problem for medical applications because it contains more sensitive medical records of patients which can cause severe ill effects on slight modification. In order to resolve the confidentiality and integrity issues of telemedicine applications, medical image encryption and watermarking comes into play. The security issues in telemedicine applications is to be given higher importance and thus choosing a reliable and effective approach or framework is more essential.

Health monitoring plays a vital role to overcome the health issues of the patients. According to research, approximately 2000 people die due to carelessness of monitoring their health. Wearable monitoring systems record the activities of daily life. A 24-hour wearable monitoring system was developed and changes were identified. This project is designed for helping the soldiers to maintain their health conditions and to identify their health issues at war's end. Different health parameters are monitored using sensors, and the data are transmitted through GSM to the receiver, and the received data are analyzed using convolutional neural networks, which is performed in cloud IoT. If any abnormalities are found during the analyzing process, the message is sent to military personnel and the doctor at the camp so that they could take necessary actions to recover the ill soldier from the war field and provide emergency assistance on time. The location of the soldier is also shared using the input from GPS modem in the smart jacket.

Remote medical health management is the most attractive research field in the domain of WSN. Wireless body area network (WBAN) produces constant, unbroken observation of the patient. Basically, WBAN acts as the appliance of internet of things (IoT) which offers an opportunity to a medical examiner to supervise chronic disease. Dissimilar protocols, guidelines, policies have been developed and developing in the last decade. In WBAN, minute power sensor nodes deployed toward capturing unusual essential signs of patients at home, hospitals in support of analysis purpose and furthermore advise suitable procedures. The main goal of this chapter is to introduce a complete and advanced understanding of WBANs, energy savings methods, human activity monitoring procedures, challenges and research issues, applications, and a comprehensive literature survey.

Elderly monitoring has become essential to provide comfort and flexible life for the aged. Internet of things is a field that aids in providing accurate information through communication. Using these devices, emergency alerts can be raised. The chapter provides an assistance model that aids the caretakers and doctors to provide appropriate action during emergencies. Different conditions of the patient are considered to analyze the working of the system. The work shows considerable amount of flexibility from the previous system.

In this chapter, the major enhanced techniques of internet of healthcare things (IoHT) with wearable sensor technologies (WST), stationary medical devices (SMD), and integrated system technologies (IST) for heterogeneous healthcare professionals are explored. A detailed view of the system architecture for developing IoHT device and a lot of issues are also described. The latest innovative technologies are realistic to specific purposes in the field of healthcare assessment. Analysis, sensor, and data studies approach the opportunities to improve personal healthcare and benefits for the medical industry. The ultimate aim of succeeding superior healthcare practice is to competently combine with information from diverse bases, to allocate the accumulated data, to retrieve the collected data. Effective data analysis tools from data with initialed conception services are needed while maintaining their security and privacy. Healthcare professionals, patients, and clients can take benefit of the IoHT for giving personalized smart care guidelines or solutions for existing technologies.

Epilepsy is a disorder that affects the life of the patient. In this neurological disorder, patients may suffer from different types of seizures. From epileptic patients, we may acquire electroencephalogram (EEG) data using various kinds of sensors and transmit them through the cloud. In this chapter, the authors have discussed various platforms related to IoT-enabled cloud for sharing the information and to get quick response in form suggestion. Use of smartphone applications for real-time monitoring of patients and for other applications is presented here. Various wearable devices may provide huge benefits for taking care of seizures and patients. The authors proposed a system model based on IoT-enabled cloud for sharing the information with various sensors and other devices to make a proper judgment about seizures, which will be able to provide improved e-health service. With the increasing rate of improvement in both IoT and e-health field, it is now a challenge to upgrade ourselves and work with the digital world to provide low cost, accurate, and quick solutions.

The emergence of internet of things allows the integration of health systems by enabling real-time monitoring with a low cost. Therefore, one of the essential targets in this work is the realization of a new smart real-time electrocardiogram remote monitoring system based on cloud networks. This health wireless system allows the acquisition of electrocardiogram signal with the temperature and acceleration measurement of the patient's body using the inertial measurement unit module sensor. A strong access schemes is employed to transfer the data from sensors to cloud environment by keeping the protection of e-health information. The second objective in this chapter is designing a flexible and stretchable health circuit basing on design considerations, aiming the combination of flexible, elastic, and rigid materials around minimal constraints and maximum mechanical dependability in the structures. The flexible fabrication part was inspired from the biocompatible process technology.

Foreword

I am pleased to write the foreword for this edited book on *Smart Medical Data Sensing and IoT Systems Design in Healthcare*. This book concisely describes the methods to handle and process the sensed medical data, and finally, the processed information is accessible to health practitioner/doctors at any place and at any time with the help of Internet of Thing (IoT) healthcare system.

Healthcare is the maintenance or improvement of health via the prevention, diagnosis, and treatment of disease, illness, injury, and other physical and mental impairments in human beings. To accomplish this task, many data are gathered about a patient. These data are either generated manually by regular and repeated observation or may be by digital means by using various machines. These data are of various type and format. Some are image-based; some are text, some are sound, some are electrical signals, etc. To extract the information about a patient from such heterogeneous data is a vast and complicated task and requires many tools and techniques.

Furthermore, the book divides into two sections, which provide the complete steps for an end to end solution in the healthcare domain. First section deals with the different medical data handling, gathering and classification techniques, and later part discuss the IoT healthcare system and its security.

This book handles different types of data records for analysis of patient's health condition and transmission of patient's health condition information with security. This is one of the unique features of this book, which makes it stand apart.

The book also describes the algorithms on how to deal with high dimensional medical data and how to store in the cloud and how to keep this data securely. It also focuses on the different types of data security algorithms for data stored in the cloud and during the transmission of medical information.

This book provides an exposure toward the challenges and solution towards healthcare IoT system. This book also provides an application for handling epileptical seizure and ECG signal through IoT system. This book helps in the field of analysis of medical and healthcare data gathering, classification and study in a comprehensive way and enumerates the evolutions of such tools and techniques to make the data available at any point of time and any place through the IoT healthcare platform.

In this new age of global interconnectivity and interdependence, it is necessary to provide medical information to health practitioners and patients, with state-of-the-art knowledge in the field of healthcare monitoring. This book is a good step in that direction.

It is my hope and expectation that this book will provide a useful learning experience and referenced resource for all healthcare professionals.

Bharat Gupta
National Institute of Technology, Patna, India

Preface

Smart healthcare technology can be defined as using smartphone and electronic technology for good diagnosis of the diseases, improves treatment of the patients, and enhanced quality of lives. Technology-enabled healthcare provides the current and future needs of medical organizations, providers, telemedical agents, patients, and doctors. This is the most emerging and demanding platform for the population. This technology gives easy to access facility, supports emergency care service, expanded usage, enhanced impact, and extended communications. This technology is used to minimize the gaps between major medical facilities such as clinics and providers such as general practitioners. The end-to-end clinical data connectivity involves the development of many technologies that should enable reliable and location-agnostic communication between a patient and a healthcare provider. Mhealth and eHealth are the major components of the smart healthcare system for medical data sharing between patients and healthcare providers. Smart healthcare can reduce the time, cost, and risk of Internet of Things (IoT) deployments in healthcare, and gives superior efficiency and patient care. The medical data protection is one of the main challenges nowadays for end-to-end delivery. Internet of Medical Things is the major technological innovation which has included the element of "smartness" in the healthcare industry and also identifying, monitoring and informing service providers about the patient's clinical information with faster delivery of care services. Big Data helps to build a smart healthcare system for the machine-to-machine and machine-to-home large volumes of medical data processing. The cloud-assisted medical framework is used to enhance the strength of the smart healthcare system because of cost savings, scalability, and system flexibility.

OBJECTIVE

The aim of this book is to provide innovation in healthcare technology and the recent trends on the phenomena of smart medical data sensing and processing. This book focuses on robust and easy solutions in the delivery of medical information from patients-to-doctors with an accurate diagnosis. This book will be focused to publish the original research outcomes towards healthcare using various useful technological developments. The objective is to initiate conversations among technologists, engineers, scientists, and clinicians to synergize their efforts in producing low-cost, high-performance, highly efficient, deployable IoT systems in healthcare systems. The book will additionally investigate the potential for making faster advances in many scientific disciplines and improving the profitability and success of different enterprises.

BOOK ORGANISATION

The book content is organized as follow:

The book is structured into two main sections: (1) Smart Medical Data and (2) IoT Healthcare System. The summary of the chapters is presented here briefly. This book consists of 11 excellent chapters in the field of smart healthcare technology.

Section 1: Smart Medical Data

Section 1 of this book compromises five chapters that highlight the performance of smart medical data.

mHealth: A Low-Cost Approach for Effective Disease Diagnosis, Prediction, Monitoring, and Management

This chapter discusses the Mobile health (mHealth) system for healthcare services. The aim of this chapter is to identify the scope and range of studies on mHealth used as low-cost tools for effective disease diagnosis, prediction, monitoring, and management. The findings revealed that low-cost mHealth approaches such as text messaging and mobile applications developed using artificial intelligence algorithms have been used for disease diagnosis, prediction, monitoring, and management. The findings of this scoping review present information regarding different mHealth approaches which can be used by researchers and practitioners interested in the application of low-cost mHealth solutions in low-resource settings.

Electronic Health Record Security in Cloud: Medical Data Protection Using Homomorphic Encryption Schemes

This chapter deals with sensitive medical data protection using robust encryption schemes. Here one of the most feasible methods for maintaining privacy is Homomorphism Encryption. According to the type of operations and a limited number of operations performed on encrypted data, it is categorized into three types like Partially Homomorphic Encryption (PHE), Somewhat Homomorphic Encryption (SWHE), and Fully Homomorphic Encryption (FHE). The homomorphism Encryption algorithm is very suitable for the EHR which requires data privacy and security.

Blended Models for Nearest Neighbor Algorithms for High Dimensional Smart Medical Data

This chapter mainly deals with a blending technique for evaluation of Nearest neighbor algorithms based on various parameters such as the size of data, dimensions of data, window size and number of nearest neighbors to make it suitable for massive datasets. Nearest neighbor algorithms like kNN and Parzen Window are generative algorithms which are used extensively for medical diagnosis and classification of diseases. The data generated or collected in health care is high dimensional and cannot be assumed to follow a particular distribution. The conventional approaches fail due to computational complexity, the curse of dimensionality and varying distributions. Dimensionality reduction and clustering are combined with the nearest neighbor classifier such as kNN and Parzen window to observe the performance of the blended models on various types of datasets. Experimental results on 15 real datasets with various models reveal the efficacy of the proposed blends.

Developing Security Solutions for Telemedicine Applications: Medical Image Encryption and Watermarking

This chapter presents the security solutions for telemedicine application, mainly for sensed medical data protection. Telemedicine is mainly useful in overcoming the obstacles of distance and provide an enhancement in the access to medical services that would not be easily available in different rural areas. Telemedicine security includes issues such as confidentiality, integrity, and authentication that are also present in other systems involving information and data. Maintaining the integrity of data stored and used is a huge problem for medical applications because it contains more sensitive medical records of patients which can cause severe ill effects on slight modification. In order to resolve the confidentiality and integrity issues of telemedicine applications, medical image encryption and Watermarking comes into play. The security issues in telemedicine applications are to be given higher importance and thus choosing a reliable and effective approach or framework is more essential.

Smart Healthcare Monitoring System for War-End Soldiers Using CNN

This chapter is designed for helping the soldiers to maintain their health conditions and to identify their health issues at war end. Different health parameters are monitored using sensors and the data are transmitted through GSM to the receiver and the received data are analyzed using Convolutional Neural Networks which is performed in cloud IoT. If any abnormalities are found during the analyzing process the message is sent to military personnel and the doctor at the camp, so that they could take necessary actions to recover the ill soldier from the war field and provide emergency assistance on time. The location of the soldier is also shared using the input from the GPS modem in the smart jacket. A 24-hour wearable monitoring system was developed and changes were identified.

Section 2: IoT Healthcare System

Section 2 of this book compromises six chapters that focus on presenting the role of IoT in the healthcare system.

Wireless Body Sensor Networks for Patient Health Monitoring: Security, Challenges, Applications – IoT Healthcare Management

The chapter discusses the recent trends of Wireless body area networks (WBANs) for patients monitoring. Remote medical health management is the most attractive research field in the domain of WSN. Basically WBAN act as the appliance of IoT which offer an opportunity to a medical examiner to supervise chronicle disease. Dissimilar protocols, guidelines, policies have been developed and developing from the last decade. In WBAN minute power sensor nodes deployed toward capturing unusual essential signs of patients at home, hospitals in support of analysis purpose furthermore advise suitable procedures. The main goal of this chapter is to introduce a complete and advanced understanding of WBANs, energy savings methods, Human activity monitoring procedures, challenges and research issues, applications, comprehensive literature survey and a small introduction to Next-generation wireless sensor networks.

Methodical IoT-Based Information System in Healthcare

This chapter describes various challenges and limitations of IoT-based healthcare information systems. Elderly monitoring hence has become essential to provide comfort and flexible life for the aged ones. IoT is a field that aids in providing accurate information by communicating with each other. Using these devices emergency alert can be raised and alerted the respective. This chapter provides an assistance model that aids the caretakers and doctors to provide appropriate action during emergencies. Different conditions of the patient are considered to analyze the working of the system. The work shows a considerable amount of flexibility from the previous system.

Feasible Challenges and Applications of IoT in Healthcare: Essential Architecture and Challenges in Various Fields of Internet of Healthcare Things

In this chapter, the major enhanced techniques of Internet of Healthcare Things (IoHT) with Wearable Sensor Technologies (WST), Stationary Medical devices (SMD) and Integrated System Technologies (IST) for heterogeneous healthcare professionals. A detailed view of the system architecture for developing IoHT device, a lot of issues, impugns of trending IoHT, to researchers are also described. The latest innovative technologies are realistic to specific purposes in the field of healthcare assessment, analysis, Sensor and data studies approach the opportunities to improve personal healthcare and benefits for the medical industry. The ultimate aim of succeeding superior healthcare practice is to competently combine with information from diverse bases, to allocate the accumulated data, to retrieve the collected data. So effective data analysis tools from data with initialed conception services are needed while maintaining their security and privacy. Healthcare professionals, patients, and clients can take benefit of the IoHT for giving personalized smart care guidelines or solutions for existing technologies.

Role of Sensors in Medical and Industrial Perspective Under IoT

This chapter highlights the recent advancement of IoT for medical and industry perspective. The two things (sensors and actuators) are playing a vital role in an IoT ecosystem. This chapter focuses on the role of different sensors in the medical field for human health status monitoring and the Industrial Internet of Things (IIoT) to monitor production processes and reduces the complexity of the process. In this chapter, we are going to discuss how to connect different sensors to these prototype boards and how to interact with them for medical and industrial applications. Further, it is very important to read the sensor data set carefully before connecting it to apply to avoid damage. This chapter is to explore the technological advancement of sensors-IoT using various sensors used in medical and industrial fields for data collection, processing, storage, and manipulation.

Sensing and Monitoring of Epileptic Seizure Under the IoT Platform

Epilepsy is a kind of disorder which affects the life of the patient. In this neurological disorder, patients may suffer from different types of seizures. From epileptic patients, we may acquire Electroencephalogram (EEG) data using various kinds of sensors and transmit them through the cloud. In this chapter, we have discussed various platforms related to IoT enabled cloud for sharing the information and to get a quick response in the form suggestion. Use of smartphone applications for real-time monitoring of patients and for other applications is going to present here. Various wearable devices may provide huge benefits for taking care of seizures and patients. We proposed a system model based on IoT enabled cloud for sharing the information with various sensors and other devices to make a proper judgment about seizures, which will be able to provide improved e-health service. With the increasing rate of improvement in both IoT and e-health field, it is now challenging to upgrade our self and work with the digital world, to provide low cost, accurate and quick solutions.

Smart ECG Monitoring Through IoT

The emergence of IoT allows the integration of health systems in the significant domain by enabling real-time monitoring at a low cost. Therefore, one of the essential targets in this work is the realization of a new smart Real-Time Electro-Cardio-Gram (ECG) remote monitoring system based on Cloud networks. This health wireless system allows the acquisition of the ECG signal with the temperature and acceleration measurement of the patient's body using the Inertial Measurement Unit module sensor. A strong access scheme is employed to transfer the data from sensors to the Cloud environment by keeping the protection of e-health information. The second objective in this chapter is designing a flexible and stretchable health circuit basing on design considerations, aiming the combination of flexible, elastic and rigid materials around minimal constraints and maximum mechanical dependability in the structures. The flexible fabrication part was inspired by the biocompatible process technology.

TARGET AUDIENCE

The target audience is constituted by students of Engineering and allied branches; Engineers, Research Scientists, Academicians, technology developers will benefit from reading this book. This book will be a collective resource with comprehensive knowledge in the field of medical imaging and healthcare technology. Contributions to this publication will be made by innovation and technology management practitioners and academics throughout the world.

Acknowledgment

I would like to acknowledge the help of all the people involved in this project and, more specifically, to the authors and reviewers that took part in the review process. Without their support, this book would not have become a reality.

First, the editors would like to thank each one of the authors for their contributions. Our sincere gratitude goes to the chapter's authors who contributed their time and expertise to this book.

Second, the editor wishes to acknowledge the valuable contributions of the reviewers regarding the improvement of quality, coherence, and content presentation of chapters.

I would like to express my gratitude to the global manager team of IGI global for their suggestions and helps in order to make this work much less painful than it could be.

Thank you finally to the authors who will recognize themselves here, for their participation so precious and especially for their availability which allowed me to realize in good conditions this project.

Chinmay Chakraborty
Birla Institute of Technology, India
August 2019

Chapter 1
mHealth:
A Low-Cost Approach for Effective Disease Diagnosis, Prediction, Monitoring and Management - Effective Disease Diagnosis

Gloria Ejehiohen Iyawa
Namibia University of Science and Technology, Namibia

Collins Oduor Ondiek
United States International University, Kenya

Jude Odiakaosa Osakwe
Namibia University of Science and Technology, Namibia

ABSTRACT

Mobile health (mHealth), the application of mobile technologies for healthcare services, has been the driving force in healthcare in the last few decades; from healthcare service delivery to low-cost tools for effective disease diagnosis, prediction, monitoring, and management. The main purpose of this chapter was to identify the scope and range of studies on mHealth used as low-cost tools for effective disease diagnosis, prediction, monitoring, and management. The authors identified 55 papers that met the inclusion and exclusion criteria after searching different academic databases. The findings revealed that low-cost mHealth approaches such as text messaging and mobile applications developed using artificial intelligence algorithms have been used for disease diagnosis, prediction, monitoring, and management. The findings of this scoping review present information regarding different mHealth approaches that can be used by researchers and practitioners interested in the application of low-cost mHealth solutions in low-resource settings.

DOI: 10.4018/978-1-7998-0261-7.ch001

INTRODUCTION

According to Iyawa, Herselman and Botha (2016, p.246), digital health can be defined as "an improvement in the way healthcare provision is conceived and delivered by healthcare providers through the use of information and communication technologies to monitor and improve the wellbeing and health of patients and to empower patients in the management of their health and that of their families." This definition suggests that digital health goes beyond the traditional approach of providing care with the use of certain technologies, but encompasses the outcome of the use of these digital technologies for healthcare. As such, there must be an improvement in health outcomes after adopting these technologies for the management of patients' health. Mesko et al. (2017, p.1) define digital health as "the cultural transformation of how disruptive technologies that provide digital and objective data accessible to both caregivers and patients leads to an equal level doctor-patient relationship with shared decision-making and the democratization of care." This definition suggests that technologies can enable patients to take part in the healthcare delivery process. Some of these digital health technologies include mobile technologies for healthcare, also referred to as mobile health (mHealth), wearables and sensors (Iyawa, Botha and Herselman, 2016). The literature adequately captures how these technologies have been used for improved health outcomes (Teng et al., 2019; Shabut et al., 2018; Seppala et al., 2019).

mHealth

mHealth has gained attention recently because of its capabilities and applicability in low-resource settings (Heimerl et al., 2015). The World Health Organisation (2011, p. 6) describes mHealth as a "component of e-health". Electronic health (e-health) presents a broader view on the use of computer technologies as Oh et al. (2005) emphasizes that e-health supports activities relating to providing healthcare services. Chakraborty (2019, p. 99) explains that e-health services are "driven by computers." mHealth, thus, relates to supporting activities relating to providing healthcare services through the use of mobile technologies (Park, 2016). Some studies have been specific about what constitutes mobile technologies. For example, Singh and Panjwani (2016) describe wearable technologies as a type of mobile technology. According to Wilson and Liang (2018, p.1), a wearable technology consists of "items (often with electronic capabilities) worn with acceptable function and aesthetic properties, consisting of a simple interface to perform set tasks to satisfy needs of a specific group." In addition, Kamisalic et al. (2018) suggest that wearable technologies can be linked to mobile phones to support engagement with the user. Wearable technologies are usually linked to sensors to gather data about the patients' health (Wilson and Liang, 2018). This suggests that mHealth does not only support healthcare processes but can also be used to gather information related to patients' health.

mHealth, Sensors and Internet-of-Things (IoT)

Wireless sensor networks (WSNs) can be defined as "a network of devices, denoted as nodes, which can sense the environment and communicate the information gathered from the monitored field" (Burrati et al., 2009). Manisha and Nandal (2015) also suggest that mobile devices are part of WSNs. The inclusion of mobile technologies such as mobile phones as sensor devices have been useful in diagnosing and predicting health conditions of patients (Munos et al., 2016). Ali et al. (2015, p.38) describe Internet-of-Things (IoT) as the inclusion of "Internet" technology and "wireless sensor networks." This suggests that sensing devices in a networked mode can transmit information to other locations with the use of the Internet, thereby extending the capabilities of WSNs to a larger platform. Almotiri et al. (2016) provdes instances on how mHealth devices have been connected to IoT. Almotiri et al. (2016) also suggest that data gathered from mHealth devices can be kept in a platform which can be accessed by health care practitioners to keep track of diabetes, heart rate of patients, hypertension and asthma. Examples of mHealth sensors include microphone sensors for diagnosing certain diseases from a distant location, camera sensors for diagnosisng diseases through pictures which are sent to medical practitioners at distant locations, and location-based sensor for detecting patients' activities (Stankevich et al., 2012).

There is an upsurge in the use of mobile technologies for disease diagnosis, prediction, monitoring and management (Jonas et al., 2015; Hosu et al., 2017; Calabria et al., 2017;Carrera et al., 2016; Park et al., 2019). This includes mHealth in different areas such as mental health (Teng et al., 2019, Stamate et al., 2017, Seppala et al., 2019), maternal health (Muller et al., 2019; Tang et al., 2019, Chan et al., 2019), asthma (Kagen and Garland, 2019; Cook et al., 2016) and diabetes (Agarwal et al., 2019; Istepanian and Al-anzi, 2018; Holtz and Lauckner, 2012; Iyawa, Velusamy and Palanisamy, 2019). The reason for this development is the adoption of mobile technologies especially rural communities (Afolayan et al., 2015; Iyawa and Coleman, 2015). The use of mobile technologies for disease diagnosis has proven to be beneficial, especially in low-resource settings (Chin et al., 2013). In less developed areas, access to healthcare services can be challenging for reasons such as, not being able to afford medical services and health centres located in distant locations (Peters et al., 2008). mHealth presents a platform in which low-cost tools can be used in accessing medical services, which could be through the use of mobile phones to diagnose certain diseases (Wood et al., 2019) and receiving health-related information (Karazs et al., 2013).

Empirical studies have been conducted on the use of mobile technologies for disease diagnosis, prediction, monitoring and management (Oyelami, 2012, Hosu et al., 2017; Calabria et al., 2017; Gandhi et al., 2017; Alloghani et al., 2016), reviews have also been conducted on the subject (Bates and Zumla, 2015; Mohammadzadeh and Safdari, 2014; Jutel and Lupton, 2015). A missing link in the literature is the scope and range of studies on the use of mobile technologies for disease diagnosis, prediction, monitoring and management. It is important to understand what already exists in the literature regarding the use of mobile technologies for disease diagnosis, prediction, monitoring and management in order to identify the benefits of this approach as well as the gap in the current research. This chapter contributes to the existing body of literature on the use of mobile technologies for diagnosing, predicting, monitoring and managing diseases. The findings of this chapter present information regarding different mHealth approaches which can be used by researchers and practitioners interested in the application of low-cost mHealth solutions in low-resource settings.

The purpose of this chapter was to identify the scope and range of studies on the use of mobile technologies for disease diagnosis, prediction, monitoring and management. This chapter is structured as follows: the methodology section is presented, then the findings of the scoping review and discussion are presented in line with the guidelines of a scoping review. The chapter ends with the conclusion and future work.

METHODOLOGY

Munn et al. (2018) state that a scoping review is necessary when there is a need to provide a summary of existing literature on a specific topic. While Peterson et al. (2017) explain that there is no single definition of a scoping review, they admit that a scoping review presents an overview of the literature. A scoping review was, therefore, appropriate for this study as it aimed to provide an overview of studies on mHealth as low-cost tools for disease diagnosis, prediction, monitoring and management.

The guidelines for conducting a scoping review as presented by Arksey and O'Malley (2005) were followed in this chapter. The scoping review was conducted in five stages which are presented below.

Identifying the Research Question

The research questions posed in this chapter are outlined as follows:

- What is being discussed about mHealth as an approach for disease diagnosis in the current literature?
- What is being discussed about mHealth as an approach for disease prediction in the current literature?
- What is being discussed about mHealth as an approach for disease monitoring in the current literature?
- What is being discussed about mHealth as an approach for disease management in the current literature?

Identifying Relevant Studies

We searched three academic databases including IEEE Xplore, ACM Digital Library and Science Direct. We also searched Google Scholar and Google Search Engine. We used keywords "mobile health", "mobile health", mHealth", "mhealth", "mobile phones", "mobile technology", "disease", "diagnosis". "prediction", "monitoring" and "management". The search was conducted from 2009 to 2019.

Our inclusion and exclusion criteria were based on the following:

- We excluded papers that were not related to mobile technologies
- We excluded papers that did not explain how mobile technologies can be used for disease diagnosis, prediction, monitoring or management
- We excluded papers that were not published in English
- We excluded paper that focused on frameworks
- We included papers published between 2009 and 2019
- We included journal and conference papers

Study Selection

We identified an initial number of 1383 papers. However, after we removed duplicate publications, 1083 papers remained. We looked at the paper titles for relevance and in this process, we removed 538 irrelevant papers. We read the abstract of the remaining 545 papers and we only found 87 relevant papers. 87 full-text publications were read, however, only 55 papers met the inclusion and exclusion criteria.

Charting the Data

The summary of our findings is presented in Table 1 below.

Table 1. mHealth for disease diagnosis, prediction, monitoring and management

Author(s)	Year of publication	Technology/approach used	Disease type	Diagnosis	Prediction	Monitoring	Management
Lewinski et al.	2019	• Text messaging	• Diabetes • Hypertension	-	-	-	✓
Salimien et al.	2019	• Mobile app	• Cancer	-	-	-	✓
Almeida et al.	2019	• Mobile app	• Schizophrenia	-	-	-	✓
Fraiwan et al.	2019	• Mobile app	• Diabetic foot ulcer	✓	-	-	-
Park et al.	2019	• Mobile app	• Advanced lung cancer	-	-	-	✓
Anand et al.	2018	• Cheap peak flow meter device • Machine learning	• Asthma • Chronic obstructive pulmonary disease (COPD)	✓	-	-	-
Lopez et al.	2018	• Wearable device	• High blood pressure	-	-	✓	-
Petersen et al.	2018	• Mobile app	• Sarcopenia	-	-	-	✓
Hamrioui et al.	2018	• Mobile app	• Heart disease	-	-	-	✓
Castensøe-Seidenfaden et al.	2018	• Mobile app • Smart phone	• Diabetes	-	-	-	✓
Lefler et al.	2018	• Android health tablet	• Heart failure	-	-	✓	-
Vagg et al.	2018	• SMS • Game	• Cystic fibrosis	-	-	✓	-
Reyes et al.	2018	• Mobile app • Smart phone	• Pneumonia	✓	-	-	-
Shabut et al.	2018	• Mobile phone • Expert system	• Tuberculosis	✓	-	-	-
Honkoop et al.	2017	• Mobile app	• Asthma attacks	-	✓	-	-
Khan et al.	2017	• Mobile app • Machine learning	• Diabetes	-	✓	-	-
Kosse et al.	2017	• Mobile app	• Asthma	-	-	✓	-
Simpson et al.	2017	• Mobile technology	• Asthma	-	-	-	✓
Saeb et al.	2017	• Mobile phone	• Depression • Anxiety	✓	-	-	-
Gandhi et al.	2017	• Mobile app	• Diseases	-	✓	-	-
Tsiouris et al.	2017	• Smartphone • Mobile app • Commercial wrist • Insole sensors • Machine learning	• Parkinson's disease	✓	-	-	-
Lakshminarayana et al.	2017	• Smart phone	• Parkinson's disease	-	-	-	✓

continued on the following page

Table 1. Continued

Author(s)	Year of publication	Technology/approach used	Disease type	Diagnosis	Prediction	Monitoring	Management
Isinkaye et al.	2017	• Mobile app • Expert system	• Various diseases	✓	-	-	-
Cushing et al.	2016	• Mobile app	• Asthma	-	-	✓	-
Frederix et al.	2016	• Mobile app • Smartphone	• Coronary artery disease	-	-	✓	-
Quintiliani et al.	2016	• Text messaging	• Cancer	-	-	-	✓
Martin et al.	2016	• Mobile app	• Weight management	-	-	-	✓
Alloghani et al.	2016	• Mobile app	• Obesity	-	-	-	✓
Carrera et al.	2016	• Mobile app	• Hypertension	-	-	✓	-
Chakraborty et al.	2016	• Smartphone • Telemedicine	• Chronic wound	-	-	✓	-
Kaur et al.	2015	• Smartphones • Neural networks	• Cataract	✓	-	-	-
Abiola et al.	2015	• Mobile app	• Infectious disease	-	-	✓	-
Juen et al.	2015	• Mobile phone • Machine learning	• COPD	-	-	✓	-
Dobson et al.	2015	• Text messaging	• Hypertension	-	-	-	✓
Knowlton et al.	2015	• Smartphone • Mobile app	• Sickle cell disease	✓	-	-	-
Dallet et al.	2014	• Mobile app	• Malaria	✓	-	-	-
Zennifa et al.	2014	• Mobile app	• Heart disease	✓	-	-	-
Yu et al.	2014	• Mobile app	• Chronic diseases	-	-	-	✓
Springer et al.	2014	• Mobile phone	• Rheumatic heart disease	✓	-	-	-
Chakraborty et al.	2014	• Smartphone	• Chronic wound	-	-	✓	-
Cheng et al.	2013	• Text Messaging	• Sickle cell disease	-	-	-	✓
Al-Dowaihi et al.	2013	• Mobile app	• Asthma	-	-	✓	-
Rodrigues et al.	2013	• Mobile app	• Pressure ulcer	-	-	✓	-
Ashrafuzzaman et al.	2013	• Smartphone	• Heart attack	✓	-	-	-
Panyasoponlert et al.	2012	• Mobile app	• Flu	-	-	✓	-
Aliev et al.	2012	• Mobile phones	• Cardiovascular diseases	-	-	✓	-
Lv et al.	2012	• Text messaging	• Asthma	-	-	-	✓
Dongre and Dongre	2012	• Mobile app	• Different diseases	-	-	-	✓
Piette et al.	2012	• Mobile app	• Chronic diseases	-	-	-	✓
Sirikham	2011	• Mobile phones • Short message service (SMS)	• Heart attack	✓	-	-	-
Adnan et al.	2011	• Mobile app	• Alzheimer disease	-	✓	-	-
Petrie et al.	2011	• Text messaging	• Asthma	-	-	-	✓
Sufi et al.	2010	• Mobile phone-based electrocardiography system • Text messaging	• Cardiovascular diseases	✓	-	-	-
LeMoyne et al.	2010	• iPhone	• Parkinson's disease	✓	-	-	-
Garcia et al.	2010	• Mobile phone	• Cardiovascular diseases	-	-	-	✓

Collating, Summarizing and Reporting the Results

Mobile technologies have been used for diagnosing diseases. Gall et al. (2017) describe disease diagnosis as a means of identifying the presence of an ailment by following scientific procedures. mHealth technologies have been used in identifying different diseases which are explained below.

- **Detection of Cataract**: Artificial intelligence techniques have been used for the detection and prediction of diseases. Rashid et al. (2019, p.113) further point these techniques which include "Support Vector Machine, Fuzzy C-means, Principal Component Analysis, Navies Bayes Classifier, Decision Trees and Artificial Neural Networks." Kaur et al. (2015) developed a low-cost mobile solution for detecting cataract with artificial intelligence techniques such as neural networks.
- **Detection of Heart Attack**: With the use of SMS, Sirikham (2011) facilitated notifications sent to mobile phones of medical practitioners and relatives of patients with an impending heart attack. The technology used for detecting heart attack included an electronic signal data receiver, a chest string with an electrocardiogram (ECG). The data was sent to a microcontroller in order to determine the heartbeat rate. Ashrafuzzaman et al. (2013) also applied fuzzy logic to detect a potential heart attack.
- **Diagnosis of Asthma, COPD and Allergic Rhinitis (AR):** Anand et al. (2018) explained that misdiagnosis of asthma, COPD and AR is a common problem; as such, they developed a mobile application to resolve this problem. Anand et al. (2018) developed a mobile application using machine learning algorithms and a cheap peak flow meter device to segregate asthma, COPD and AR symptoms effectively.
- **Diagnosis of Cardiovascular Diseases**: A mobile phone-based electrocardiography system was developed by Sufi et al. (2010). The system incorporated algorithms to detect the presence of cardiovascular activities and alert the healthcare provider through text messaging.
- **Categorizing Parkinson's Disease Tremor**: Classifying Parkinson's disease tremor through the use of an iPhone was an approach proposed by LeMoyne et al. (2010). This represents the use of mobile phones as a low-cost tool in place of a wireless accelerometer. This is important in low-resource settings where acquiring expensive medical equipment is limited.
- **Diagnosis of Malaria**: Diagnosis of malaria has been implemented through a mobile application (Dallet et al., 2014). The mobile application is also able to detect the level of malaria infection using the Annular Ring Ratio Method. The Annular Ring Ratio Method is an approach used for the segregation of blood cells (Kareem et al., 2012).
- **Diagnosis of Heart Disease**: Zennifa et al. (2014) developed a rule-based mobile app to detect the presence of heart diseases in patients. The app is also able to categorise the type of heart disease present.
- **Diagnosis of Rheumatic Heart Disease**: Springer et al. (2014) explained how a mobile phone can be used as a diagnostic tool to detect the presence of rheumatic heart disease in patients.
- **Diagnosis of Depression:** Saeb et al. (2017) explored using specific locations to determine the presence of depression and anxiety through the use of mobile phones.

- **Diagnosis of Sickle Cell Disease:** Smartphones have been used in the diagnosis of sickle cell disease. For example, Knowlton et al. (2015) developed a mobile application which can be run on a smartphone to support in diagnosing sickle cell disease.
- **Diagnosis of Diabetic Foot Ulcer:** Fraiwan et al. (2018) developed a mobile application to diagnose the presence of diabetic foot ulcer in patients. The mobile application used factors such as the Mean Temperature Difference to determine the presence of foot ulcer.
- **Diagnosis of Pneumonia in Patients:** With the aid of a mobile application, pneumonia can be detected in patients using the time-varying autoregressive modeling (Reyes et al., 2018). The mobile application captures sounds into the mobile application and is analysed using the time-varying autoregressive modeling for the presence of pneumonia in patients.
- **Diagnosis of Parkinson's Disease:** Tsiouris et al. (2017) developed a mobile app to help clinicians diagnose the progression of Parkinson's disease and send alerts to medical practitioners.
- **Diagnosis of Various Diseases**: Isinkaye et al. (2017) developed an expert mobile application to diagnose various diseases. The application was evaluated by 13 participants who found the application to be useful.
- **Diagnosis of Tuberculosis:** Shabut et al. (2018) developed an expert mobile phone-based diagnostic tool for diagnosing tuberculosis.

These findings suggest that diseases can be diagnosed with the use of mobile technologies as well as the incorporation of artificial intelligence techniques such as machine learning and neural networks.

In terms of predicting diseases, different diseases have been predicted using mobile technologies and are described below:

- **Prediction of Alzheimer's Disease (AD):** Adnan et al. (2011) explored the use of a mobile application to determine the chances of AD being present in a patient. The application was developed using Java.
- **Prediction of Asthma Attacks**: Honkoop et al. (2017) developed a mobile application, MyAirCoach, to predict asthma attacks.
- **Prediction of Diabetes**: Khan et al. (2017) developed a mobile application based on machine learning algorithms for the prediction of diabetes in patients.
- **Prediction of Diseases**: Gandhi et al. (2017) described the development of a mobile app to predict different diseases.

Mobile technologies have been used for actively monitoring patients with diseases which are explained in the next section.

- **Monitoring of Infectious Diseases**: Abiola et al. (2015) developed a mobile app to monitor infectious diseases in real time.
- **Monitoring of Asthma Patients**: A mobile app was developed to determine if medication adherence can be maintained among asthma patients (Cushing et al., 2016; Kosse et al., 2017).

- **Monitoring of High Blood Pressure in Pregnant Women**: A wearable device was developed for monitoring the presence of high blood pressure in pregnant women (Lopez et al., 2018). The findings from the evaluation of the app showed that wearable technologies can be used to control blood pressure in pregnant women. Other apps such as BPControl have been used to monitor blood pressure in patients (Carrera et al., 2016)
- **Monitoring of Flu**: Panyasoponlert et al. (2012) developed a mobile application that allows people to report flu incidences.
- **Monitoring of Cardiovascular Diseases:** Aliev et al. (2012) applied mobile phones for monitoring cardiovascular diseases.
- **Monitoring of Patients with Coronary Artery Disease**: Frederix et al. (2016) developed a mobile application to support the monitoring of patients with coronary artery disease in distant locations.
- **Monitoring of Heart Failure**: A mobile device connected to a cloud platform was used to monitor patients with heart failure on a daily basis based on information provided by patients (Lefler et al. 2018).
- **Monitoring of Cystic Fibrosis**: A game app was developed for cystic fibrosis patients and based on poor performance, patients were alerted via SMS (Vagg et al., 2018).
- **Monitoring of Asthma:** Al-Dowaihi et al. (2013) developed a mobile application for monitoring asthma patients and notifying medical practitioners when the need arises.
- **Monitoring of Pressure Ulcer:** Rodrigues et al. (2013) developed a mobile platform to keep track of people with pressure ulcer.
- **Monitoring of Chronic Wound:** Chakraborty et al. (2014; 2016) explored the use of smartphones for monitoring chronic wound in patients from a distant location.

Faxon et al. (2004, p. 2651) define disease management as an "effort to improve the quality and cost-effectiveness of care for selected patients suffering from chronic diseases." The main aim of disease management is to improve the quality of healthcare services patients receive. Mobile technologies have been used to achieve not only the quality of care but also in reducing the cost of receiving such care. mHealth has been used for the cost-effective management of diseases in the following ways:

- **Management of Sarcopenia:** Sarcopenia is a health condition that causes disability due to the muscles, often found in aged people (Santilli et al., 2014). Petersen et al. (2018) developed a mobile application to help physicians detect when exercises are done by patients outside the hospital premises. The mobile application helped physicians determine if patients followed exercise plans. This approach helps doctors monitor their patients through the app, without the need to physically monitor the patient; hence, this provides a cost-effective approach in disease management through the use of mHealth.
- **Rehabilitation of Patients with Cardiovascular Diseases:** Garcia et al. (2010) proposed mobile phones as pedometers for keeping track of the number of steps taken by cardiovascular disease patients rather than a standard pedometer device.

- **Management of Asthma:** Text messaging is a low-cost method for reaching patient and it has been used to improve the uptake of asthma preventer medications by asthma patients (Petrie et al., 2011) and health outcomes for asthma sufferers (Lv et al., 2012). Patients are also in support of mobile technologies for managing asthma (Simpson et al., 2017). Text messaging has a method for prompting asthma patients in sending their peak flow reading, which is used for monitoring the signs of asthma in asthma patients (Holtz and Whitten, 2009).
- **Management of Heart Diseases:** Hamrioui et al. (2018) developed a mobile application to enable patients manage heart diseases.
- **Disease Management:** While other mobile applications focused on managing specific diseases (Peterson et al., 2018), Dongre and Dongre (2012) developed a mobile application to manage different diseases.
- **Management of Chronic Diseases:** Piette et al. (2012) evaluated the use of mobile applications for managing non-communicable diseases in four North American countries. The findings of the study suggest that it is cost-effective in using these apps for managing chronic diseases. Yu et al. (2014) also developed a mobile app to support patients with chronic diseases.
- **Management of Diabetes:** A mobile app was developed for managing young patients with diabetes (Castensøe-Seidenfaden et al., 2018). The evaluation of the mobile app found that it can be used to manage diabetes in young patients. Text messaging has also been used to support patients with diabetes and high blood pressure (Lewinski et al., 2019; Dobson et al., 2015). Although the findings suggest that this approach did not improve health outcomes for these patients (Lewinski et al., 2019), text messaging can be used as a platform for disseminating health information to patients (Lewinski et al., 2019) and can be used by patients with diabetes to support healthy lifestyles (Dobson et al., 2015).
- **Management of Cancer:** Text messaging has also been used to support patients with cancer in order for them to receive information about maintaining their weight (Quintiliani et al. 2016). Mobile applicationshave also been developed to support health management among patients with cancer (Salimien et al., 2019). Park et al. (2019) also developed a mobile app to support patients who have undergone advanced lung cancer treatment.
- **Weight Management:** A mobile application was developed to support people with weight management and provide a tailored approach to managing these patients (Martin et al., 2016).
- **Management of Schizophrenia:** A mobile app was developed to help schizophrenia patients manage their health (Almeida et al., 2019).
- **Management of Obesity:** A mobile application can be used to support patients with obesity to enhance diets and provide healthy living plans (Alloghani et al., 2016).
- **Management of HIV:** Dillingham et al. (2018) did not only develop a mobile app for patients with HIV but also proved that a mobile app can improve health outcomes for HIV patients.
- **Management of Parkison's Disease:** Parkinson's diseases have also been managed through the use of smartphones (Lakshimarayana et al., 2017).
- **Management of Patients with Sickle Cell Disease:** Cheng et al. (2013) developed a text messaging platform for providing therapy sessions for patients with sickle cell disease.

In general, different mHealth technologies have been used ranging from mobile apps, text messaging/SMS, mobile phones, Android devices, wearable technologies and games. It is important to diagnose diseases at an early stage, this will facilitate treatment mechanisms which will prevent diseases from spreading. This is especially useful in impoverished settings where access to medical services are limited. In locations where medical facilities are not available, it will be useful to provide care to patients through mobile apps and technologies where they can manage their health without traveling long distances to receive certain healthcare services.

Non-communicable diseases (NCD) such as cataract, asthma, COPD, diabetes, cancer as well as infectious diseases have been managed with mobile technologies (Quintiliani et al. 2016; Park et al., 2019). The mHealth approach is relatively cheaper, especially when providing health promotion services through text messaging and SMS interventions. However, for future work, it is recommended in line with the findings of Iyawa and Hamunyela (2019) that voice messages can be used as well as text messaging and SMS interventions converted to local languages in areas where literacy is a problem.While this study found mobile applications that support mental health, there was a dearth of applications to support the mental health of sexual and gender based violence (SGBV) victims which is in line with the findings of Iyawa et al. (2019) which also identified that there was a lack of published research focused in this area. For future work, mobile applications, specific to the mental health of SGBV victims should be developed.

CONCLUSION

In conclusion, this chapter presented an overview of mHealth for disease diagnosis, prediction, monitoring and management. Majority of the approaches are based on low-cost technologies. This provides a cost-effective solution for patients in low-resource settings. The findings of the scoping review present a platform for further in-depth systematic literature review on mHealth technologies for tackling diseases.

Despite our findings, this chapter might have been limited based on the inclusion and exclusion criteria. As such,we might have excluded relevant papers on the use of mHealth technologies for disease diagnosing, prediction, monitoring and managing diseases. However, we recommend that for a systematic in-depth literature review, the inclusion criteria should be broadened and a wide range of databases should be used in searching for academic publications. As such our future work includes conducting a systematic literature review on the subject.

REFERENCES

Abelson, J. S., Symer, M., Peters, A., Charlson, M., & Yeo, H. (2017). Mobile health apps and recovery after surgery: What are patients willing to do? *American Journal of Surgery*, *214*(4), 616–622. doi:10.1016/j.amjsurg.2017.06.009 PMID:28666581

Abiola, S. O., Portman, E., Kautz, H., & Dorsey, E. (2015). *Node view: a mHealth real-time infectious disease interface disease interface-2014 Ebola outbreak case study*. Paper presented at the International Joint Conference on Pervasive and Ubiquitous Computing and International Symposium on Wearable Computers, Osaka, Japan. 10.1145/2800835.2800851

Adnan, S. F. S., Hashim, H., & Pasya, I. (2011). *Implementation of MIDlet application on probability of Alzheimer's disease via mobile phone.* Paper presented at the IEEE International Conference on Computer Applications and Industrial Electronics, Penang, Malaysia. 10.1109/ICCAIE.2011.6162115

Afolayan, T., Aiterebhe, E. F., & Mejabi, V. (2015). Mobile phone usage in rural communities in Kwara state, Nigeria. *Inform Technolt, 12*(2), 1–15.

Agarwal, P., Mukerji, G., Desveaux, L., Ivers, N. M., Bhattacharyya, O., Hensel, J. M., ... Cooper, M. (2019). Mobile app for improved self-management of type 2 diabetes: Multicenter pragmatic randomized controlled trial. *JMIR mHealth and uHealth, 7*(1), e10321. doi:10.2196/10321 PMID:30632972

Al-Dowaihi, D., Al-Ajlan, M., Al-Zahrani, N., Al-Quwayfili, N., al-Jwiser, N., & Kanjo, E. (2013). *Mbreath: Asthma monitoring system on the go.* Paper presented at the International Conference on Computer Medical Applications, San Francisco, CA. 10.1109/ICCMA.2013.6506169

Ali, Z. H., Ali, H. A., & Badawy, M. M. (2015). Internet of Things (IoT): Definitions, challenges and recent research directions. *International Journal of Computers and Applications, 128*(1), 37–47. doi:10.5120/ijca2015906430

Aliev, T., Babayev, T., Sabziev, E., Pashayev, A., & Alizada, T. (2012). *Monitoring of condition of the cardiovascular system by means of mobile phones using ECG noise variance.* Paper presented at the 4th International Conference of Problems of Cybernetics and Informatics, Baku, Azerbaijan. 10.1109/ICPCI.2012.6486303

Alloghani, M., Hussain, A., Al-Jumeily, D., Fergus, P., Abuelma'Atti, O., & Hamden, H. (2016). *A mobile health monitoring application for obesity management and control using the internet-of-things.* Paper presented at the Sixth International Conference on Digital Information Processing and Communications, Piscataway, NJ. 10.1109/ICDIPC.2016.7470785

Almeida, R. F., Sousa, T. J., Couto, A. S., Marques, A. J., Queirós, C. M., & Martins, C. L. (2019). Development of weCope, a mobile app for illness self-management in schizophrenia. *Archives of Clinical Psychiatry (São Paulo), 46*(1), 1–4. doi:10.1590/0101-60830000000182

Almotiri, S. H., Khan, M. A., & Alghamdi, M. A. (2016). *Mobile health (m-health) system in the context of IoT.* Paper presented at the 4th International Conference on Future Internet of Things and Cloud Workshops, Vienna, Austria.

Anand, A., Chamberlain, D., Kodgule, R., & Fletcher, R. R. (2018). *Pulmonary screener: A mobile phone screening tool for pulmonary and respiratory disease.* Paper presented at the IEEE Global Humanitarian Technology Conference, San Jose, CA. 10.1109/GHTC.2018.8601821

Arksey, H., & O'Malley, L. (2005). Scoping studies: Towards a methodological framework. *International Journal of Social Research Methodology, 8*(1), 19–32. doi:10.1080/1364557032000119616

Ashrafuzzaman, M., Huq, M. M., Chakraborty, C. M., Khan, R. M., Tabassum, T., & Hasan, R. (2013). Article. *International Journal of Technology Enhancements and Emerging Engineering Research, 1*(3), 23–27.

Bates, M., & Zumla, A. (2015). Rapid infectious diseases diagnostics using Smartphones. *Annals of Translational Medicine*, *3*(15). PMID:26488011

Buratti, C., Conti, A., Dardari, D., & Verdone, R. (2009). An overview on wireless sensor networks technology and evolution. *Sensors (Basel)*, *9*(9), 6869–6896. doi:10.339090906869 PMID:22423202

Calabria, D., Caliceti, C., Zangheri, M., Mirasoli, M., Simoni, P., & Roda, A. (2017). Smartphone-based enzymatic biosensor for oral fluid L-lactate detection in one minute using confined multilayer paper reflectometry. *Biosensors & Bioelectronics*, *94*, 124–130. doi:10.1016/j.bios.2017.02.053 PMID:28267667

Carrera, A., Pifarré, M., Vilaplana, J., Cuadrado, J., Solsona, S., Mateo, J., & Solsona, F. (2016). BP-control: A mobile app to monitor hypertensive patients. *Applied Clinical Informatics*, *7*(04), 1120–1134. doi:10.4338/ACI-2015-12-RA-0172 PMID:27924346

Castensøe-Seidenfaden, P., Husted, G. R., Jensen, A. K., Hommel, E., Olsen, B., Pedersen-Bjergaard, U., & Teilmann, G. (2018). Testing a smartphone app (Young with Diabetes) to improve self-management of diabetes over 12 months: Randomized controlled trial. *JMIR mHealth and uHealth*, *6*(6), e141. doi:10.2196/mhealth.9487 PMID:29945861

Chakraborty, C. (2019). Mobile health (m-Health) for tele-wound monitoring: Role of m-Health in wound management. In C. Chakraborty (Ed.), *Mobile Health Applications for Quality Healthcare Delivery*. IGI Global. doi:10.4018/978-1-5225-8021-8.ch005

Chakraborty, C., Gupta, B., & Ghosh, S. K. (2014). Mobile metadata assisted community database of chronic wound images. *Wound Medicine*, *6*, 34–42. doi:10.1016/j.wndm.2014.09.002

Chakraborty, C., Gupta, B., & Ghosh, S. K. (2016). Mobile telemedicine systems for remote patient's chronic wound monitoring. In A. Moumtzoglou (Ed.), *M-Health Innovations for Patient-Centered Care*. IGI Global. doi:10.4018/978-1-4666-9861-1.ch011

Chan, K. L., & Chen, M. (2019). Effects of Social Media and Mobile Health Apps on Pregnancy Care: Meta-Analysis. *JMIR mHealth and uHealth*, *7*(1), e11836. doi:10.2196/11836 PMID:30698533

Cheng, C., Brown, R. C., Cohen, L. L., Venugopalan, J., Stokes, T. H., & Wang, M. D. (2013). *iACT- An interactive mHealth monitoring system to enhance psychotherapy for adolescents with sickle cell disease*. Paper presented at the Annual International Conference of the IEEE Engineering in Medicine and Biology Society, Osaka, Japan. 10.1109/EMBC.2013.6609992

Chin, C. D., Cheung, Y. K., Laksanasopin, T., Modena, M. M., Chin, S. Y., Sridhara, A. A., & Karita, E. (2013). Mobile device for disease diagnosis and data tracking in resource-limited settings. *Clinical Chemistry*, *59*(4), 629–640. doi:10.1373/clinchem.2012.199596 PMID:23327782

Cook, K. A., Modena, B. D., & Simon, R. A. (2016). Improvement in asthma control using a minimally burdensome and proactive smartphone application. *The Journal of Allergy and Clinical Immunology. In Practice*, *4*(4), 730–737. doi:10.1016/j.jaip.2016.03.005 PMID:27107690

Cushing, A., Manice, M. P., Ting, A., & Parides, M. K. (2016). Feasibility of a novel mHealth management system to capture and improve medication adherence among adolescents with asthma. *Patient Preference and Adherence, 10*, 2271–2275. doi:10.2147/PPA.S115713 PMID:27853357

Dallet, C., Kareem, S., & Kale, I. (2014). *Real time blood image processing application for malaria diagnosis using mobile phones.* Paper presented at the International Symposium on Circuits and Systems, Melbourne, Australia. 10.1109/ISCAS.2014.6865657

Dillingham, R., Ingersoll, K., Flickinger, T. E., Waldman, A. L., Grabowski, M., Laurence, C., ... Cohn, W. F. (2018). PositiveLinks: A Mobile health intervention for retention in HIV care and clinical outcomes with 12-month follow-up. *AIDS Patient Care and STDs, 32*(6), 241–250. doi:10.1089/apc.2017.0303 PMID:29851504

Dobson, R., Carter, K., Cutfield, R., Hulme, A., Hulme, R., McNamara, C., & Whittaker, R. (2015). Diabetes text-message self-management support program (SMS4BG): A pilot study. *JMIR mHealth and uHealth, 3*(1), e32. doi:10.2196/mhealth.3988 PMID:25830952

Dongre, D., & Dongre, E. (2012). *Mobile multi sense disease management platform.* Paper presented at the International Conference on Green Technologies, Trivandrum, India.

Faxon, D. P., Schwamm, L. H., Pasternak, R. C., Peterson, E. D., McNeil, B. J., Bufalino, V., & Smaha, L. A. (2004). Improving quality of care through disease management: Principles and recommendations from the American Heart Association's Expert Panel on Disease Management. *Circulation, 109*(21), 2651–2654. doi:10.1161/01.CIR.0000128373.90851.7B PMID:15173048

Fraiwan, L., Ninan, J., & Al-Khodari, M. (2018). Mobile application for ulcer detection. *The Open Biomedical Engineering Journal, 12*(1), 16–26. doi:10.2174/1874120701812010016 PMID:30069252

Frederix, I., Sankaran, S., Coninx, K., & Dendale, P. (2016). *MobileHeart, a mobile smartphone-based application that supports and monitors coronary artery disease patients during rehabilitation.* Paper presented at the 38th Annual International Conference of the IEEE Engineering in Medicine and Biology Society, Lake Buena Vista, FL. 10.1109/EMBC.2016.7590752

Gall, T., Valkanas, E., Bello, C., Markello, T., Adams, C., Bone, W. P., & Davis, J. (2017). Defining disease, diagnosis, and translational medicine within a homeostatic perturbation paradigm: The national institutes of health undiagnosed diseases program experience. *Frontiers in Medicine, 4*, 62. doi:10.3389/fmed.2017.00062 PMID:28603714

Gandhi, B., Singh, L., & Gupta, L. (2017). Disease predictor: A disease prediction app. *International Journal for Research in Applied Science and Engineering Technology, 5*(4), 1509–1512. doi:10.22214/ijraset.2017.4265

Garcia, E., Ding, H., Sarela, A., & Karunanithi, M. (2010). *Can a mobile phone be used as a pedometer in an outpatient cardiac rehabilitation program?* Paper presented at the IEEE/ICME International Conference on Complex Medical Engineering, Gold Coast, Australia. 10.1109/ICCME.2010.5558833

Hamrioui, S., Gonzalez, J. H., Castillo, G., de la Torre-Diez, I., & Lopez-Coronado, M. (2018). *Development and QoE evaluation of an iOS mHealth app for self-controlling and education of patients with heart diseases*. Paper presented at the 13th Iberian Conference on Information Systems and Technologies, Cáceres, Spain. 10.23919/CISTI.2018.8398633

Heimerl, K., Menon, A., & Hasan, S. (2015). *Analysis of smartphone adoption and usage in a rural community cellular network*. Paper presented at the Seventh International Conference on Information and Communication Technologies and Development, Singapore, Singapore. 10.1145/2737856.2737880

Holtz, B., & Lauckner, C. (2012). Diabetes management via mobile phones: A systematic review. *Telemedicine Journal and e-Health*, *18*(3), 175–184. doi:10.1089/tmj.2011.0119 PMID:22356525

Holtz, B., & Whitten, P. (2009). Managing asthma with mobile phones: A feasibility study. *Telemedicine Journal and e-Health*, *15*(9), 907–909. doi:10.1089/tmj.2009.0048 PMID:19919198

Honkoop, P. J., Simpson, A., Bonini, M., Snoeck-Stroband, J. B., Meah, S., Chung, K. F., & Sont, J. K. (2017). MyAirCoach: The use of home-monitoring and mHealth systems to predict deterioration in asthma control and the occurrence of asthma exacerbations; study protocol of an observational study. *BMJ Open*, *7*(1), e013935. doi:10.1136/bmjopen-2016-013935 PMID:28119390

Hosu, O., Ravalli, A., Piccolo, G. M. L., Cristea, C., Sandulescu, R., & Marrazza, G. (2017). Smartphone-based immunosensor for CA125 detection. *Talanta*, *166*, 234–240. doi:10.1016/j.talanta.2017.01.073 PMID:28213228

Isinkaye, F. O., Awosupin, S. O., & Soyemi, J. (2017). A mobile based expert system for disease diagnosis and medical advice provisioning. *International Journal of Computer Science and Information Security*, *15*(1), 568–572.

Istepanian, R. S., & Al-anzi, T. M. (2018). m-Health interventions for diabetes remote monitoring and self management: Clinical and compliance issues. *mHealth*, *4*(4), 1–3. PMID:29552566

Iyawa, G. E., Botha, A., & Herselman, M. (2016). Identifying and defining the terms related to a Digital Health Innovation Ecosystem. In M. Herselman & A. Botha (Eds.), *Strategies, Approaches and Experiences: Towards Building a South African Digital Health Innovation Ecosystem*. Pretoria: CSIR.

Iyawa, G. E., & Coleman, A. (2015). Improving health care delivery in rural communities through the use of mobile phones: A case study in Windhoek. *International Science and Technology Journal of Namibia*, *8*, 1–21.

Iyawa, G. E., & Hamunyela, S. (2019). *mHealth apps and services for maternal healthcare in developing countries*. Paper presented at IST Africa, Nairobi, Kenya.

Iyawa, G. E., Herselman, M., & Botha, A. (2016). Digital health innovation ecosystems: From systematic literature to conceptual framework. *Procedia Computer Science*, *100*, 244–252. doi:10.1016/j.procs.2016.09.149

Iyawa, G. E., Langan-Martin, J., Seville, S., & Masikara, W. (2019). mHealth as tools for development in mental health. In Impacts of Information Technology on Patient Care and Empowerment. In R. W. McHaney, I. Reychev, J. Azuri, M. E. McHaney & R. Moshonov. IGI Global.

Iyawa, G. E., Velusamy, V., & Palanisamy, P. (2019). Wearable technologies for glucose monitoring: A systematic mapping study of publication trends. In D. Goyal, S. Balamurugan, S. Peng, & D. S. Jat (Eds.), *The IoT and the Next Revolutions Automating the World*. IGI Global. doi:10.4018/978-1-5225-9246-4.ch007

Jonas, S. M., Deserno, T. M., Buhimschi, C. S., Makin, J., Choma, M. A., & Buhimschi, I. A. (2015). Smartphone-based diagnostic for preeclampsia: An mHealth solution for administering the Congo Red Dot (CRD) test in settings with limited resources. *Journal of the American Medical Informatics Association*, *23*(1), 166–173. doi:10.1093/jamia/ocv015 PMID:26026158

Juen, J., Cheng, Q., & Schatz, B. (2015). A natural walking monitor for pulmonary patients using mobile phones. *IEEE Journal of Biomedical and Health Informatics*, *19*(4), 1399–1405. doi:10.1109/JBHI.2015.2427511 PMID:25935052

Jutel, A., & Lupton, D. (2015). Digitizing diagnosis: A review of mobile applications in the diagnostic process. *Diagnosis*, *2*(2), 89–96. doi:10.1515/dx-2014-0068 PMID:29540025

Kagen, S., & Garland, A. (2019). Asthma and Allergy Mobile Apps in 2018. *Current Allergy and Asthma Reports*, *19*(1), 6. doi:10.100711882-019-0840-z PMID:30712150

Kamišalić, A., Fister, I., Turkanović, M., & Karakatič, S. (2018). Sensors and functionalities of non-invasive wrist-wearable devices: A review. *Sensors (Basel)*, *18*(6), 1714–1747. doi:10.339018061714 PMID:29799504

Karasz, H. N., Eiden, A., & Bogan, S. (2013). Text messaging to communicate with public health audiences: How the HIPAA Security Rule affects practice. *American Journal of Public Health*, *103*(4), 617–622. doi:10.2105/AJPH.2012.300999 PMID:23409902

Kareem, S., Kale, I., & Morling, R. C. (2012). *Automated P. falciparum detection system for post-treatment malaria diagnosis using modified annular ring ratio method*. Paper presented at the UKSim 14th International Conference on Computer Modelling and Simulation, Cambridge, UK.

Kaur, M., Kaur, J., & Kaur, R. (2015). *Low cost cataract detection system using smart phone*. Paper presented at theInternational Conference on Green Computing and Internet of Things, Delhi, India. 10.1109/ICGCIoT.2015.7380724

Khan, N. S., Muaz, M. H., Kabir, A., & Islam, M. N. (2017). *Diabetes predicting mHealth application using machine learning*. Paper presented at the International WIE Conference on Electrical and Computer Engineering, Dehradun, India. 10.1109/WIECON-ECE.2017.8468885

Knowlton, S. M., Sencan, I., Aytar, Y., Khoory, J., Heeney, M. M., Ghiran, I. C., & Tasoglu, S. (2015). Sickle cell detection using a smartphone. *Scientific Reports*, *5*(1), 15022. doi:10.1038rep15022 PMID:26492382

Kosse, R. C., Bouvy, M. L., de Vries, T. W., Kaptein, A. A., Geers, H. C., van Dijk, L., & Koster, E. S. (2017). mHealth intervention to support asthma self-management in adolescents: The ADAPT study. *Patient Preference and Adherence*, *11*, 571–577. doi:10.2147/PPA.S124615 PMID:28356720

Lakshminarayana, R., Wang, D., Burn, D., Chaudhuri, K. R., Galtrey, C., Guzman, N. V., ... Steiger, M. (2017). Using a smartphone-based self-management platform to support medication adherence and clinical consultation in Parkinson's disease. *MPJ Parkinson's Disease*, *3*(1), 2. doi:10.103841531-016-0003-z PMID:28649602

Lefler, L. L., Rhoads, S. J., Harris, M., Funderburg, A. E., Lubin, S. A., Martel, I. D., ... Beverly, C. J. (2018). Evaluating the use of mobile health technology in older adults with heart failure: Mixed-methods study. *JMIR Aging*, *1*(2), e12178. doi:10.2196/12178

LeMoyne, R., Mastroianni, T., Cozza, M., Coroian, C., & Grundfest, W. (2010, August). Implementation of an iPhone for characterizing Parkinson's disease tremor through a wireless accelerometer application. In *2010 Annual International Conference of the IEEE Engineering in Medicine and Biology* (pp. 4954-4958). IEEE. 10.1109/IEMBS.2010.5627240

Lewinski, A. A., Patel, U. D., Diamantidis, C. J., Oakes, M., Baloch, K., Crowley, M. J., ... Bosworth, H. B. (2019). Addressing diabetes and poorly controlled hypertension: Pragmatic mHealth self-management intervention. *Journal of Medical Internet Research*, *21*(4), e12541. doi:10.2196/12541 PMID:30964439

Lopez, B. D. B., Aguirre, J. A. A., Coronado, D. A. R., & Gonzalez, P. A. (2018). *Wearable technology model to control and monitor hypertension during pregnancy*. Paper presented at the 13th Iberian Conference on Information Systems and Technologies, Cáceres, Spain. 10.23919/CISTI.2018.8399200

Lv, Y., Zhao, H., Liang, Z., Dong, H., Liu, L., Zhang, D., & Cai, S. (2012). A mobile phone short message service improves perceived control of asthma: A randomized controlled trial. *Telemedicine Journal and e-Health*, *18*(6), 420–426. doi:10.1089/tmj.2011.0218 PMID:22667695

Manisha, N. D. (2015). Fault detection in wireless sensor networks. *International Journal of Computer Science, 3*(3), 6-10.

Martin, C. K., Gilmore, L. A., Apolzan, J. W., Myers, C. A., Thomas, D. M., & Redman, L. M. (2016). Smartloss: A personalized mobile health intervention for weight management and health promotion. *JMIR mHealth and uHealth*, *4*(1), e18. PMID:26983937

Meskó, B., Drobni, Z., Bényei, É., Gergely, B., & Győrffy, Z. (2017). Digital health is a cultural transformation of traditional healthcare. *mHealth*, *3*(38), 1–8. PMID:29184890

Mohammadzadeh, N., & Safdari, R. (2014). Patient monitoring in mobile health: Opportunities and challenges. *Medicinski Arhiv*, *68*(1), 57. doi:10.5455/medarh.2014.68.57-60 PMID:24783916

Muller, N., Emmrich, P. M. F., Rajemison, E. N., De Neve, J. W., Bärnighausen, T., Knauss, S., & Emmrich, J. V. (2019). A Mobile Health Wallet for Pregnancy-Related Health Care in Madagascar: Mixed-Methods Study on Opportunities and Challenges. *JMIR mHealth and uHealth*, *7*(3), e11420. doi:10.2196/11420 PMID:30457972

Munn, Z., Peters, M. D., Stern, C., Tufanaru, C., McArthur, A., & Aromataris, E. (2018). Systematic review or scoping review? Guidance for authors when choosing between a systematic or scoping review approach. *BMC Medical Research Methodology*, *18*(1), 143. doi:10.118612874-018-0611-x PMID:30453902

Munos, B., Baker, P. C., Bot, B. M., Crouthamel, M., de Vries, G., Ferguson, I., & Ozcan, A. (2016). Mobile health: The power of wearables, sensors, and apps to transform clinical trials. *Annals of the New York Academy of Sciences*, *1375*(1), 3–18. doi:10.1111/nyas.13117 PMID:27384501

Oh, H., Rizo, C., Enkin, M., & Jadad, A. (2005). What is eHealth (3): A systematic review of published definitions. *Journal of Medical Internet Research*, *7*(1), e1. doi:10.2196/jmir.7.1.e1 PMID:15829471

Oyelami, O. M. (2012). A Mobile Phone-Based Expert System for Disease Diagnosis. In E-Healthcare Systems and Wireless Communications: Current and Future Challenges. IGI Global. doi:10.4018/978-1-61350-123-8.ch011

Panyasoponlert, N., Piboonudompornkul, P., Rudahl, K. T., & Goldin, S. E. (2012). *Flu incident reporting on mobile phone*. Paper presented at the International Conference on Communication, Networks and Satellite, Bali, Indonesia.

Park, S., Kim, J. Y., Lee, J. C., Kim, H. R., Song, S., Kwon, H., ... Choi, C. M. (2019). Mobile phone app–based pulmonary rehabilitation for chemotherapy-treated patients with advanced lung cancer: Pilot study. *JMIR mHealth and uHealth*, *7*(2), e11094. doi:10.2196/11094 PMID:30714943

Park, Y. T. (2016). Emerging new era of mobile health technologies. *Healthcare Informatics Research*, *22*(4), 253–254. doi:10.4258/hir.2016.22.4.253 PMID:27895955

Peters, D. H., Garg, A., Bloom, G., Walker, D. G., Brieger, W. R., & Hafizur Rahman, M. (2008). Poverty and access to health care in developing countries. *Annals of the New York Academy of Sciences*, *1136*(1), 161–171. doi:10.1196/annals.1425.011 PMID:17954679

Petersen, C. L., Wechsler, E. V., Halter, R. J., Boateng, G. G., Proctor, P. O., Kotz, D. F., & Batsis, J. A. (2018). *Detection and monitoring of repetitions using an mHealth-enabled resistance band.* Paper presented at the IEEE/ACM International Conference on Connected Health: Applications, Systems and Engineering Technologies, Washington, DC.

Peterson, J., Pearce, P. F., Ferguson, L. A., & Langford, C. A. (2017). Understanding scoping reviews: Definition, purpose, and process. *Journal of the American Association of Nurse Practitioners*, *29*(1), 12–16. doi:10.1002/2327-6924.12380 PMID:27245885

Petrie, K. J., Perry, K., Broadbent, E., & Weinman, J. (2012). A text message programme designed to modify patients' illness and treatment beliefs improves self-reported adherence to asthma preventer medication. *British Journal of Health Psychology*, *17*(1), 74–84. doi:10.1111/j.2044-8287.2011.02033.x PMID:22107110

Piette, J. D., Blaya, J. A., Lange, I., & Sanchis, J. B. B. (2011). *Experiences in mHealth for chronic disease management in 4 countries.* Paper presented at the 4th International Symposium on Applied Sciences in Biomedical and Communication Technologies, Barcelona, Spain. 10.1145/2093698.2093868

Quintiliani, L. M., Mann, D. M., Puputti, M., Quinn, E., & Bowen, D. J. (2016). Pilot and feasibility test of a mobile health-supported behavioral counseling intervention for weight management among breast cancer survivors. *JMIR Cancer, 2*(1), e4.

Rashid, T. A., Hassan, M. K., Mohammadi, M., & Fraser, K. (2019). Improvement of variant adaptable LSTM trained with metaheuristic algorithms for healthcare analysis. In C. Chakraborty (Ed.), *Advanced Classification Techniques for Healthcare Analysis*. IGI Global. doi:10.4018/978-1-5225-7796-6.ch006

Reyes, B., Olvera-Montes, N., Charleston-Villalobos, S., González-Camarena, R., Mejía-Ávila, M., & Aljama-Corrales, T. (2018). A Smartphone-Based System for Automated Bedside Detection of Crackle Sounds in Diffuse Interstitial Pneumonia Patients. *Sensors (Basel)*, *18*(11), 3813. doi:10.339018113813 PMID:30405036

Rodrigues, J. J., Pedro, L. M., Vardasca, T., de la Torre-Díez, I., & Martins, H. M. (2013). Mobile health platform for pressure ulcer monitoring with electronic health record integration. *Health Informatics Journal*, *19*(4), 300–311. doi:10.1177/1460458212474909 PMID:24255053

Saeb, S., Lattie, E. G., Kording, K. P., & Mohr, D. C. (2017). Mobile phone detection of semantic location and its relationship to depression and anxiety. *JMIR mHealth and uHealth*, *5*(8), e112. doi:10.2196/mhealth.7297 PMID:28798010

Salimien, N., Ehteshami, A., & Talouki, M. A. (2019). Developing Ghasedek: A mobile application to improve the quality of cancer palliative care. *Acta Medica Informatica*, *27*(1), 19–22. doi:10.5455/aim.2019.27.19-22

Seppala, J., De Vita, I., Jamsa, T., Miettunen, J., Isohanni, M., Rubinstein, K., ... Bulgheroni, M. (2019). Mobile phone and wearable sensor-based mHealth approaches for psychiatric disorders and symptoms: systematic review. *JMIR Mental Health, 6*(2), 1-14.

Shabut, A. M., Tania, M. H., Lwin, K. T., Evans, B. A., Yusof, N. A., Abu-Hassan, K. J., & Hossain, M. A. (2018). An intelligent mobile-enabled expert system for tuberculosis disease diagnosis in real time. *Expert Systems with Applications*, *114*, 65–77. doi:10.1016/j.eswa.2018.07.014

Simpson, A. J., Honkoop, P. J., Kennington, E., Snoeck-Stroband, J. B., Smith, I., East, J., & Usmani, O. (2017). Perspectives of patients and healthcare professionals on mHealth for asthma self-management. *The European Respiratory Journal*, *49*(5), 1601966. doi:10.1183/13993003.01966-2016 PMID:28461291

Singh, P., & Panjwani, M. (2016). mHealth: Meaning, purpose and outcome. *International Journal of Computer Science and Information Technologies*, *7*(5), 2216–2221.

Sirikham, A. (2011). *Abnormal heart rate detection device warning via mobile phone network*. Paper presented at the International Conference on Multimedia Computing and Systems, Ouarzazate, Morocco. 10.1109/ICMCS.2011.5945590

Sonderman, K. A., Nkurunziza, T., Kateera, F., Gruendl, M., Koch, R., Gaju, E., ... Riviello, R. (2018). Using mobile health technology and community health workers to identify and refer cesarean-related surgical site infections in rural Rwanda: A randomised controlled trial protocol. *BMJ Open*, *8*(5), e022214. PMID:29739786

Springer, D. B., Zuhike, L. J., Mayosi, B. M., Tarassenko, L., & Clifford, G. D. (2014). *Mobile phone-based rheumatic heart disease diagnosis*. Paper presented at the Appropriate Healthcare Technologies for Low Resource Settings, London, UK. 10.1049/cp.2014.0761

Stamate, D., Katrinecz, A., Alghamdi, W., Stahl, D., Delespaul, P., van Os, J., & Guloksuz, S. (2017). *Predicting Psychosis Using the Experience Sampling Method with Mobile Apps*. Paper presented at the IEEE International Conference on Machine Learning and Applications, Cancun, Mexico. 10.1109/ICMLA.2017.00-84

Stankevich, E., Paramonov, I., & Timofeev, I. (2012). *Mobile phone sensors in health applications*. Paper presented at the 12th Conference of Open Innovations Association, Oulu, Finland.

Sufi, F., Khalil, I., & Tari, Z. (2010). *A cardiod based technique to identify cardiovascular diseases using mobile phones and body sensors*. Paper presented at theIEEE Engineering in Medicine and Biology, Buenos Aires, Argentina. 10.1109/IEMBS.2010.5626578

Tang, S., Ghose, B., Hoque, M. R., Hao, G., & Yaya, S. (2019). Women Using Mobile Phones for Health Communication Are More Likely to Use Prenatal and Postnatal Services in Bangladesh: Cross-Sectional Study. *JMIR mHealth and uHealth*, *7*(2), e10645. doi:10.2196/10645 PMID:30816850

Teng, M. H., Hou, Y. M., Chang, S. H., & Cheng, H. J. (2019). Home-delivered attention bias modification training via smartphone to improve attention control in sub-clinical generalized anxiety disorder: A randomized, controlled multi-session experiment. *Journal of Affective Disorders*, *246*, 444–451. doi:10.1016/j.jad.2018.12.118 PMID:30599367

Tsiouris, K. M., Gatsios, D., Rigas, G., Miljkovic, D., Seljak, B. K., Bohanec, M., & Fotiadis, D. I. (2017). PD_Manager: an mHealth platform for Parkinson's disease patient management. *Healthcare Technology Letters*, *4*(3), 102-108.

Vagg, T., Tan, Y. Y., Shortt, C., Hickey, C., Plant, B. J., & Tabirca, S. (2018). *MHealth and serious game analytics for cystic fibrosis adults*. Paper presented at the 31st International Symposium on Computer-Based Medical Systems, Karlstad, Sweden. 10.1109/CBMS.2018.00025

Wilson, S., & Liang, R. (2018). *Wearable technology: Present and future*. Paper presented at the 91st World Conference of the textile institute, Leeds, UK

Wood, C. S., Thomas, M. R., Budd, J., Mashamba-Thompson, T. P., Herbst, K., Pillay, D., ... Stevens, M. M. (2019). Taking connected mobile-health diagnostics of infectious diseases to the field. *Nature*, *566*(7745), 467–474. doi:10.103841586-019-0956-2 PMID:30814711

World Health Organisation. (2011). mHealth: New horizons for health through mobile technologies. WHO Press.

Yu, D. X., Parmanto, B., Dicianno, B. E., Watzlaf, V. J., & Seelman, K. D. (2014). *Accessible mHealth for patients with dexterity impairments*. Paper presented at the 16th International ACM SIGACCESS Conference on Computers & Accessibility, Rochester, NY. 10.1145/2661334.2661402

Zennifa, F., Filtrilina, H. &Iramina, K. (2014). *Prototype early warning system for heart disease detection using android application*. Paper presented at the Annual International Conference of the IEEE Engineering in Medicine and Biology Society, Chicago, IL. 10.1109/EMBC.2014.6944369

Chapter 2
Electronic Health Record Security in Cloud:
Medical Data Protection Using Homomorphic Encryption Schemes

Desam Vamsi
VIT-AP, India

ABSTRACT

Security is the primary issue nowadays because cybercrimes are increasing. The organizations can store and maintain their data on their own, but it is not cost effective, so for convenience they are choosing cloud. Due to its popularity, the healthcare organizations are storing their sensitive data to cloud-based storage systems, that is, electronic health records (EHR). One of the most feasible methods for maintaining privacy is homomorphism encryption (HE). HE can combine different services without losing security or displaying sensitive data. HE is nothing but computations performed on encrypted data. According to the type of operations and limited number of operations performed on encrypted data, it is categorized into three types: partially homomorphic encryption (PHE), somewhat homomorphic encryption (SWHE), fully homomorphic encryption (FHE). HE method is very suitable for the EHR, which requires data privacy and security.

DOI: 10.4018/978-1-7998-0261-7.ch002

INTRODUCTION

The "Internet of things" (IoT) is becoming an increasing subject of discussion in the latest technology advancements. It means the interconnection of physical devices, applications, sensors and objects that communicate and share information among them. The distinguishing feature of the IOT in the medical system is the patient's continuous monitoring of different parameters, and the history of such continuous surveillance also yields excellent results. In past times, despite 24 hours of monitoring, the doctor cannot be notified about an emergency on time and also sharing of patient's real time data with specialists, family members, and friends was difficult. Currently, all the instruments in the hospital's ICU are fitted with medical sensors to avoid hurdles faced in the past. The technology that enhances such hurdles is available, but most of them are expensive and not accessible. IoT plays an important role in providing improved medical facilities to patients and also facilitates physicians & hospitals with better monitoring methods. A health surveillance system is composed of a wearable device which monitors patients' health continuously. This wearable unit comprises of various sensors like a sensor for temperature, heart rate, blood pressure etc. This device not only collects the data in bio-signals from sensors and transfers it to the hospital cloud server, which is used for further storage and processing accordingly. This information is accessible from anywhere on the IOT to physicians on the Cloud. Wireless and wearable sensors have become standard instruments for monitoring patients at risk for certain chronic diseases.

Researchers have found many applications using IOT technology over the time. For example, BSN (Body Sensor Network) is a network for particular purposes designed to connect with several medical sensors and implants inside and outside the human body autonomously (Vippalapalli & Ananthula, 2016). Using this, we can monitor human's physiological social information, to monitor hospital patients, to administer drugs at clinics, etc. The progress of bio instructors (Kale & Khandelwal, 2013) and telecommunications techniques make it easier for a home-based monitoring system to collect, display, record and communicate physiological information from a human body to any place. (Chakraborty, Gupta, & Ghosh, 2016) using a smartphone explains telemedicine system for a chronic wound (CW) monitoring. The primary purpose of this study is to design and create a Tele-wound technology network (TWTN) system to capture process and track issues associated with CW using a low-cost smartphone and improve general system efficiency. (Chakraborty, & Kumari, 2016) identified that iris recognition is one of the essential biometric technique to identify a person based on iris. In (Chakraborty, Gupta, & Ghosh, 2014), a low-cost integrated smartphone and an efficient quality-based metadata creation process for acquiring chronic wound image and provide a smooth interaction between doctor and patient.

This paper covers healthcare data aggregation approaches using IOT systems and its applications in medical field. The main focus of this chapter is to identify the methods that provide security storage systems to healthcare records using several cryptographic frameworks. The rest of the paper is covered as follows. Section 1 gives an idea of cloud computing importance and its characteristics, cloud service models, deployment models. Section 2 covers a quick review of cloud computing architecture and its components. Section 3 deals with security concerns of the cloud and controls methods to ensure data protection. Section 4 explains importance of cryptography and several encryption methods. HE schemes along with related work are covered in detail in this section. Section 5 ends the paper with a conclusion

APPROACHES OF DATA AGGREGATION IN SENSOR NETWORKS

The data aggregation is described as the method by which data from various sensors are aggregated to remove redundancy and provide the base station with complete information. Data aggregation usually includes the fusion of data at medium nodes from multiple sensors and the transfer of such aggregated data to the base station (sink). In this section, the data aggregation in Sensor Networks and the methodologies used are discussed. The data aggregation is performed in four ways, namely centralized, tree-based approach, cluster-based approach, and in-network aggregation.

1. **Centralized Approach**: In this strategy, each node transmits its sensed information to the primary node, generally the mote node (e.g., power, bandwidth, etc.). Central address routing along with multi-hop algorithms is used in every intermediate node by considering the cost. The primary node task is to add the data received from other nodes to the base station and to report that data. Traffic is the main issue in this data gathering methodology. In the paper (Fouchal, Herbin, & Blanchard, 2015) a centralized approach that monitors energy usage of all nodes (about their principal activities: communication) is discussed. The authors present a network-based model that assesses how the residual energy of every node is handled. The primary aim is to estimate the energy consumption of all nodes (after a learning phase). Many methods could be used to discover a cure for such disorders (wake up sleeping neighboring nodes, increasing radio ranges of some neighboring nodes).
2. **In-Network Aggregation:** Data is processed at intermediate nodes in this methodology in order to reduce the consumption of critical resources such as energy, computation time, etc. This strategy also improves the network lifetime of each node by decreasing its energy consumption. There are two more ways of aggregation within the network: Loss aggregation with a reduction in packet size or lossless data aggregation without a reduction in packet size. Data is collected from different sources and certain group functions, for example, sum, count, maximum, and minimum, are then applied over the collected information in loss aggregation. In Networked sensors, if they have worn on the body or embedded in our living environments, provide ample data of the physical and mental health (Hassanalieragh et al., 2015). Such data is continuously collected, aggregated, and efficiently mined, which can bring a significant variation in the health environment. In particular, the accessibility of information on unimaginable scales and time lengths combined with a present generation of smart processing algorithms likely to promote the development of medical practice, from its current post-facto reactive paradigm to the proactive prevention, cure, and illness diagnosis framework.
3. **Tree-Based Approach:** In this approach, a composite tree is usually a minimum threaded tree is built first. The root node acts as a base station, leaf nodes act as a source node, and middle nodes act as parent nodes within this tree. Leaf node sends your sensed node in a path found between the leaf node and the base station. In (Habib et al., 2016), the authors discussed various approaches of tree-based data aggregation techniques right from data management framework for biosensors to decision making. Initially, the authors suggested a biosensor-level adaptive information collection method. Secondly, they present a coordinator-level information fusion model with a choice matrix and fuzzy set theory. The findings demonstrate that this strategy decreases the number of redundancy of information gathered and preserves data integrity.

4. **Cluster-based Approach:** This approach divides the nodes into several groups called clusters. A cluster head is chosen within each group and the primary task of the cluster head is to aggregate the data. Each node senses and reports the required information to the cluster head of the same cluster instead of sending the information to the base station because of which it saves a lot of energy. Authors (Nie & L, 2011), addressed the application of Structured Health Monitoring [SHM] using Cluster based Data Aggregation approach and shown the results that this Cluster based technique of data aggregation reduces computing tasks and saves energy of sensors while monitoring patients data.

CLOUD COMPUTING

An increasing number of businesses have already adapted and started working on the cloud atmosphere due to its inherent benefits of flexibility, accessibility, security, and cost-effectiveness. Resources like services, infrastructure, software are shared among all stakeholders in Cloud computing. Hence, cryptography plays an important role in cloud computing because the data is to be secured from all kinds of threats or misuse when it is placed over the cloud. There are various cryptographic techniques evolved for this reason which ensures the security of data on the cloud environment. Security strategy no longer uses a single encryption method rather it makes utilization of multiple encryption methods. These security measures involve encryption of the information, converting the information to unreadable format and decoding at the end with the key which is unique. Currently, various encryption methods are in usage for ensuring the safety of data in different applications. Hence utilizing the cryptographic strategies inside the cloud will guarantee the integrity and information security to users which form essential characteristics of the cloud.

Cloud computing is portable in nature where end users have the flexibility to handle the data from anywhere when connected to the cloud. It uses a network of a large group of servers connected both publicly and privately, thereby providing massive infrastructure for data storage and application. Cloud Computing permit platform independence to users so as to rely on shared computing services like hardware and software rather than having a local infrastructure set-up. During pre-cloud computing days, companies used to manufacture their own servers for meeting various demands, which were highly capital intensive and time taking. With the advent of cloud computing, companies can offer their virtual machines and distribute information to anyone on the cloud with ease. This way, many firms drifted towards the variable priced model from a capital intensive model.

Cloud computing is a broadly utilized strategy for storing information on-demand but it also faces several risk factors including but not limited to data confidentiality, security, access-controls, privacy protection, etc. In the current study, several encryption methods that are used to protect sensitive data on the cloud are examined in detail. Various encryption strategies are analyzed and studied to distinguish enhancement highlights for cloud security. The research in cryptography has become widely and popularly known in the advent of computers. A lot of scopes is there for the researchers and academicians in this area.

CLOUD CHARACTERISTICS

The five important characteristics of cloud computing defined by the National Institute of Standards and Technology's (NIST) (Mell & Grance, 2011) are:

1. **On-demand Self-Service:** A consumer can unilaterally access computing resources, such as server time and network storage, as needed automatically without requiring any human interaction with each service provider. Services such as email, social networking applications are provided without any intervention with service providers. Salesforce.com, Gmail, Facebook, Amazon Web Services are some examples falls under this characteristic.
2. **Broad Network Access**: Cloud computing resources are accessible through multiple devices. User can access by not only using common devices like laptops and personal computers, but they can also be accessed via mobiles, tablets and so on.
3. **Resource Pooling:** Consumers are served by pooling of the service provider's computing resources using a multi-tenant model. It involves allocation and reallocation of different physical and virtual resources as per users demand. The user may not be able to identify the exact coordinates of resources thereby having a sense of location independence. However, the user may be able to specify the location at a broad level of abstraction (e.g. country, state, core data center). Storage-space, memory, e-mail services, and network bandwidth form some examples of cloud computing resources.
4. **Rapid Elasticity:** Resources can be elastically provisioned when needed, and removed when not required. Resources can be scaled up/down basis the requirements (or) in some cases automatically, to commensurate with demand. To the consumer, the services available for usage often appear unlimited and can be appropriated in any quantity at any time.
5. **Measured Service:** The usage of resources (e.g. storage, applications, and hardware) is monitored, controlled and sent to the users. This usage is metered and companies pay as per it, for what they have used. It maintains transparency in terms of utilization rates and costs.

CLOUD SERVICE MODELS

Depending on the business objectives, work requirements and storage needs, companies decide on a specific service model or a combination of models. There are 3 types of service models discussed (Kavis & M. J, 2014), and those are represented in Figure 1:

1. **Infrastructure as a Service (IaaS):** A service provider gives customers pay-as-you-go access to systems administration, storage, servers, and other assets in the cloud. IaaS rapidly scales all over with interest, giving a chance to customer, to pay just for what they use. It helps the client to evade the cost and multifaceted nature of purchasing and dealing with their own physical servers and other data center infra. Every asset is offered as a different segment, and they just need to lease a specific one for whatever duration of time that they need it.
    a. Key Features:
        i. Instead of purchasing hardware completely, users pay for IaaS on demand.
        ii. Infrastructure is scalable depending on processing and storage needs.

    iii. Saves enterprises the costs of buying and maintaining their own hardware.
    iv. Because data is on the cloud, there can be no single point of failure.
    v. Enables the virtualization of administrative tasks, freeing up time for other work.
  b. IaaS Business Scenarios:
    i. Test and advancement: Companies can rapidly set up test conditions, put up new applications for sale to the public user with ease. Also, IaaS makes it brisk and efficient to scale up device-test situations.
    ii. Site facilitating: Running sites utilizing IaaS can be more affordable than customary web facilitating.
    iii. Web applications: IaaS gives all the resources to help web applications, including storage-space, web & application servers, and systems administration resources. Companies can customize the web applications on IaaS and scale up the framework as and when required.

2. **Platform as a Service (PaaS):** It empowers the cloud consumer to convey everything from straight-forward cloud-based applications to complex cloud-empowered advance applications. The consumer buys the assets they need from a cloud specialist on a pay per use model and accesses them over a protected internet association. PaaS is intended to help the total web application lifecycle like building, testing, sending, managing, and restoring. PaaS enables the consumer to evade the cost and multifaceted nature of purchasing and managing programming licenses, the hidden application framework, and hardware or advanced machines. The consumer deal with the applications and administrations they create and the cloud provider usually manages everything else.
  a. Key Highlights:
    i. PaaS gives resources to test, create applications in a similar situation.
    ii. Empowers companies to concentrate on advancement without agonizing over hidden framework.
    iii. Suppliers oversee security, working frameworks, server programming and reinforcements.
    iv. Encourages community-oriented work regardless of whether groups work remotely.
  b. PaaS Business Scenarios:
    i. Improvement system: PaaS gives a system that designers can expand upon to create or alter cloud-based applications. Like the manner in which the client make an Excel spreadsheet, PaaS gives designers a chance to make applications utilizing programming segments decrease the measure of coding that designers must do.
    ii. Examination or business knowledge: PaaS enable companies to break down and extract their information, discovering bits of knowledge, designs and see results to improve company returns, and different business choices.
    iii. Extra administrations: PaaS suppliers may offer different administrations that upgrade applications, for example, work process and security.

3. **Software as a Service (SaaS):** It is a distributed computing offering where clients access to a provider's cloud-based programming. Clients don't develop applications on their gadgets rather the applications dwell on a remote cloud which can be accessed through the web or an API. Through the application, clients can store and investigate information and team up on activities. SaaS gives a total programming arrangement that the customer buys on a pay per use model from the cloud service providers. Customer leases the utilization of an application for their companies and to their clients interface with it over the Internet, more often than not with an internet browser. The

majority of the basic hardware, application programming, and application information are situated with the cloud service provider's server. The service provider company deals with equipment and programming. With the proper administration, they will guarantee the accessibility and the security of the application.

a. Key Highlights:
   i. SaaS sellers give programming and applications to clients by means of a membership display.
   ii. Clients don't need to manage, develop or update programming; SaaS suppliers deal with this.
   iii. Utilization of software can be scaled relying upon company needs.
   iv. Applications are accessible from practically any web associated gadget, from any place on the planet.
b. Regular SaaS Situations:
   i. If the cloud consumer utilizes an electronic email administration such as Outlook, Hotmail, or Yahoo! Mail, at that point they are using a type of SaaS. With these applications, they can sign into their record over the internet, regularly from an internet browser.
   ii. Email programming is situated on the cloud providers system. Users can get to their email and place messages through an internet browser on any PC or Internet-associated gadget.
   iii. For organizational use SaaS provides profitability applications, for example, email, and calendaring; and advanced business applications, like, customer relationship management (CRM), Enterprise Resource Planning (ERP) which helps in organizational growth. Companies pay for the utilization of these applications by membership or as per the utilization.

Figure 1. Cloud service models

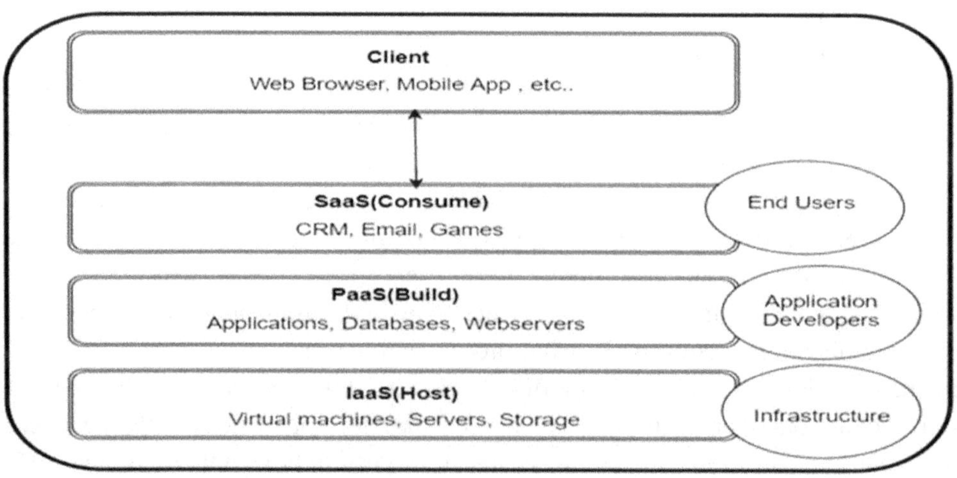

CLOUD DEPLOYMENT MODELS

Basis the configuration of cloud factors like accessibility, storage space, and ownership certain cloud deployment models are available. Depending on the business objectives, work requirements, storage needs companies to decide on specific cloud deployment model (Furht & Escalante, 2010). There are 4 common cloud deployment models shown in Figure 2:

1. **Public Cloud:** As the name indicates, the clouds infrastructure is available for open use to everyone. The responsibility of the creation and routine maintenance of the cloud and its IT infrastructure lies with the cloud owner/the third party. Users can't be guaranteed for information security & integrity because of dependence on an external party for monitoring the cloud. This model is preferred by industries with low-security concerns.
2. **Private Cloud:** The design of a private cloud is similar to public cloud technically. The only difference is that the cloud resources are provisioned for selective use by a company having many users (e.g., business divisions). The cloud can be managed by a third party though it is being used by an organization on a private basis. Only selective persons will be able to access the information, thereby avoiding common public accessing it. This model is preferred by companies with high-security concerns.
3. **Community Cloud:** This cloud resembles a private cloud to a major extent. Unlike only single company owns resources in a private cloud, in community cloud, companies with common backgrounds share the resources on the cloud. This model is preferred by companies that involve joint projects.
4. **Hybrid Cloud:** The hybrid cloud model is a combination of at least two above-mentioned deployment models (private, public and community) as per the requirements. For instance, a company can manage its workload by placing critical ones on private cloud and locating less sensitive ones on the public cloud.

Figure 2. Cloud Deployment Models

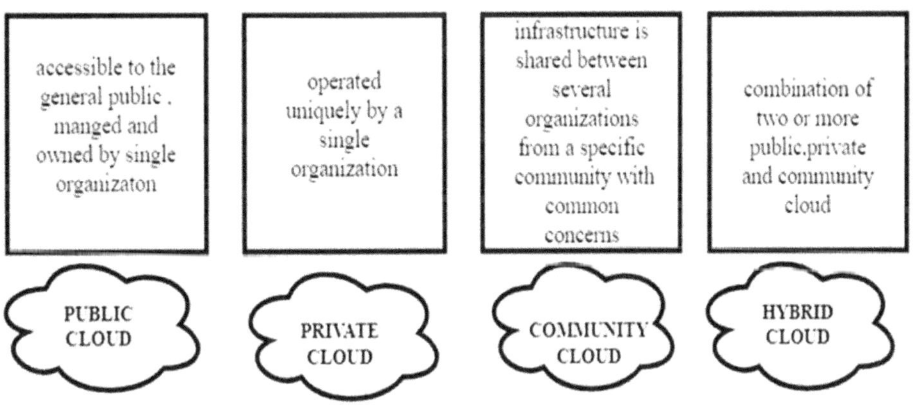

Figure 3. Cloud Architecture

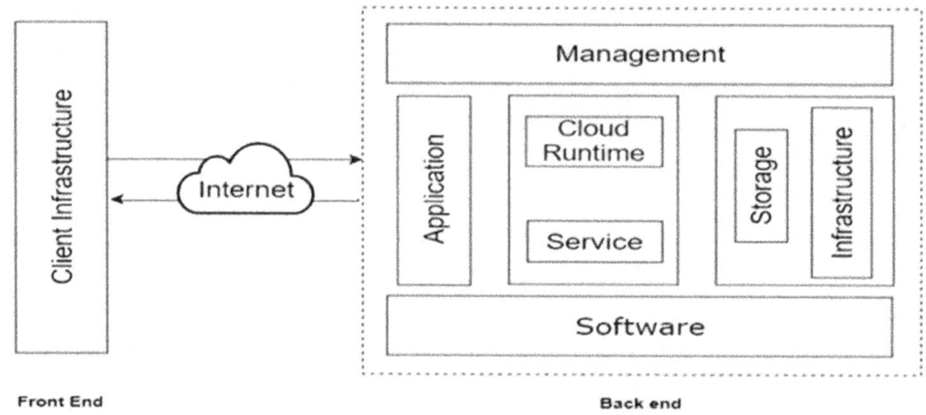

CLOUD COMPUTING ARCHITECTURE

The cloud computing architecture is broadly divided into two parts: front end and back end which are connected through the internet or virtual network. Both Front end and Back end connects by means of the internet.

a) **Front-End:** The interface that is visible to the computer users or clients defines the front end. User interface and user's network which is used for connecting the cloud system form the components of Front End. Various user interfaces are available for various cloud computing systems. For instance, users have a category of web browsers (chrome, internet explorer, firefox) to choose from, but the salesforce interface is not quite the same as that of Google Docs.

b) **Back-End**: On the other side, where the service provider operates the back end. Comprising all the resources including computers, virtual machines, data storage systems, servers and programs required for cloud-computing services forms components of Back end. It is the obligation of back end to provide an inherent security & management mechanisms, protocols and traffic control to all users.

Components of Cloud Computing Architecture

The relationship of components in cloud Architecture is shown in Figure 3, and the components are discussed in this section.

1. **Management Software:** The performance of the cloud can be enhanced by using different plans and methodologies of Management software. Some features of this software include timely delivery of data, security and anytime access. Critical characteristics of Management Software include backup plans, compliance auditing, and disaster management.
2. **Deployment Software:** Deployment software helps in initiating the task (SaaS, PaaS, and IaaS) that can be accessed by users. It involves mandatory installations and configurations of the cloud

3. **Route of Connectivity:** It is an essential part of the design through which the entire cloud gets linked. The speed of exchange relies upon the internet connection. With the assistance of this virtual route, all the cloud servers get connected. Also, users can customize the flow and protocol using this.
4. **A Server of the Cloud:** It is a virtual server which is hosted using a cloud computing platform via the internet. These servers are stable, fast and safe which can be accessed from everywhere. Businesses prefer cloud servers over physical servers to escape from hardware issues and increase options of scalability to optimize cost.
5. **Storage of Cloud:** This is the place where all the data is placed, monitored and protected from outsiders. The data can be accessed from any place and they act as offsite storage for organizations with options for automatic scalability.

SECURITY ISSUES RELATED WITH THE CLOUD

Both the traditional data center environment and cloud environment experience similar threats at a higher level. Cloud computing depends on software which is vulnerable to several attacks. These attackers attempt to misuse those vulnerabilities. In cloud computing, unlike IT systems in the traditional data center, the onus of controlling risks is shared between cloud user and cloud service provider. Hence, users must perceive the responsibilities and work in coordination with cloud service providers. With most of the companies migrated to cloud, the security threat is a major concern for everyone. The following are some of the major risks identified by (Cameron Coles, 2019) are explained.

1. **Theft or Misuse of Company's Intellectual Property:** Many researchers found that around 20% of the files transferred to cloud-based storage services have sensitive and patented information such as licenses, blueprints, strategies, etc. Cybercriminals attack the cloud servers for obtaining such critical information of the companies and try to misuse them. In certain cases, some cloud services are prone to risk which claim ownership of the information on the cloud through terms and agreements signed during the early contractual stage.
2. **Less Control on Insiders:** Organizations have trust in their employees who are given access to cloud on a daily routine. However, there is a risk of privacy from some workers who give importance to personal benefits over organizational values. For example, a sales representative who is going to leave from the organization could download a report of all client contacts, transfer the information to personal storage, and share that information to the competitor. This way insiders misuse their authorized access.
3. **Incomplete Data Deletion:** Consumers are not aware of the physical location of own data and also not sure of the complete deletion of their data without any traces. This risk is concerning because the information is spread over various storage devices inside the cloud service provider's infrastructure. Companies are not in a position to confirm that their information was safely erased and that leftovers of the information are not available to attackers.
4. **Loss of Client's Trust in Cloud**: Users trust is being diminished due to data breaches in large volumes over the world. In one of the largest breakages of credit card information, cyber lawbreakers stole more than 40 million customer card information from cloud servers. This made clients to maintain distance from the cloud, thereby reducing the company's revenue

5. **Stolen Credentials:** If the credentials fall in the hand of attackers, then they could use cloud resources to target the company's administrative users and also other companies using services of the same providers. If the attacker gets the credentials of the cloud service provider administrator, they will be able to exploit the agency's data & systems. The role of administrator varies between a company and a cloud service provider. The cloud administrator has access to network, applications and other resources on the cloud, however, the company's administrator access is limited to the company's cloud usage.
6. **Authoritative Ruptures with Clients or Colleagues:** Contracts among business parties define the usage of data and authorized persons who can access it. At the point when worker moves some confidential information into the cloud without approval, then it is a violation of the contract and has legal implications. If in case cloud service provider sells data on the cloud to outsiders as per the terms and conditions, this will further complicate the situation and result in breach of confidentiality under business contract.
7. **Breach Intimation to Victims and Disclosures:** Certain regulations in an industry require disclosure of any information breach related to stakeholders. Such companies are required to publish and send notifications to exploited people. Regulators can impose fines against an organization after mandated disclosures. Also, it's rightful for customers whose information was breached to file legal suits.
8. **Reduced Client Base:** Clients may take their business to another company in the event they presume that their information isn't completely secure by security controls. It is suggested to maintain distance from cloud providers who don't ensure client security.
9. **Incomplete Due Diligence:** Before migrating to the cloud, companies should perform detailed due diligence. Incomplete due diligence results in moving information to the cloud without understanding the full scope, the safety methods used by the cloud service provider, and their own obligation to give safety mechanisms. This way some companies choose lower secured cloud services without giving detailed attention to them.

CLOUD SECURITY CONTROLS

It is often believed by many that cloud service provider (CSP) is solely responsible for the security of the cloud. Though cloud providers, deal with security for their server hardware and data centers, they rely on individuals for ensuring the security of virtual machines and applications. CSP's provide various security tools to ensure the safety mechanisms in place, but the users have to really execute the essential defenses. Hence it is non-beneficial if the users do not ensure safety for their own networks and applications, there is no use of having numerous security defenses from cloud service providers.

Irrespective of who is using it such as security team, administrator and service provider, many people do not have a comprehensive understanding of how to configure the cloud. Organizations shall implement the following security control measures by (Rashid, 2017) to ensure the safety of applications, data and cloud form hackers.

1. **Data Protection:** Data transiting channels should be safeguarded against any kind of altering or stealing through encryption methods. It is considered as highly insecure to keep data unencrypted on cloud. Cloud security intelligence discovered that around 82 percent of databases in the open

the cloud is not encoded. Voter data and government confidential documents were stolen on the grounds that the information was not encoded and the servers were open to unauthorized groups. Hence, storing confidential information on a cloud without proper security encryptions is dangerous.

2. **Security Mechanisms:** Deploying best security mechanisms at every stage helps in securing cloud environment. If one security feature fails, there is always another control which protects the network, data, and applications in cloud architecture. For example, Multiple factor authentication (MFA) is always more secure than single or double factor authentication making it difficult for hackers to break in. Many researchers suggest that around 60 percent of users do not have MFA enabled to their accounts makes them vulnerable to attacks.
3. **Infrastructure Protection:** All physical components in cloud system which store and process the information should be secured from any seizure, theft, fire, damage and physical altering. The locations of the storage servers, data center buildings should be monitored with physical protection including video surveillance. The hardware should be disposed of in a way that does not compromise the security of the user stored, once its life is over.
4. **Continuous Monitoring:** The responsibility of monitoring the services and infrastructure lies with cloud service providers and the monitoring of applications and virtual machines are with end users. CSPs play a major role in identifying any unauthorized access of applications and systems using security tools. Consumers also should take responsibility to escalate the issue of any unexpected behavior observed while using cloud services without any delay. Both CSP and consumer should coordinate with each other to ensure the security of data systems.
5. **Supply Chain Security Control:** As most of the cloud services are provided by third parties, they can affect the general security of the services. Companies should generate a list of approved vendors after a review process and they are to be complied with security policies before granting them access to information systems and facilities. If this control is not followed, it might compromise the security of service and effects the implementation of other security controls.

For implementing cloud security controls, cloud users should develop a comprehensive understanding of the services they are using. Threats or unauthorized access shall be avoided by using tools supplied by cloud service providers like multi-factor authentication, configured access control. Small & medium companies can avoid risks associated with moving data to the cloud by approaching renowned and established cloud service providers. These cloud service providers should not just provide services, but they should come along with best security practices, encrypting methods and good governance.

FUNDAMENTALS OF CRYPTOGRAPHY

Fundamentals of Cryptography

Cryptography plays an important role in many organizations all around the world because the data is to be secured from threats or misuse when it is placed over the cloud. Initially, from Caesar cipher to Enigma machines and AES to RSA, where the confidentiality is needed so, the cryptography has occurred. To maintain the confidentiality of the information shared, encryption techniques are designed. The secrecy of the key used in the encryption process helps the security of encryption techniques. Encryption methods are categorized into two types: symmetric and asymmetric encryption method.

Symmetric Encryption Method

In this approach, both sender and receiver of data share a single key. This is a secret key which will be used by both for encryption as well as decryption of the messages. Only one secret key is used in Symmetric encryption as shown in Figure 4. Hence, every time different keys are needed for communicating with different persons. This method becomes more complex for generating and managing a huge number of keys. This technique is used in applications, where high efficiency of execution is required. The popular symmetric encryptions are Snow (Ekdahl & Johansson, 2002) and AES (Daemen & Rijmen, 2000; Daemen & Rijmen, 2002).

Asymmetric Encryption Schemes

Unlike symmetric encryption where a single key is used, Asymmetric encryption uses two keys as shown in Figure 5. One key for the encryption and is publically available while the other is for the decryption and is secret. The private key is assigned for the person itself and the public key is meant for every person of the group. Thus this application provides the establishment of secure communication among the groups, which does not require the prior acceptance before communication. The two well-known asymmetric encryption schemes are ElGamal (ElGamal, 1985) and RSA (Rivest et al., 1978b).

Figure 4. Symmetric encryption technique

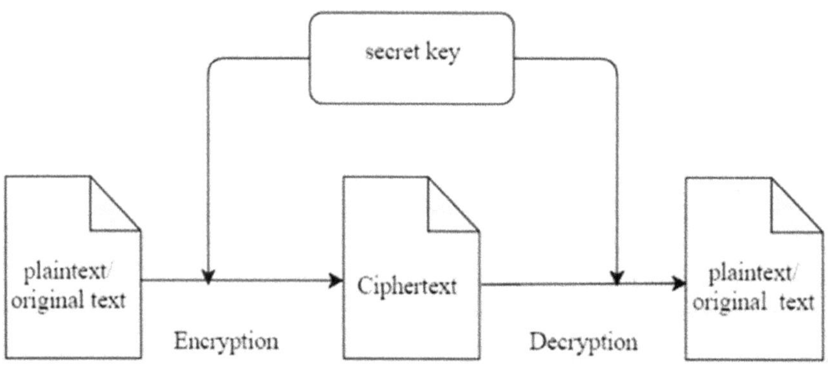

Figure 5. Asymmetric encryption technique

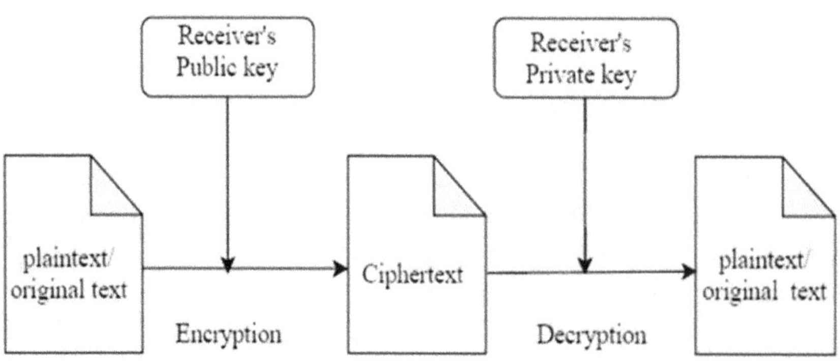

HOMOMORPHIC ENCRYPTION SCHEMES

In ancient Greece, the word *homo* refers to as "same", *morphe* refers as "shape". The word homomorphism is originated in many areas such as cryptography, medical science, and abstract algebra by Malik et.al in (Malik et al., 2007). In cryptography, a homomorphism is one of the encryption type used to secure the data. Homomorphic Encryption (HE) gives the output data in encrypted form. When a third party performs computations on ciphertext, results in the encrypted data. When decryption is performed the output matches the operations as if they had performed on plaintext to maintain the privacy of the data. The multiplicative HE schema example is performed on two messages t_1 and t_2, the result is $E(t_1*t_2)$ by using $E(t_1)$ and $E(t_2)$ without knowing t_1 and t_2 explicitly. Where E refers to Encryption function.

The security is provided for electronic health record that is stored in the cloud by using homomorphic encryption techniques. The patient's medical and personal data is stored in EHR. The healthcare organizations are storing these records in the cloud. There are many privacy issues as EHR information is exposed to unauthorized parties and third-party servers. So, the best method is to encrypt the Electronic Health Record before storing it to cloud to provide confidentiality, security, and efficiency. Based on attributes and roles the patient's data can be accessed.

In cryptology, the word homomorphism is coined by Rivest, Adleman, and Dertouzos in 1978, which allows encrypted data to be computed on, without initial decryption of the operands they named it as "***privacy homomorphism***". They give some simple and modest examples of homomorphism scheme to explain the validity of the idea. After (Rivest et al., 1978a) there is plenty of work done by many researchers around the globe represented with a huge set of operations called homomorphic scheme. The main motive of this HE surveys is that there are many further enhancements in the HE schemes like Partially, Somewhat, Fully HE schemes. Figure 6 gives a clear example of HE for a cloud application.

The early attempt of Yao's 'garbled circuit' proposed a two-party communication which solved the millionaire's problem. It compares a wealth of 2 rich people without showing the exact amount to each other. In Yao's proposal, the size of ciphertext grows linearly with the computations and hence it results in too much complexity in communication protocol and very poor computational efficiency (Yao, 1982). For the next three decades, there is no secure homomorphism scheme is obtained.

Figure 6. Client-server HE scheme, where U is user and C is cloud

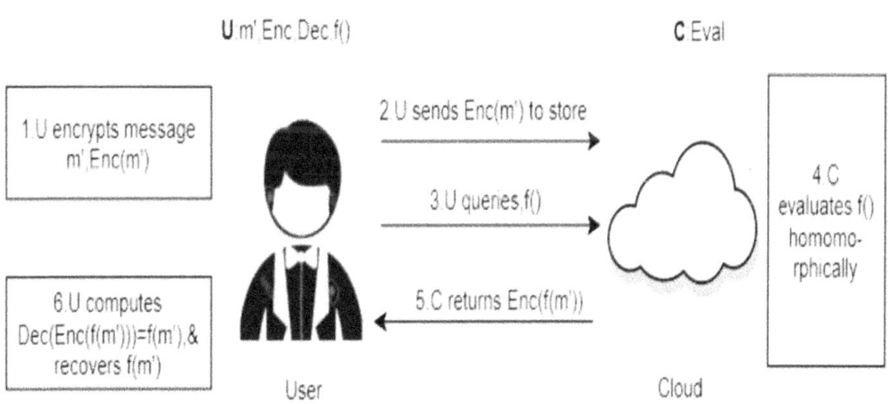

Until Gentry's innovation (Gentry & Boneh, 2009), all the researchers performed either one type of operations or a very limited number of operations on the ciphertext. All these attempts are categorized into three types based on type and number of operations that are performed. 1. Partially Homomorphic Encryption (PHE), 2. Somewhat Homomorphic Encryption (SWHE). 3. Fully Homomorphic Encryption (FHE).

Definition: An encryption scheme has to satisfy the following equation in order to call it as homomorphic.

$$E\left(t_1\right)+E\left(t_2\right)=E\left(t_1+t_2\right),\ \forall t_1,t_2 \in M. \tag{1}$$

where E - encryption algorithm and M - set of all messages

In Homomorphic Encryption schemes, the same key can be used for encryption and decryption (secret key encryption) or different keys to encrypt and decrypt (public key encryption). H is a set of four functions in Homomorphic Encryption. H = {$KeyGen_H$, Enc_H, Dec_H, $Eval_H$}, where $KeyGen_H$ is the function which generates a single key for secret key encryption and secret, public key pair for public key encryption. Enc_H (Encryption) and Dec_H (Decryption) are as same as they performed in Conventional encryption schemes. However, $Eval_H$ is the function where it takes the ciphertext as input and generates a ciphertext according to a functioned plaintext as output. The ciphertext obtained as output after the evaluation is preserved in order to decrypt it correctly. To support the unlimited number of operations, the size of the ciphertext has to be constant. Otherwise, it restricts the number of operations as it requires additional resources. Either additive or multiplicative operations are supported by $Eval_H$ function in PHE schemes, and the only limited number of operations are supported by SWHE schemes, while FHE schemes support the evaluation of arbitrary functions with the unlimited number of times over ciphertext. After Gentry's work, the significance of the HE has gained momentum to a great extent. Figure 7 displays the overall view of the HE schemes until Gentry's first FHE scheme. These homomorphic encryption algorithms can apply on electronic health records to secure the data which is to be stored in a cloud.

Figure 7. A graphical representation of time-period of HE Schemes.

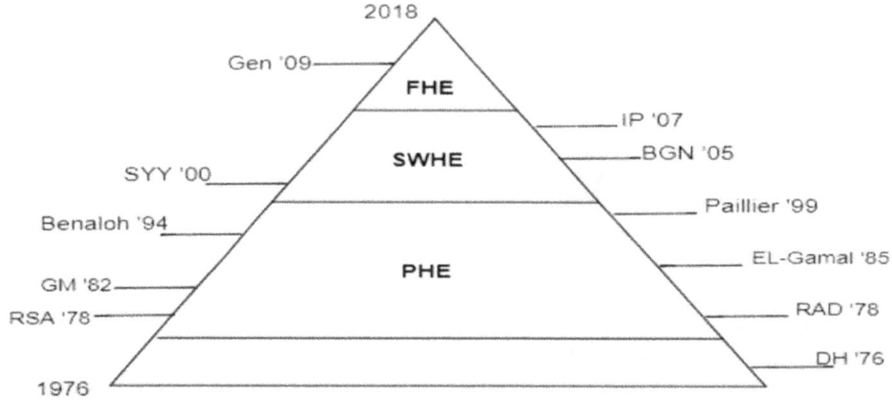

Steps for Homomorphic Encryption Scheme

The encryption needs four functions, key Generation algorithm, Encryption algorithm, Decryption algorithm, Evaluation function (Homomorphic additive and multiplicative).

Step 1: The key generation algorithm $KeyGen_H$, generates the public and secret key pair (pu_k, pr_k);
Step 2: The algorithm of encryption Enc_H (pu_k, x) which encrypts the plaintext x with the public key pu_k;
Step 3: The algorithm of decryption Dec_H (pr_k, c) which decrypts the ciphertext c using private key pr_k;
Step 4: The homomorphic additive function Add (c_1, c_2) where, the inputs c_1, c_2 are the ciphertexts of message x_1 and x_2, it gives the output as ciphertext by encrypting the addition of two plaintexts x_1 and x_2 ;
Step 5: The homomorphic multiplicative function Mul (c_1, c_2) where, the inputs c_1, c_2 are the ciphertexts of message x_1 and x_2, it gives the output as ciphertext by encrypting the product of two plaintexts x_1 and x_2;

Partially Homomorphic Encryption

Various popular and useful instances of PHE schemes will be elaborated in this section, which are the foundations for other PHE schemes. The notation *E(t)* is used to encrypt the message '*t* '.

a. RSA: The RSA Cryptosystem is the initial paradigm of PHE presented by Rivest, Shamir, and Adleman (Rivest et al., 1978b) after the invention of asymmetric cryptography by Diffie and Hellman (Diffie and Hellman, 1976). The RSA Homomorphic property was done by Rivest, Adleman, and Dertouzos (Rivest et al., 1978a), shortly after the invention of the RSA (Rivest et al., 1978b). The decryption key which is kept secret (private) is different from the encryption key that is public. The RSA cryptosystem is based on the difficulty of factorization problem of the product of two large prime numbers. In RSA, the Homomorphic property $E(t_1 * t_2)$ is directly calculated from $E(t_1)$ and $E(t_2)$ without decrypting them. The homomorphic addition is not performed on ciphertexts and only homomorphic multiplication is performed in RSA.

To encrypt the message t in RSA, $E(t) = t^e \bmod n$, where e is exponent and the public key is modulus n. The *Homomorphic property* of RSA Cryptosystem is:

$$\begin{aligned} E\left(t_1\right) * E\left(t_2\right) &= t_1^e t_2^e \bmod n, \\ &= \left(t_1 t_2\right)^e \bmod n, \\ &= E\left(t_1 * t_2\right). \end{aligned} \tag{2}$$

b. Goldwasser-Micali: The GM Cryptosystem is a two-pair key encryption algorithm developed by (Goldwasser and Micali, 1982). It is the first probabilistic asymmetric key encryption scheme based on the hardness of the quadratic residuosity problem. In GM there is only homomorphic over addition and homomorphic multiplication on ciphertexts is not possible.

To encrypt the bit b in GM Cryptosystem, $E(b) = p^b r^2 \bmod n$ for some random variable $r \in \{0,\ldots,n\text{-}1\}$, where p is quadratic non-residue, and the public key is modulus n, $\oplus$ indicates addition modulo 2.

The *Homomorphic property* of GM Cryptosystem is:

$$\begin{aligned} E(b_1) * E(b_2) &= p^{b_1} r_1^2 p^{b_2} r_2^2 \, mod\, n, \\ &= p^{b_1+b_2} (r_1 r_2)^2 \, mod\, n, \\ &= E(b_1 \oplus b_2) \end{aligned} \quad (3)$$

c. El-Gamal: The Taher Elgamal developed a new asymmetric key encryption algorithm in (Elgamal, 1985). It is an upgraded version of the authentic Diffie-Hellman Key Exchange [7] based on the discrete logarithm. The Digital signature algorithm is a slightly different form of the Elgamal signature scheme that should not be confused with Elgamal encryption. The Homomorphic property of El-Gamal supports over multiplication and homomorphic addition operation over ciphertext is not supported here.

To encrypt the message x in El-Gamal Cryptosystem, $E(x)=(g^r, x, p^r)$, for some random variable $r \in \{0,\ldots,p\text{-}1\}$, where a cyclic group G of order p with generator g, the public key is (G, p,g,q), and $q=g^c$ where, c is a secret key.

The *Homomorphic property* of El-Gamal Cryptosystem is:

$$\begin{aligned} E(x_1) * E(x_2) &= (g^{r_1}, x_1 . q^{r_1})(g^{r_2}, x_2 . q^{r_2}), \\ &= (g^{r_1+r_2}, (x_1 * x_2) q^{r_1+r_2}), \\ &= E(x_1 * x_2) \end{aligned} \quad (4)$$

d. Benaloh: In 1994, Benaloh proposed a scheme which is an addition of GM cryptosystem. Instead of encrypting bit by bit it encrypts long blocks of the message (Benaloh, 1994). Mainly this algorithm is based on higher residuosity problem, where it is a generalization of quadratic residuosity problems used in GM cryptosystem. The additive homomorphic property of Benaloh is calculated directly from the encrypted messages $E(t_1)$ and $E(t_2)$ so, it is additively homomorphic.

To encrypt a message $m$in Benaloh Cryptosystem, $E(m) = g^m r^b \text{mod} n$, for some random variable $r \in \{0,\ldots,n\text{-}1\}$, where the public key is modulus n, base g with block size b.

The *Homomorphic property* of Benaloh Cryptosystem is:

$$E(m_{1)} * E\left(m_2\right) mod\, n = \left(g^{m_1} r_1^{\,b}\right)\left(g^{m_2} r_2^{\,b}\right) mod\, n, \\ = g^{m_1+m_2}\left(r_1 r_2\right)^b, \\ = E\left(m_1 + m_2\right) \tag{5}$$

e. Paillier: The Pascal Paillier in 1999, introduced a probabilistic asymmetric algorithm based on composite residuosity problem for public key cryptosystem (Paillier, 1999). Quadratic and higher residuosity problem that is used in GM & Benaloh is very identical to composite residuosity problem. The homomorphic property in Paillier Cryptosystem is homomorphic over addition.

To encrypt the message *m* in Paillier Cryptosystem, $E(m)=g^m r^n \mathrm{mod} n^2$, for some random variables $r\in \{0,\ldots,n\text{-}1\}$, where the public key is modulus *n*, the base *g*.

The *Homomorphic property* of Paillier Cryptosystem is:

$$E\left(m_1\right) * E\left(m_2\right) = \left(g^{m_1} r_1^{\,n}\right)\left(g^{m_2} r_2^{\,n}\right) mod\ n^2, \\ = g^{m_1+m_2}\left(r_1 r_2\right)^n mod\, n^2, \\ = E\left(m_1 + m_2\right) \tag{6}$$

f. Others: Later there are few PHE algorithms proposed based on the previous algorithms. By changing the set of functions, they introduced a new PHE scheme and improved the computational efficiency explained in (Okamoto and Uchiyama, 1998). Later, Naccache-Stern (Naccache & Stern, 1998) introduced another PHE, where the security rests on higher residuosity problem and this algorithm is generalization of Benaloh Cryptosystem to enhance computational performance. Damgard and Jurik (DJ), proposed a PHE algorithm that is the generalization of Paillier is explained in (Damgard & Jurik, 2001). The security of DJ that has been shown to be true by decisional composite residuosity assumption. Galbraith (Galbraith, 2002), introduced a Cryptosystem by performing elliptic curves even though the homomorphic property is still preserving. It is a more real generalization of Paillier Cryptosystem. All these PHE algorithms are additively homomorphic.

Somewhat Homomorphic Encryption

In SWHE only a limited number of operations are performed. SWHE can only be operated to assess lower degree polynomial over ciphertext data. It is constrained mainly due to noisy nature of ciphertext. Further, this noise gets augmented on performing addition and multiplication operations on ciphertext. This complex nature makes the deciphering of ciphertext cumbersome. The main pillar behind the FHE scheme is SWHE scheme and can be applied to real time applications like medical, electronic voting, financial etc. SWHE is much faster than FHE and are replacing FHE schemes, to increase the performance.

Before Gentry's work, there were some well-known SWHE schemes that were developed. Yao's (Yao, 1982), the evaluating size is arbitrary over 'garbled circuit' where the ciphertext size grows linearly. The (Sander et al. 1999) SWHE scheme on the semi-group is supported by only one OR/NOT gate and many polynomially many ANDing of encrypted data. The size of ciphertext grows exponentially with each OR/NOT gate evaluation. In (Boneh et al., 2005), the 2-DNF (Disjunctive Normal Form) formulas on ciphertext are evaluated and performed operations on encrypted data with one multiplication and unlimited additions keeping the ciphertext constant. In (Yuval Ishai and Paskin, 2007) they presented a public key encryption and evaluated branching program on the ciphertext. The size of ciphertext size doesn't depend on the size of the function. The unique characteristic of this protocol is that in a server-client relationship, the client cannot see the size of server's input. In BGN (Boneh et al., 2005), the size of the ciphertext stays constant whereas, with each homomorphic operation in (Sander et al., 1999; Yuval Ishai & Paskin, 2007; Yao, 1982), the ciphertext size grows. However, in homomorphic addition the ciphertext size is constant while the ciphertext grows exponentially in homomorphic multiplication. Because of constant size of the ciphertext in BGN (Boneh et al., 2005) cryptosystem, it is further used to obtain FHE schemes.

Fully Homomorphic Encryption

Almost 30 years from the institution of privacy homomorphism idea by (Rivest et al., 1978a), Gentry (Gentry, 2009) proposed the first viable scheme in his PhD thesis to a longstanding open issue, which acquires a scheme called FHE. The Fully Homomorphic Encryption (FHE) performs unlimited number of operations on the ciphertext and gives the resultant output within the ciphertext space. In Figure 8 there are mainly four FHE families after Gentry's innovation are represented.

Gentry's scheme acts as a framework to obtain an FHE scheme. After his work, many researchers have tried to design a secure FHE scheme. Gentry (Gentry, 2009) introduced Ideal lattice-based FHE scheme showing signs of future success and had a lot of hindrances like the cost to implement in real life and executing advanced mathematical functions. Later many of them work on Gentry's proposal addressing the hindrances. All the work done till now is to achieve a new secure FHE scheme which solves the hardships on lattices. Later the work done on lattices becomes popular for the cryptographic researchers, after gentry scheme. Firstly, a small work is done by the researchers (Smart and Vercauteren, 2010) to

Figure 8. Fully Homomorphic Encryption (FHE) categories

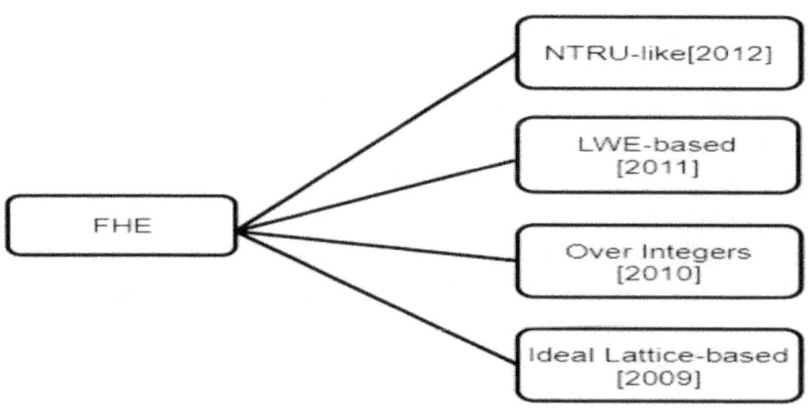

enhance the Gentry's ideal lattice-based FHE scheme and later they introduced the FHE scheme over integers. The main motive behind this scheme is to make it more conceptually understandable based on Approximate-GCD problems by (Van Dijk et al., 2010). Then, (Brakerski and Vaikuntanathan, 2011) suggested another FHE scheme based on the hardness of Ring Learning with Error problems which assure some efficiency characteristics. At last, NTRU-like FHE is presented by (Lopez-Alt et al., 2012), is an old systematic lattice-based-encryption scheme with good efficiency and standardized homomorphic properties.

RELATED WORK DONE ON HE SCHEMES

The homomorphic encryption scheme has its application in many areas and has already given the best results. In ideal lattice-based FHE, bootstrapping and squashing techniques are included. The latest work that has been done in (Zhou et al., 2018), where they accelerated the bootstrapping by three improvements which gave the better performance in data protection. In (Chatterjee & Sengupta, 2018), by using FHE, encrypting the sensitive data and storing on the cloud for confidentiality, they obtained a way to translate algorithms and handling the termination between client and server by passing the message. In bioinformatics for providing privacy (Dowlin et al., 2017) proposed a Homomorphic Encryption for sensitive health and genomic data using a Simple Encrypted Arithmetic Library (SEAL) which made it publicly accessible. Secret sharing of data is one of the important components in cryptography, a novel HE scheme is proposed (Zhang et al., 2017) for outsourcing secret sharing data. By applying ring-LWE and ideal-lattice homomorphic encryption (Yasuda, 2017) developed secure maintenance of the biometric system in (Yasuda, 2017). The first multi-hop homomorphic identity-based proxy re-encryption scheme is discussed in (Li et al., 2017a), it can be useful for many applications like securing e-mail forwarding, data sharing, and access control systems. In (Cheon & Kim, 2015) constructed a hybrid scheme by concatenating Goldwasser-Micali and ElGamal schemes. In (Wu et al., 2018) the server builds an inverted encryption index structure to reduce the single keyword search time complexity without query trapdoor mechanism. Not only the confidentiality but also the integrity protections are proposed in (Tsoutsos & Maniatakos, 2018), which gives encrypted computations efficiently using additive HE. Based on Homomorphic Encryption (Yang et al., 2018), proposed a secure verifiable e-voting system in which they used ElGamal cryptosystem.

HElib, which is termed as 'assembly language for HE, without using commands and functions of programming language deals with the hardware constraints of the computer. Microsoft has released other HE library named Simple Encrypted Arithmetic Library -SEAL (Laine et al. 2017) with an aim to provide a well-documented HE library. It can be accessed by both crypto and non-crypto experts including practitioners in bioinformatics. It acts independently using automatic parameter selection and noise eliminator tools. Fastest Homomorphic Encryption in the West - FHEW, a major application is developed by Ducas and Micciancio documented in (Ducas and Micciancio 2015). The time required to bootstrap the ciphertext is reduced to "in less than a second" claiming homomorphic evaluation of a NAND gate. There are some publicly accessible FHE implementations which can be used by the researchers. A few implementations that are publicly accessible are displayed in the Table 1.

Table 1. Publicly accessible FHE applications

Name	Language	Authors
SEAL	C++	Laine et al .,2017
TFHE	C++	Chillotti et al .,2017
HElib	C++	Halevi and Shoup, 2015
FHEW	C++	Ducas and Micciancio, 2014

FURTHER RESEARCH DIRECTIONS

FHE can be still explored to different applications like multi-party FHE, multikey FHE and also in designing Attribute Based Encryption (ABE) and Identity Based Encryption (IBE) with FHE. These ABE and IBE are suitable for access control to data that is stored in the cloud. Some works are done on these applications, but their performance doesn't match with traditional approaches so, these problems can lead to promising research applications. FHE also solves Functional Encryption (i.e., ABE, IBE). FE restricts the access of data but allows operations on it based on their attribute or identity characteristics. Later a standard model, an efficient identity based FHE scheme is designed in two-levels in (Hu et al., 2018) i.e. first-level is multi-bit IBE and the second level is batch identity-based fully homomorphic encryption (IBFHE). In FHE, one of the processes that increases the computational cost is bootstrapping, which is helpful in decreasing the noise in evaluated ciphertext, and these are still an open issue. Another important application of FHE is multi-party computation which takes multiple inputs from different users and makes the computation function by keeping the inputs hidden. In (Clear & McGoldrick, 2015) the multi-identity and key based FHE from learning with errors are reported. This multi-key FHE with the unlimited number of users is one of the new promising approaches in the future. These attribute and identity based encryptions are used to secure the sensitive data of the patient health records. Using attribute based encryption the personal health records are securely shared in the cloud (Li et al., 2013b).

Challenges

1. IoT systems capture and communicate real-time information. Data Security and privacy is one of the most important threat for IoT System Design in Healthcare.
2. Multiple device integration and protocols also creates hindrance in the healthcare industry IoT applications.
3. IoT devices keep recording a ton of information. The information gathered by IoT devices is used to obtain vital signs. However, the quantity of information is so huge that it becoming highly hard for physicians to give treatment from it, which eventually impacts decision-making quality.
4. IoT has not yet made healthcare affordable to the ordinary man. The boom in healthcare expenses is a worrying sign for the developed countries in particular.

CONCLUSION

IoT technologies are evolving around the world than ever before. So, protecting the data plays a key role. Many applications based on IOT technology found its usage in medical field and all the patient's information is gathered and stored in cloud. The significance increases for sensitive industries like healthcare, where the documents stored in the cloud must be protected from both malign and benign third parties. Security is one of the most important tasks nowadays. In a smart healthcare system, the Electronic Health Records are the major modules which share the medical data between healthcare providers and patients. Encryption is the main means to protect the privacy of the data. Its performance is evaluated by security, speed, and understandability. Homomorphic Encryption is the special kind of encryption scheme where the computations are done on ciphertext without deciphering it. Applying this encryption algorithm for EHR data will provide better security when it is stored in the cloud.

REFERENCES

Benaloh, J. (1994, May). Dense probabilistic encryption. In *Proceedings of the workshop on selected areas of cryptography* (pp. 120-128). Academic Press.

Boneh, D., Goh, E. J., & Nissim, K. (2005, February). Evaluating 2-DNF formulas on ciphertexts. In *Theory of Cryptography Conference* (pp. 325-341). Springer.

Brakerski, Z., & Vaikuntanathan, V. (2011, August). Fully homomorphic encryption from ring-LWE and security for key dependent messages. In *Annual cryptology conference* (pp. 505-524). Springer. 10.1007/978-3-642-22792-9_29

Cameron, C. (2019). *Cloud computing security risks every company faces*. Retrieved from https://www.skyhighnetworks.com/cloud-security-blog/9-cloud-computing-security-risks-every-company-faces/

Chakraborty, C., & Kumari, S. (2016). Bio-metric Identification using Automated Iris Detection Technique. *IEEE: 3rd International Conference on Microelectronics, Circuits, and Systems*, 113-17.

Chakraborty, C., Gupta, B., & Ghosh, S. K. (2014). Mobile metadata assisted community database of chronic wound images. *Wound Medicine*, *6*, 34–42. doi:10.1016/j.wndm.2014.09.002

Chakraborty, C., Gupta, B., & Ghosh, S. K. (2016). Mobile telemedicine systems for remote patient's chronic wound monitoring. In *M-Health innovations for patient-centered care* (pp. 213–239). IGI Global. doi:10.4018/978-1-4666-9861-1.ch011

Chatterjee, A., & Sengupta, I. (2018). Translating algorithms to handle fully homomorphic encrypted data on the cloud. *IEEE Transactions on Cloud Computing*, *6*(1), 287–300. doi:10.1109/TCC.2015.2481416

Cheon, J. H., & Kim, J. (2015). A hybrid scheme of public-key encryption and somewhat homomorphic encryption. *IEEE Transactions on Information Forensics and Security*, *10*(5), 1052–1063. doi:10.1109/TIFS.2015.2398359

Chillotti, I., Gama, N., Georgieva, M., & Izabachène, M. (2017). *TFHE: Fast FullyHomomorphicEncryptionLibraryovertheTorus*. Retrieved from https://github.com/tfhe/tfhe

Clear, M., & McGoldrick, C. (2015, August). Multi-identity and multi-key leveled FHE from learning with errors. In *Annual Cryptology Conference* (pp. 630-656). Springer. 10.1007/978-3-662-48000-7_31

Daemen, J., & Rijmen, V. (2000). The Block Cipher Rijndael. In *Proceedings of International Conference on Smart Cards Research and Applications (CARDS'98), Lecture Notes in Computer Science* (Vol 1820, pp. 247-256). Springer-Verlag. 10.1007/10721064_26

Daemen, J. & Rijmen, V. (2002). *The Design of Rijndael.* AES- The Advanced Encryption.

Damgård, I., & Jurik, M. (2001, February). A generalisation, a simpli. cation and some applications of paillier's probabilistic public-key system. In *International Workshop on Public Key Cryptography* (pp. 119-136). Springer. 10.1007/3-540-44586-2_9

Diffie, W., & Hellman, M. (1976). New directions in cryptography. *IEEE Transactions on Information Theory*, *22*(6), 644–654. doi:10.1109/TIT.1976.1055638

Dowlin, N., Gilad-Bachrach, R., Laine, K., Lauter, K., Naehrig, M., & Wernsing, J. (2017). Manual for homomorphic encryption for bioinformatics. *Proceedings of the IEEE, 105*(3), 552–567.

Ducas, L., & Micciancio, D. (2015, April). FHEW: bootstrapping homomorphic encryption in less than a second. In *Annual International Conference on the Theory and Applications of Cryptographic Techniques* (pp. 617-640). Springer. 10.1007/978-3-662-46800-5_24

Ducas & Micciancio. (2014). *A Fully Homomorphic Encryption library*. Retrieved from https://github.com/ lducas/FHEW

Ekdahl, P., & Johansson, T. (2002, August). A new version of the stream cipher SNOW. In *International Workshop on Selected Areas in Cryptography* (pp. 47-61). Springer.

ElGamal, T. (1985). A public key cryptosystem and a signature scheme based on discrete logarithms. *IEEE Transactions on Information Theory*, *31*(4), 469–472. doi:10.1109/TIT.1985.1057074

Fouchal, H., Herbin, M., & Blanchard, F. (2015, August). Centralized energy monitoring over wireless sensor networks. In *2015 International Wireless Communications and Mobile Computing Conference (IWCMC)* (pp. 788-792). IEEE. 10.1109/IWCMC.2015.7289183

Furht, B., & Escalante, A. (2010). *Handbook of cloud computing* (Vol. 3). New York: Springer. doi:10.1007/978-1-4419-6524-0

Galbraith, S. D. (2002). Elliptic curve Paillier schemes. *Journal of Cryptology*, *15*(2), 129–138. doi:10.100700145-001-0015-6

Gentry, C., & Boneh, D. (2009). A fully homomorphic encryption scheme: Vol. 20. *No. 09.* Stanford, CA: Stanford University.

Goldwasser, S., & Micali, S. (1982, May). Probabilistic encryption & how to play mental poker keeping secret all partial information. In *Proceedings of the fourteenth annual ACM symposium on Theory of computing* (pp. 365-377). ACM. 10.1145/800070.802212

Habib, C., Makhoul, A., Darazi, R., & Salim, C. (2016). Self-adaptive data collection and fusion for health monitoring based on body sensor networks. *IEEE Transactions on Industrial Informatics*, *12*(6), 2342–2352. doi:10.1109/TII.2016.2575800

Halevi & Shoup. (2013). *An Implementation of homomorphic encryption*. Retrieved from https://github.com/ shaih/HElib

Hassanalieragh, M., Page, A., Soyata, T., Sharma, G., Aktas, M., Mateos, G., & Andreescu, S. (2015, June). Health monitoring and management using Internet-of-Things (IoT) sensing with cloud-based processing: Opportunities and challenges. In *2015 IEEE International Conference on Services Computing* (pp. 285-292). IEEE. 10.1109/SCC.2015.47

Hu, M., Ye, Q., & Tang, Y. (2018). Efficient batch identity-based fully homomorphic encryption scheme in the standard model. *IET Information Security*, *12*(6), 475–483. doi:10.1049/iet-ifs.2017.0567

Ishai, Y., & Paskin, A. (2007, February). Evaluating branching programs on encrypted data. In *Theory of Cryptography Conference* (pp. 575-594). Springer. 10.1007/978-3-540-70936-7_31

Kale, S., & Khandelwal, C. S. (2013, March). Design and implementation of real time embedded telehealth monitoring system. In *2013 International Conference on Circuits, Power and Computing Technologies (ICCPCT)* (pp. 771-774). IEEE. 10.1109/ICCPCT.2013.6528842

Kavis, M. J. (2014). *Architecting the cloud: design decisions for cloud computing service models (SaaS, PaaS, and IaaS)*. John Wiley & Sons. doi:10.1002/9781118691779

Laine, K., Chen, H., & Player, R. (2017). *Simple Encrypted Arithmetic Library*. Retrieved from https:// sealcrypto. codeplex.com/

Li, M., Yu, S., Zheng, Y., Ren, K., & Lou, W. (2013b). Scalable and secure sharing of personal health records in cloud computing using attribute-based encryption. *IEEE Transactions on Parallel and Distributed Systems*, *24*(1), 131–143. doi:10.1109/TPDS.2012.97

Li, Z., Ma, C., & Wang, D. (2017a). Towards multi-hop homomorphic identity-based proxy re-encryption via branching program. *IEEE Access: Practical Innovations, Open Solutions*, *5*, 16214–16228. doi:10.1109/ACCESS.2017.2740720

López-Alt, A., Tromer, E., & Vaikuntanathan, V. (2012, May). On-the-fly multiparty computation on the cloud via multikey fully homomorphic encryption. In *Proceedings of the forty-fourth annual ACM symposium on Theory of computing* (pp. 1219-1234). ACM. 10.1145/2213977.2214086

Malik, D. S., Mordeson, J. N., & Sen, M. K. (2007). *MTH 581-582 Introduction to Abstract Algebra*. Academic Press.

Mell, P., & Grance, T. (2011). *The NIST definition of cloud computing*. Academic Press.

Naccache, D., & Stern, J. (1998, November). A new public key cryptosystem based on higher residues. In *Proceedings of the 5th ACM conference on Computer and communications security* (pp. 59-66). ACM. 10.1145/288090.288106

Nie, P., & Li, B. (2011, July). A cluster-based data aggregation architecture in WSN for structural health monitoring. In *2011 7th International Wireless Communications and Mobile Computing Conference* (pp. 546-552). IEEE. 10.1109/IWCMC.2011.5982592

Okamoto, T., & Uchiyama, S. (1998, May). A new public-key cryptosystem as secure as factoring. In *International conference on the theory and applications of cryptographic techniques* (pp. 308-318). Springer. 10.1007/BFb0054135

Paillier, P. (1999, May). Public-key cryptosystems based on composite degree residuosity classes. In *International Conference on the Theory and Applications of Cryptographic Techniques* (pp. 223-238). Springer. 10.1007/3-540-48910-X_16

Rashid, F. Y. (2017). Top cloud security controls you should be using. *InfoWorld*. Retrieved from https://www.csoonline.com/article/3208905/top-cloud-security-controls-you-should-be-using.html

Rivest, R. L., Adleman, L., & Dertouzos, M. L. (1978a). On data banks and privacy homomorphisms. *Foundations of Secure Computation, 4*(11), 169-180.

Rivest, R. L., Shamir, A., & Adleman, L. (1978b). A method for obtaining digital signatures and public-key cryptosystems. *Communications of the ACM, 21*(2), 120–126. doi:10.1145/359340.359342

Sander, T., Young, A., & Yung, M. (1999). Non-interactive cryptocomputing for NC/SUP 1. In *Foundations of Computer Science, 1999. 40th Annual Symposium on* (pp. 554-566). IEEE.

Standard. Information Security and Cryptography. (2002). New York, NY: Springer.

Tsoutsos, N. G., & Maniatakos, M. (2018). Efficient Detection for Malicious and Random Errors in Additive Encrypted Computation. *IEEE Transactions on Computers, 67*(1), 16–31. doi:10.1109/TC.2017.2722440

Van Dijk, M., Gentry, C., Halevi, S., & Vaikuntanathan, V. (2010, May). Fully homomorphic encryption over the integers. In *Annual International Conference on the Theory and Applications of Cryptographic Techniques* (pp. 24-43). Springer.

Vippalapalli, V., & Ananthula, S. (2016, October). Internet of things (IoT) based smart health care system. In *2016 International Conference on Signal Processing, Communication, Power and Embedded System (SCOPES)* (pp. 1229-1233). IEEE. 10.1109/SCOPES.2016.7955637

Wu, D. N., Gan, Q. Q., & Wang, X. M. (2018). Verifiable Public Key Encryption With Keyword Search Based on Homomorphic Encryption in Multi-User Setting. *IEEE Access: Practical Innovations, Open Solutions, 6*, 42445–42453. doi:10.1109/ACCESS.2018.2861424

Yang, X., Yi, X., Nepal, S., Kelarev, A., & Han, F. (2018). A Secure Verifiable Ranked Choice Online Voting System Based on Homomorphic Encryption. *IEEE Access: Practical Innovations, Open Solutions, 6*, 20506–20519. doi:10.1109/ACCESS.2018.2817518

Yao, A. C. (1982, November). Protocols for secure computations. In *Foundations of Computer Science, 1982. SFCS'08. 23rd Annual Symposium on* (pp. 160-164). IEEE. 10.1109/SFCS.1982.38

Yasuda, M. (2017). Secure Hamming distance computation for biometrics using ideal-lattice and ring-LWE homomorphic encryption. *Information Security Journal: A Global Perspective, 26*(2), 85-103.

Zhang, E., Peng, J., & Li, M. (2017). Outsourcing secret sharing scheme based on homomorphism encryption. *IET Information Security, 12*(1), 94–99. doi:10.1049/iet-ifs.2017.0026

Zhou, T., Yang, X., Liu, L., Zhang, W., & Li, N. (2018). Faster bootstrapping with multiple addends. *IEEE Access: Practical Innovations, Open Solutions, 6*, 49868–49876. doi:10.1109/ACCESS.2018.2867655

Chapter 3
Blended Models for Nearest Neighbour Algorithms for High Dimensional Smart Medical Data

Sandhya Harikumar
Department of Computer Science and Engineering, Amrita School of Engineering, Amrita Vishwa Vidyapeetham, Amritapuri, India

ABSTRACT

Nearest neighbor algorithms like kNN and Parzen Window are generative algorithms that are used extensively for medical diagnosis and classification of diseases. The data generated or collected in healthcare is high dimensional and cannot be assumed to follow a particular distribution. The conventional approaches fail due to computational complexity, curse of dimensionality, and varying distributions. Hence, this chapter deals with a blending technique for evaluation of nearest neighbor algorithms based on various parameters such as the size of data, dimensions of data, window size, and number of nearest neighbors to make it suitable for massive datasets. Dimensionality reduction and clustering are combined with nearest neighbor classifier such as kNN and Parzen Window to observe the performance of the blended models on various types of datasets. Experimental results on 15 real datasets with various models reveal the efficacy of the proposed blends.

DOI: 10.4018/978-1-7998-0261-7.ch003

INTRODUCTION

The capability of machine learning to learn from data without being explicitly programmed has accelerated medical domain in diagnosing and classifying diseases. Datasets about patients, diseases, and medicines are so massive that human beings find it difficult to analyze and come to a conclusion, given a task of prescribing a medicine to a patient or of diagnosing a disease given the symptoms in a patient. Hence the power of machine learning is leveraged in healthcare domain so as to enable hospitals to provide better services, improvise the care given to patients, generate more revenue, and improve risk management. Most of the use cases of healthcare domain congregate towards classification algorithms to solve the problems such as diagnosing a disease, prescribing a medicine, side effects of medicines, and readmission of a patient to the hospital. With huge volume of data being generated in healthcare domains, classification problems such as disease diagnosis, medicine prescription, genes identification etc. have become inevitable for proper visualization and interpretation. A single classifier may not efficiently output results in a timely manner for voluminous data due to the storage and processing limitations of conventional algorithms. The performance of any classifier adopted, are highly dependent on the problem domain. Nearest neighbor algorithms are preferable due to its simplicity, ease of implementation and effectiveness in classification. However, the complexity of these classifiers is dependent on the size of data, dimensions of data as well as parameters such as k in kNN (Murphy, 2013; Cover & Hart, 2006) and window size in Parzen window (Parzen, 1962). As a result, a system may not perform optimally in spite of best performance of a single classifier. In practical applications, a single classifier may not give required accuracy, precision, or recall. In such cases, it is better to integrate various classifiers in an appropriate manner and find an optimal model (Kittler, Hatef & Matas, 1998) suitable for the domain context. The other need for integrating different classifiers is the varying probability distributions of the data that may not be well known ahead. Furthermore, high dimensions of the data also throw challenges towards classification algorithms to learn and classify the data optimally. Hence, combining dimensionality reduction (Xie, Liu & Xue, 2017) and clustering (Anil, 2010) with classifiers such as kNN and Parzen window, may help in improving performance when compared with any other single classifiers (Chakraborty, 2017). One of the main advantages of kNN and Parzen window over other algorithms is that they can be applied to data following any distributions (Aggarwal, 2014; Cover & Hart, 2006; Anava & Levy, 2016). But since these algorithms do not understand the data, the successful execution requires careful choice of parameters 'k', feature weights 'w', window size and distance measure (Murphy, 2013). Most of the works focus on the setting of 'k' and 'w' irrespective of structure and distribution of data whose labels are to be found. Furthermore, kNN suffers from 'Curse of dimensionality' and sparsity in higher dimensions that lead to expensive computational cost and high storage requirements for voluminous data (Aggarwal, 2014; Anava & Levy, 2016; Koppen, 2008). Hence there is a crucial need for the classification of high dimensional data.

In practical datasets, data points may be skewed and most of them may belong to one class (majority class) than other classes (minority class) (Murphy, 2013). With a fixed high value for 'k', kNN algorithm has high bias towards the majority class. Hence, finding best 'k' value using cross validation or pruning the execution of the search algorithm, or combining the eager and lazy learning method (Wu, Cai & Gao, 2010; Ougiaroglou, & Nanopoulos et. al. 2007; Duda, Stork, & Hart, 2001) are effective strategies. The most common distance measure used by conventional kNN to find nearest neighbors of a sample from a training set, is the Euclidean measure (Murphy, 2013; Aggarwal, 2014). This measure gives equal weight to each of the attributes of a sample. However, in high dimensional data, when datasets have a huge number of irrelevant attributes, the value of distance function becomes inaccurate and inappropriate. An effective approach to deal with this issue is to give a measure of importance in the form of some values to each attribute differently (Han, Karypis, and Kumar, 2001). Another approach adopted in (Song, Huang, Zhou, Zha, & Giles, 2007) is to assign different weights to nearest neighbors according to their distance from test instance. Based on the weights of the neighbors, class of a test sample is inferred.

Nearest neighbor classifiers predict the class of a sample just by the class of its neighbors that is highly similar to it. These are non-parametric models that do not try to come up with a general model by learning the data. The execution time of these classifiers depends on the underlying search technique and the distance measure used to find the similarity between the instances. Linear search on large training sets is quite inefficient especially when the data is high dimensional. A solution to this problem is to design suitable index structures like kd-tree (Friedman, Bentley & Finkel, 1977) but kd-tree fails for very high dimensions. Reducing the size of training dataset without loss of information also helps in decreasing the execution time of kNN classification. Computing centroids of each class and finding nearest neighbors with few representatives from each class can also improve the performance of kNN algorithm (Taniar, 2008). This approach, though simple gives accurate classification for data. Data Clustering is another step for speeding up data retrieval and improving accuracy especially in a large database. The most adapted method for clustering is the K-Means clustering algorithm proposed by James MacQueen in 1967 (Chakraborty, 2017). This chapter presents evaluations of classifiers with various combinations of dimensionality reduction and clustering, on various types of datasets from medical, healthcare and other domains. The statistical techniques in this chapter include nearest neighbor algorithms (k-NN and Parzen window), K-means clustering, and dimensionality reduction technique, Principal Component Analysis (PCA). The authors in this paper blend various strategies to get optimal classification for a given dataset. Experimental analysis shows the efficacy and feasibility of this blending technique.

The organization of this chapter is as follows. Section 2 presents background on healthcare analytics and various types of machine learning algorithms used to analyze healthcare data. Section 3 describes the proposed blended models. Section 4 presents the experimental results in the form of solutions and recommendations for various types of datasets. Section 5 presents the conclusion and future work.

BACKGROUND

Due to the increase in huge volume of different types of data generated in medical and health care domain, the various issues that soar in health care domain, include diagnosing disease of a patient, forecasting the disease well ahead from clinical test results, optimized combination of medicines for disease therapy, vaccination, identifying genetic characteristics that lead to diseases like cancer, etc (Chen, Hao, Hwang, Wang & Wang, 2017). Health care analytics is the analysis of data so as to find solutions to some extent to the aforementioned issues. The other problems that health care analytics can solve, include clinical and genomic analysis where the medical data are high dimensional. Data needs to be extracted and organized properly for causal, descriptive, predictive and prescriptive analysis. This aids in better prediction and to take preventive measures (Niu, Zhao & Zhang, 2013; Islam, Hasan, Wang, Germack, Noor-E-Alam, 2018; Saleh et al, 2017; Sathya, Joshi, Padmavathi, 2017; Gutjahr, Chinju Krishna, & Nedungadi, 2018; Nedungadi, Iver, Gutjahr, et al., 2018).

Healthcare analytics has very progressive and good effects on life. Analysis of patients data can help inhibit epidemic diseases, reduce treatment costs by suggesting optimal treatment to prevent the possible diseases that the patients may suffer in future (Chen, Hao, Hwang, Wang & Wang, 2017). Thus, models of treatment can be changed and doctors can be recommended on possible signs of chronic disease in a patient thereby treating the patient at an early stage. This is very cost effective as patients will be able to plan their health insurance quite ahead of time. Thus healthcare data analytics help in predicting and solving a problem well ahead and also evaluate treatment methods to empower patients with the knowledge of diseases and possible remedies. Ensemble classifiers, artificial neural networks, genetic algorithms, have been used to diagnose diseases such as diabetic retinopathy and diabetic mellitus (Sala et al., 2017; Rashid & Abdullah, 2018; Chinmany, Gupta, Ghosh, & Chakraborty, 2016; Shesternikova, 2016). Though lots of works have been done, involvement of domain expert in the decision-making process for predictive and prescriptive analytics is still lacking. Researchers have found that thousands of patients lose their lives each year due to medical errors (Islam, Hasan, Wang, Germack & Noor-E-Alam, 2018). As a result various machine learning algorithms, especially classification algorithms need to be revisited to suit applications pertaining to health care domain. Extensive research has been done on various classification algorithms in data mining. Broadly, classifiers are of two types namely Parametric classifiers and Non-parametric classifiers. The kNN algorithm is one of the best non-parametric algorithms that has a wide range of applications for pattern classification (Wu, Kumar, Quinlan et al., 2007). Another non-parametric algorithm is based on kernel density estimation called Parzen Window (Parzen, 1962). This chapter evaluates alternative techniques for classification of high dimensional data by combining these non-parametric classifiers with dimensionality reduction and clustering algorithms.

Parametric Classifiers

Quite often, machine learning algorithms assume a simple function that can fit data so as to enable prediction or classification. But such assumptions have limitations in terms of what can be learned. Algorithms like linear regression and logistic regression are parametric classifiers that learn a set of parameters of fixed size with a presumed assumption about the data distribution. Such algorithms first decide on a model and then try to find the best coefficients for that model (Murphy, 2013; Aggarwal, 2014; Taniar, 2008). Though these classifiers are easy to interpret results and quite efficient in learning a simple model, these are based on a constrained form of function assumed before the learning process starts. Hence these are not suitable for a dataset that is quite small or quite huge in terms of samples as well as features. Such classifiers have usually high bias and low variance.

Non-Parametric Classifiers

Algorithms that classify given data samples without any assumption about the data distribution are called non-parametric classifiers. Any form of function may be learned in general by such classifiers. Hence these are good to learn voluminous data with no prior knowledge about its features. One of the best non-parametric classifiers is kNN (Murphy, 2013; Aggarwal, 2014). The algorithms for non-parametric classification are flexible and results in high performance for data with any type of distribution. However, the time required to estimate a good function is quite high and may lead to overfitting in an attempt to learn the data fully. Decision Trees, CART, non-linear SVM, kNN, Parzen window are some of the non-parametric classifiers (Aggarwal; 2014; Cover 7 Hart, 2006; Parzen, 1962).

Conventional kNN Algorithm

The conventional kNN algorithm is adopted in many domains like healthcare analysis for medical diagnose, classification of diseases, prediction of disease as well as recommendation and suggestions to doctors on required tests for available symptoms. In the traditional kNN algorithm, in order to label a test sample, all the available labeled samples are used. Given labeled dataset *D={(Xi,yi)},* a test sample *Xnew*, and a parameter *k*, the objective of kNN is to find most probable label or class for *Xnew* based on *k* neighbors. Training in kNN indicates calculation of similarities between a test sample and all the training samples to choose k nearest neighbors with largest similarities. The most common distance measure used to find nearest neighbors of a test sample *Xnew* with each of the training samples *Xi* is Euclidean distance as given in Equation 1.

$$Eulicidean_{dist}(Xnew, Xi) = \sqrt{\sum_{j=1}^{d}(Xnew_j - Xi_j)^2} \quad (1)$$

Once the distance values with each of the training samples *Xi* is computed, find *k* samples with minimum distance. For these *k* samples, search the label *C* with maximum samples. Thus, *C* is assigned as label for *Xnew.*

Manhattan distance as given in Equation 2 is preferable for high dimensional data since quite often such dataset is highly sparse. Manhattan is absolute value distance and hence is robust to outliers and do not exaggerate the noise terms like Euclidean distance. So if two samples are same on most of the features, and is just different on few of the features as in high dimensional data, Manhattan distance should be used as it will diminish such difference and will more influence the closeness of other features (Murphy, 2013)·

$$Manhattan_{dist}\left(Xnew, Xi\right) = \sum_{j=1}^{d}\left|Xnew_j - Xi_j\right| \quad (2)$$

Algorithm for kNN is given in Algorithm 1.

Algorithm 1. kNN

Input: *k*, Training data set *D={(Xi,yi)}*, Test sample *Xnew*

Output: Label for *Xnew*

1· Calculate Dist, the set of distances between pair (Xnew,Xi) using Euclidean distance
2. Pick k minimum distances with corresponding samples
3. Find label C of a majority of k samples
4. Assign label C to Xnew

Parameter '*k*' that finds neighborhood range is one of the significant aspects of classification accuracy in kNN. The value for '*k*' can be found by tuning in various values. If '*k*' chosen is too small, classification is likely to be very sensitive to noise and outliers and has high variance. Too large a value for '*k*' leads to high bias (Murphy, 2013)· Large memory requirements and high time complexity are two other crucial factors affecting the scalability of kNN. The computational complexity is O(*Nkd*), where

'*N*' is the number of samples, '*k*' is the number of nearest neighbors, and '*d*' is the number of features for each sample. The complexity of kNN is quite high, especially for high dimensional data (Murphy, 2013). due to a high value of '*d*'. So reducing dimensions of high dimensional data can reduce the time complexity. If the training data set is voluminous, linear search becomes very inefficient. So, various index structures like kdtree are available for efficient search of nearest neighbors. But such structures fail for high dimensional data since it requires 2d samples for building efficient index (Friedman, Bentley & Finkel, 1977). The other approach to reduce complexity is to delete samples from training set without loss of much information. This helps in decreasing the execution time of kNN classification algorithm. The output of the kNN algorithm is the class of *Xnew* that is calculated from the majority class of the '*k*' samples nearest to *Xnew*. This is majority voting. For example, in a binary classification problem, where the class is either 0 or 1, the probability of a test sample *Xnew* belonging to class 0 is given as in Equation 3.

$$P(class_{new} = c \mid Xnew, k, X) P(class_{new} = c \mid Xnew, k, X) = 1/k \sum_{ieNk(Xnew,X)} I(class_i = c) \qquad (3)$$

where

$$I(class_i = c) = \begin{cases} 1, & \text{if } i^{th} \text{neighbor belongs to class } c \\ 0, & \text{otherwise} \end{cases}$$

kNN performs well if the data is standardized. Normalizing the data in the range [0,1] is also a good practice. Quite often, dataset consists of missing values. Either such samples are deleted, or the missing values are imputed by replacing them with the mean, median or mode of the corresponding column.

Thus, kNN has various advantages of easy implementation, assumption-free model, insensitive to outliers, versatile, and no requirement of data distribution knowledge. However, it has disadvantages like an increased degree of local sensitivity with a too small value of '*k*', a high memory requirement for a huge dataset, high bias for a large value of '*k*' leading to classifying a sample to most frequent class in the training set, and computationally expensive for high dimensional data [1,2,3].

Parzen Window

Parzen Window Estimation method (Parzen, 1962) (also known as Parzen Rosenblatt window method) is another widely used non-parametric approach to estimate a probability density function p(x) for a specific point *x* from a data set. It does not require any knowledge or assumption about the underlying distribution. A popular application of the Parzen window technique is to estimate the class-conditional densities, (or also often called likelihoods) *p(x|Ci)* in a supervised pattern classification problem from the training dataset, where *p(x)* refers to a multi-dimensional sample that belongs to particular class *Ci*. The basic ideas behind many of the methods of estimating an unknown probability density function are very simple. The most fundamental techniques rely on the fact that the probability P that a vector *x* falls in a region *R* is given by Equation 4.

$$P = \int_R p(x^1)dx^1 \tag{4}$$

If R is so small that *p(x)* does not vary much within it, P can be written as in Equation 5.

$$P = \int_R p(x^1)dx^1 \approx p(x)V \tag{5}$$

where *V* is the volume of *R* and *x* is in *R*. Suppose that *n* samples *x1,…,xn* are independently drawn according to the probability density function *p(x)*, and there are *k* out of *n* samples falling within region *R*. So *P=k/n* and thus *p(x)* is given as in Equation 6.

$$p(x) = \frac{k/n}{V}. \tag{6}$$

Parzen Window Density Estimation

Consider that *R* is a hypercube centered at *x*. Let *h* be the length of the edge of the hypercube, then *V* = *h2* for 2-d square and *V* = *h3* for 3-d cube. Introduce a function that indicates whether a sample *xi* is inside the square centered at *x*, width *h* or not, as in Equation 7.

$$p(\frac{x_i - x}{h}) = 1; if \frac{x_{ik} - x_k}{h} \leq \frac{1}{2}; k = 1,2 \tag{7}$$

The total number of samples, *k*, falling within region *R*, out of *n*, is given by Equation 8.

$$k = \sum_{i=1}^{n} p(\frac{x_i - x}{h}) \tag{8}$$

The Parzen probability density estimation formula for 2-d is given by *p(x)=(k/n/V*. Thus,

$$p(x) = \frac{1}{n}\sum_{i=1}^{n} \frac{1}{h^2} p(\frac{x_i - x}{h}) \tag{9}$$

where $p(\frac{x_i - x}{h})$ is called a window function.

This can be generalized for multi-dimensional data as well as for other window functions such as Gaussian.

Non-parametric classifiers suffer from the curse of dimensionality due to the presence of a large number of irrelevant attributes. One of the techniques to deal with this problem is feature selection or dimensionality reduction (Kavilkrue & Boonma, 2015). These are integrated with kNN and Parzen window classifier to reduce the feature space and search space for voluminous data. This chapter explores clustering and dimensionality reduction to be integrated with non-parametric classifiers for its efficacy.

In Statistics, machine learning and information theory, dimensionality reduction is the process of reducing the number of random variables under consideration by obtaining a set of principal variables (Kavilkrue & Boonma, 2015; Cunningham & Ghahramani, 2015) . It can be divided into feature selection and feature extraction. It reduces the time and storage requirement too. It removes multi co-linearity thereby improving the performance of the machine learning model. The recent explosion of data size, in the number of records and attributes, has triggered the use of dimension reduction procedures (Xie, Liu & Xue, 2017; Cunningham & Ghahramani, 2015). Most of the machines learning algorithms are not scalable for high dimensional data. There are several techniques for reducing dimensions such as principal component analysis, factor analysis, linear multidimensional scaling, Fisher's Linear Discriminant Analysis(LDA), canonical correlations analysis (Cunningham & Ghahramani, 2015). These dimension reduction techniques improve execution time as well as the model performance of a chosen classification algorithm. High dimensionality is problematic because it often leads to overfitting while learning a model, which means that the model will perform well on the training data but poorly on test data. Dimensionality reduction addresses overfitting and learns predictive models while preserving most of the relevant information in the data. Thus, reducing the features is inevitable for a computationally efficient algorithm (Kavilkrue & Boonma, 2015; Cunningham & Ghahramani, 2015).

Dimensionality Reduction

Traditional algorithms break down due to large amounts of data samples generated quite frequently in almost all domains. However, the more crucial part is the number of features associated with each sample that keeps on increasing with the advent of big data. The number of features or random variables in a dataset is called the dimension of the dataset. For an instance, assume, a patient is required to be diagnosed as suffering from one or the other diseases such as liver, thyroid, or kidney failure. The dataset for this system consists of various symptoms and lab test results of each of the diseases. Thus, the number of features is quite high. However, some of the symptoms of one disease may overlap with the symptoms of other disease. Similarly, lab tests for one disease may overlap with the lab tests of another disease. Thus, there is redundancy in many symptoms and lab test results. If a patient has Hb count of 8 as per lab test, he is bound to have anaemia. Thus Hb and anaemia are correlated and hence can be collapsed to just one feature indicating Hb and anaemia. Hence, the number of features in such problems can be reduced. In other words, visualization and interpretation of a dataset with 100 features is difficult as compared to a 3-d, 2-d or a 1-d dataset. Thus 100-d dataset should be reduced to 3-d, 2-d, or 1-d without losing much information and retaining the correlation amongst the original features. Moreover, as the dimensions increase, the need for number of samples to learn and model the problem also increase. Figure 1 illustrates this concept, where a 3-d feature space requires a number of samples, however, 2-d feature space requires lesser and 1-d feature space requires very few samples to identify patterns.

Figure 1. Curse of Dimensionality. As dimensions increase, the number of samples should be increased to visualize patterns in the data properly.1

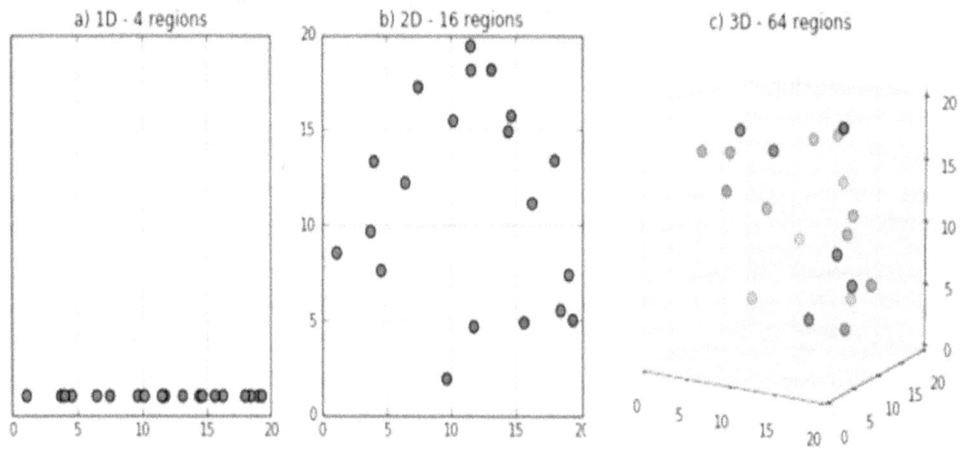

One of the major challenges of high dimensional data is that not all features are important to understanding the hidden intricate relationships amongst the samples. Hence it is necessary to do dimensionality reduction to identify important features prior to learning any type of model. Dimensionality reduction can be stated as follows. Given a *d*-dimensional data sample *X=(x1,....,xd)*, find a lower *r*-dimensional sample of *X*, *S=(s1,...,sr)*, with *r<=d* without any major loss of information. Few of the most prevalent dimensionality reduction techniques are Principal Component Analysis (PCA), LDA, and Singular Value decomposition. This chapter deals with integrating PCA with kNN.

Principal Component Analysis (PCA)

PCA is a linear dimensionality reduction technique based on the covariance of the variables or features of the dataset. It seeks to find few orthogonal linear combinations of original features with the largest variance. The main idea of PCA is to reduce the dimensionality of a data set consisting of many variables in such a way that the directions or the features where the data is mostly spread out are obtained. This is done in such a manner that the features in original dataset that are correlated with each other are captured and transformed to a new feature that gives the maximum possible variance. This transformed new feature space are called principal components (or simply, the PCs). These are orthogonal components and chosen in decreasing order. So, the first principal component retains maximum variation that was present in the original components. The principal components are the eigenvectors of a covariance matrix, and hence they are orthogonal. Importantly, the dataset on which PCA technique is to be used must be scaled. The results are also sensitive to the relative scaling. Thus, PCA projects original d-dimensional data to r-dimensional feature space and hence is a "shadow" of the data as seen from its most informative viewpoint.

Preliminaries for PCA

As discussed in previous sections, the objective of PCA is to project the data onto a lower dimensional space such that the variance of the data in projected space is maximized. In fact, it is the linear projection that minimizes the mean squared distance between the data points and their projections. Thus, given a sample X in d-dimensional space, project data using a set of orthonormal vectors U where i^{th} vector Ui is an ith principal component. Few definitions are presented here to brief PCA clearly.

Dimensionality: It is the number of random variables, or the number of features, or the number of columns present in a dataset.

Dimensionality Reduction: Given N d-dimensional data points $X= [x1,...,xN]\in R^{Nxd}$ and dimensionality $r < d$, dimensionality reduction is the process of producing a linear transformation $P \in R^{N\times r}$ which is a low dimensional projection of X onto r important dimensions.

Correlation: It shows how strongly two features are related to each other. The correlation value ranges from -1 to +1. A positive value indicates that when one variable increases, the other increases as well. A negative value indicates that when one variable increases, the other decreases. The modulus value of correlation indicates the strength of relationship between the variables.

Variance: Variance of a feature xi of a dataset is defined as the average square of the distance from the mean of the feature x' to its various values as given by following Equation 10.

$$Var(x) = \sigma^2 = 1/N\sum_{i=0}^{N}(xi - x)^2 \tag{10}$$

Covariance: Covariance is the mean value of the product of the deviations of two features x and y from their respective means. It is given as in Equation 11.

$$Cov(x,y) = 1/N\sum_{i=0}^{N}(xi - x)(yi - y) \tag{11}$$

As per Equation 11, Covariance has the following properties.

1. $Cov(x,y)=Cov(y,x)$;
2. $Cov(x,x)=Var(x)$

If x and y features are independent (uncorrelated) $Cov(x,y)=0$. If x and y are correlated (both dimensions increase together) $Cov(x,y)>0$. If x and y are anti-correlated, (one dimension increases, the other decreases) $Cov(x,y)<0$. Thus, covariance is a measure between two features. For example, if dataset is 3-dimensional (dimensions x, y, z), $cov(x,y)$, $cov(y,z)$, and $cov(x,z)$ need to be calculated. For d-dimensional data, it is required to calculate $d!/(d-2)!*2 = d(d-1)/2$ different covariance values. A dataset with N samples and d features is represented in the form of a matrix A_{Nxd}. Covariance for such dataset is represented in the form of a matrix. Following matrix is an example of covariance for a 3-dimensional dataset. An entry (i,j) in the matrix indicates the covariance between the ith and j^{th} feature.

$$C = \begin{bmatrix} Cov(x,x) & Cov(x,y) & Cov(x,z) \\ Cov(y,x) & Cov(y,y) & Cov(y,z) \\ Cov(z,x) & Cov(z,y) & Cov(z,z) \end{bmatrix}$$

Orthogonal Vectors: Two vectors are called orthogonal if they are uncorrelated to each other, i.e., the correlation between any pair of variables is 0.

Eigen Vectors: Let *A* be a square matrix. A non-zero vector v is called an eigen vector of A if $A.v$ is a scalar multiple of v as given in following Equation 12

$$Av= \lambda v \tag{12}$$

Here λ is called the Eigen value corresponding to the Eigen vector v.

Algorithm for PCA is given in Algorithm 2.

Algorithm 2. Algorithm for PCA

Input: Number of principal components r, *Dataset D with N rows and d columns. DNxd*

Output: Transformed data Dr

1. Normalize data D and do optionally feature scaling
2. Compute Covariance Matrix C_{dxd}
3. Find d eigen vectors and corresponding eigen values for C
4. U_{dxd} = Sort d eigen values and corresponding eigen vectors in decreasing order
5. Choose first r eigen vectors and eigen values

$U = [U1, U2,\ldots, Ur]$ where each $Ui \in Rd$

6. Transform *D* to *Dn= U'*D'* where *U'* and *D'* are the transpose of *U* and *D* matrices respectively.

The output of PCA is *d* principal component vectors in *U* matrix in order of significance as shown in algorithm Alg.2. In case, only r dimensions are required, initial r columns from U can be chosen. The Principal Components possess some useful properties as follows:

a) The Principal component vectors are linear combinations of the features in original space.
b) The vectors are orthogonal
c) The principal component is the eigen vector with highest eigen value obtained from the covariance matrix of the dataset. The variance of this component is highest indicating the most important feature in the dataset.

Dimensionality reduction such as PCA transforms the entire data into a new space and computes only one subspace. However, the dimensionality reduction on the entire data makes sense only if the entire data points are distributed around a single lower dimensional subspace or the data has approximately low rank. But if the data comes from different types of distribution, single low-dimensional subspace may not be sufficient. Local feature relevance and local feature correlation identify multiple subspaces that help in identifying each class separately that may exist in different subspaces (Keiegel, Kroger, & Zimek, 2009). In such scenarios, it is better to cluster the data and then apply dimensionality reduction so as to properly classify data with better models on different distributions.

Clustering

Clustering seeks to partition datasets into groups such that data points within a group have high similarity whereas data points in different groups have less similarity (Anil, 2010; Kriegel, Kroger & Zimek, 2015). Clustering is mainly used for the following three purposes (Anil, 2010):

1. *Underlying structure:* To analyse data for outlier detection, identification of important features and generate hypotheses.
2. *Natural classification:* To group data points based on similarity such that highly similar points can be naturally labeled for better classification.
3. *Compression:* To organize data points into groups based on similarity and summarize each group with centroids or few representatives from the group using cluster prototypes.

Although classification algorithms can identify labels of unknown data points effectively, provided, there are large set of historical records with proper labeling. By supervised learning, the classifier models each group. Instead, it is preferable to first divide the set of data into groups based on a good clustering mechanism, and then assign labels to the relatively small number of groups. This not only helps in dynamically capturing the distributions of the data but also helps in finding useful features that distinguish different groups. Clustering can also be used for anomaly or outlier detection, which may be more interesting than common cases. Applications of outlier detection are credit card and loan defaulters which are common applications of classification too. Clustering can also serve as a preprocessing step for dimensionality reduction and classification.

Clustering algorithms are broadly divided into 2 categories: *hierarchical* and *partitional,* as shown in Figure 2 (Rajaraman & Ullman, 2011). Hierarchical clustering recursively finds nested clusters either in agglomerative mode (bottom-up) or in divisive mode (top-down). Agglomerative mode initially assigns each data point to its own cluster and then repeatedly combines two nearest clusters into one. Divisive mode assigns all the data points into one cluster and recursively split it up into smaller clusters. Compared to hierarchical clustering algorithms, partitional clustering algorithms find all the clusters simultaneously as a partition of the points. The input to a hierarchical algorithm is a similarity matrix of size N x N, where N is the number of objects to be clustered. On the other hand, a partitional algorithm can use either a pattern matrix of size $N \times d$ or a similarity matrix of size $N \times N$.

The most popular hierarchical algorithms are single-link and complete-link, while the most popular and simplest partitional algorithm is K-means. Hierarchical algorithms are computationally expensive compared to K-means. The complexity of hierarchical algorithms is $O(N^2 log\ N)$, where N is the number of data points. So, for huge datasets that cannot fit in main memory, hierarchical algorithms are not preferable. However, the best running time of K-means clustering is linear in time, $O(NdKi)$, where N is the number of data points, d is the dimension of each data point, K is the number of clusters required and i is the number of iterations to converge (Lloyd, 1982). K-means is still one of the most preferred algorithms for clustering due to ease of implementation, simplicity, efficiency, and empirical success.

Figure 2. Clustering strategies: (a) Hierarchical clustering that is agglomerative, shown using dendrograms. (b) Partition based clustering that recursively finds centroids and assigns the data points to one of the centroids until the partitioning converges.[2]

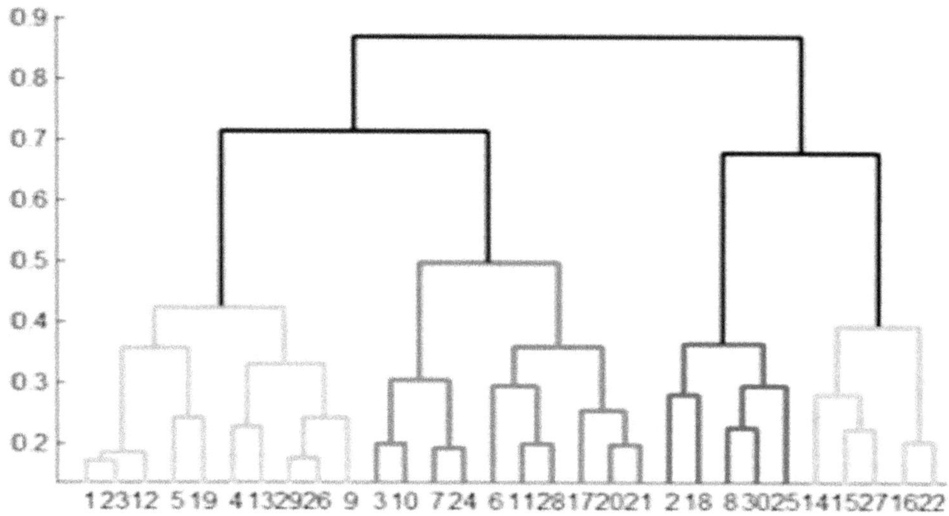

K-Means Clustering

Let $X=\{x1,\ldots,xN\}$ be a set of N data points, where each xi ϵ Rd. X is to be divided into K clusters, $C=\{c1,\ldots,cK\}$. K-Means algorithm partitions X in such a way that the squared error between empirical mean μi of a cluster ci and the data points in ci is minimized for all clusters. Thus the minimization objective is as given in the following Equation 13.

$$MinimizeF(C)=\sum_{k=1}^{K}\sum_{xi\in ck}\left\|xi-\mu k\right\|^{2} \tag{13}$$

K-means algorithm is given in Algorithm 3.

Algorithm 3. Algorithm for K-means

Input: K, Data set D with N rows and d columns. DNxd

Output: C={C1,C2,...CK)

1. *Select an initial set of K centroids.*
2. *Assign each point in D to one of the K centroids to create K partitions based on a similarity measure*
3. *Repeat until convergence*
    a. Find new centroids of each of the K partitions.
    b. Generate a new partition by assigning each point to its closest cluster centroid.

Step 1 takes only O(1). Step 2 takes distance computation of each point with K centroids using Euclidean measure as given in Eqn 1 or Eqn 2. If there are N data points and K centroids, this step takes O(NKd) since each data point is d dimensional. Repeatedly doing this until convergence for i iterations leads to complexity of O(NdKi). K-means clustering requires K as an input parameter which is difficult to specify in certain domains. If there are two highly overlapping data, K-means will not be able to resolve that there are two clusters. Different initializations of centroids can lead to different final clustering because K-means only converges to local minima. One way to overcome the local minima is to run the K-means algorithm, for a given *K*, with multiple different initial partitions and choose the partition with the smallest squared error (Anil, 2010), or apply a greedy technique to form initial partitions by choosing centroids that are farthest from each other *(Rajaraman & Ullman, 2011)*. Usually, Euclidean metric is used for computing distance between points and cluster centers to assign points to a proper centroid leading to spherical clusters. K-means with Mahalanobis distance metric has been used to detect hyper-ellipsoidal clusters (Anil, 2010; Rajaraman & Ullman, 2011), but this comes at the expense of higher computational cost. K-means is suitable only for numerical data. Hence, for categorical data, a preprocessing is required to convert into numerical before applying K-means.

Choosing K

The algorithm in Alg.4 finds clusters from a dataset for a particular *K* value. However original number of clusters in a dataset may not be known well ahead. Hence, practically, K-means algorithm is executed for different values of K and the clusters are evaluated on the basis of high intra-cluster similarity and low inter-cluster similarity. There is no universally accepted method to find proper K value for a dataset to be clustered. However, most commonly used method to compare results across different values of K is the mean distance between data points and their cluster centroid. Since increasing the number of clusters will always reduce the distance to data points, increasing *K* will always decrease this metric, to the extreme of reaching zero when K is the same as the number of data points. Thus, this metric cannot be used as the sole target. Instead, mean distance to the centroid as a function of K is plotted and the "elbow point," where the rate of decrease sharply shifts, can be used to roughly determine K, as shown in Figure 3. (Rajaraman & Ullman, 2011; Chinmay, Gupta, Ghosh, Das, & Chakraborty, 2016).

Figure 3. Choosing the right value for K using Elbow point[3]

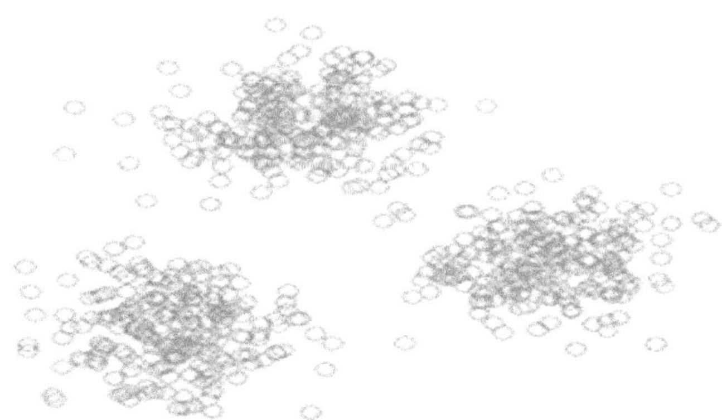

BLENDED MODELS

With the advent of voluminous and high dimensional data, a single model may not be sufficient to accurately explore data for classification. This section deals with the merits of combining various models, such as dimensionality reduction and clustering with classification algorithms. Combining multiple complementary features help to improve classification accuracy compared with one single feature. Various blended models, each consisting of various combinations of kNN, Parzen window, K-means, and dimensionality reduction algorithms, are evaluated to come up with the best combination for each type of dataset. This chapter deals with the following algorithms.

a. K-Nearest Neighbor algorithm
b. Parzen Window estimation
c. K-Means clustering algorithm
d. Dimensionality reduction algorithm (Principal Component Analysis)

Combination of non-parametric classifiers, kNN and Parzen window estimation with clustering(K-means) and dimensionality reduction algorithms are evaluated. This study is based on the comparison of their accuracy and time of execution. In the traditional kNN algorithm, all samples of a dataset are used for training. Due to the increase in a number of calculations taken between the test sample and all the training samples, the traditional method of kNN has great calculation complexity. This classifier classifies a test sample *Xnew* by assigning it to the class label that is most frequently represented among its *k* nearest samples in the training set. In the case of a tie, the test pattern is assigned the class with minimum average distance to it. Hence, this method is sensitive to the distance function. For the minimum average distance, the metric employed is the Euclidean distance. The k-nearest neighbor classifier is a conventional non-parametric classifier that is said to yield good performance for optimal values of k. kNN classification algorithm is executed for a number of times by varying the number of nearest neighbors, *k*, and compute the accuracy.

KNN Classifier With K-Means Clustering Algorithm

The first blended model combines K-means clustering algorithm with kNN classification algorithm. Dataset is initially clustered using K-means clustering algorithm. In order to classify a new sample *Xnew*, find the distance of *Xnew*with the centroid of each of the clusters. The sample is assigned to the cluster *Cnew*with the closest centroid *μnew*. Find most common class in *Cnew*to label sample *Xnew*. The overhead of finding nearest neighbors from the entire training samples is reduced to finding the nearest neighbors from one of the clusters. Thus, the combination of K-means and kNN removes the need to know all the training elements beforehand, and considerably simplifies the process. This improves accuracy and reduces the execution time. The flowchart of this blended model is shown in Figure 4. It has two phases. Phase 1 executes conventional kNN classifier on the dataset. Best k value is chosen as per the best accuracy obtained. Phase 2 executes conventional K-means clustering on the dataset. For a test sample *Xnew*, kNN is executed with the best k value from Phase 1 on one of the clusters with centroid closest to *Xnew*. The results from Phase 1 and Phase 2 are compared in terms of execution time and accuracy.

Parzen Window Estimation With K-Means Clustering

The second blended model combines the K-means clustering algorithm with Parzen window estimation. This is similar to first model with only one difference of the classifier in Phase 1. In Phase 1, the Parzen window method is used to classify test samples by varying the window size parameter. Compute the accuracy and time taken for execution for varying window sizes. The window size corresponding to maximum accuracy is chosen as the best window size. In Phase 2, dataset is clustered using K-means by varying the number of clusters. For each test sample, the nearest centroid is computed. Thereafter, the Parzen window estimation method is applied within that cluster with the best window size from Phase 1, to find the label of a test sample. This blend avoids the need of considering the entire region for density estimation for finding the label of a test sample, thereby reducing the computational complexity.

kNN Classifier With Dimensionality Reduction

The third blended model as shown in Figure 5, combines kNN algorithm with the dimensionality reduction technique, PCA. kNN is computationally expensive when dealing with high dimensional data. Irrelevant dimensions in the dataset also affect the accuracy of classifier drastically. In order to overcome this problem, the data set on which kNN has to be applied is reduced in its dimensions using PCA. On dimension reduced dataset, kNN is applied leading to reduced computational complexity of kNN on high dimensional data. This combination can be executed in different ways such as varying k value with number of principal components as constant and varying number of principal components with k value as constant(k value is chosen from best accuracy rate for conventional kNN). Results of conventional kNN are compared with results of above combination in terms of accuracy and time of execution.

Figure 4. Blended model: Non-parametric classifiers kNN/ Parzen window estimation with K-means clustering.

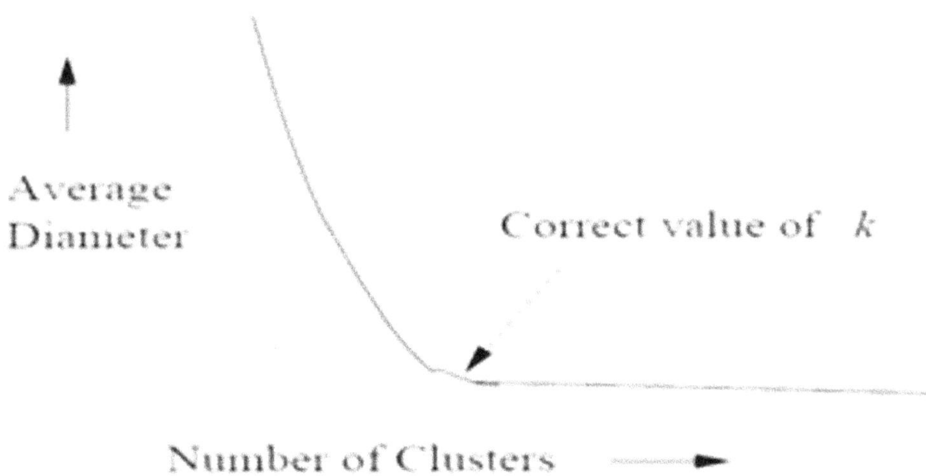

Figure 5. Blended model: Non-parametric classifiers kNN with dimensionality reduction PCA

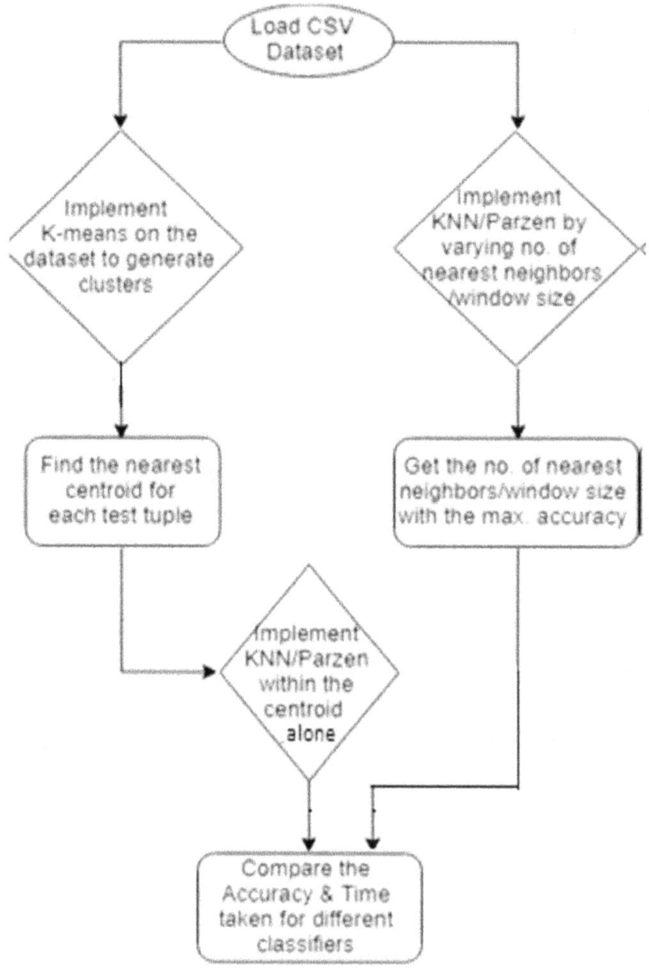

kNN Classifier With Clustering and Dimensionality Reduction

The fourth blended model as shown in Figure 6, combines the kNN algorithm with dimensionality reduction and clustering. For high dimension data, before applying classification, data is divided into clusters. Dimensionality reduction is applied to each cluster to reduce the features of samples in each cluster. Then each of the test data instances is classified using the kNN algorithm. kNN is applied only on the nearest possible cluster for a given test instance. This combination is executed for all possible variations such as varying number of clusters and principal components for a fixed value of k, varying number of clusters and k neighbors for a fixed value of r, varying number of principal components and k neighbors for a fixed number of clusters. The rate of accuracy and time of execution for all executions are evaluated to find the best ensemble.

Figure 6. Blended model: Non-parametric classifiers kNN with K-means clustering and dimensionality reduction PCA

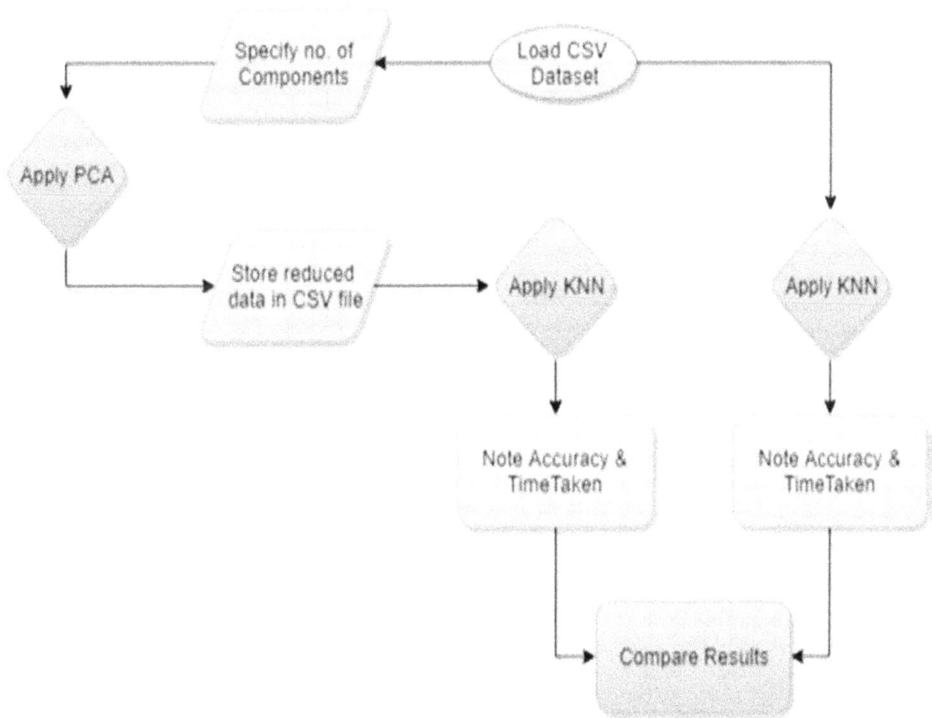

Solutions and Recommendations

This section evaluates various blended models and recommends a suitable solution for different types of datasets. Fifteen real datasets, eight of which belong to the healthcare domain, are studied to compare various models, as shown in Table 1.

The experiments were conducted on a commodity machine with 12GB main memory and X64 based processor. Blended models were implemented using Scikit-learn 0.19.1 package of python. The performance measures used were the Accuracy of classification and Execution time.

Results and Analysis

For each of the blended models, classification accuracy and execution time on various datasets were compared with basic algorithms.

Combination of kNN With K-Means

A combination of kNN and K-means algorithm for classification leads to a drastic reduction in classification time as shown in Table 2. For each dataset, the *k* value for which best accuracy is obtained is shown in bracket. Similarly, for blended model, best combination of *k* (in kNN) and *K* (in K-means) is shown

Table 1. Datasets used for evaluation of various ensemble models (UCI repository[4]). Nine datasets belong to healthcare or medical domain.

Dataset	Tuples	Dimensions	Class Labels	Category
GCM	114	16063	12	High-dimension, low tuples
B-cell2	72	4026	10	High-dimension, low tuples
B-cell3	72	4026	7	High-dimension, low tuples
Leukemia1	29	7129	2	High-dimension, low tuples
Leukemia2	32	7129	2	High-dimension, low tuples
Tumer	50	7129	2	High-dimension, low tuples
B-cell1	33	4026	2	High-dimension, low tuples
Colon	46	2000	2	High-dimension, low tuples
Bank	41188	62	2	High-dimension, high tuples
Synthetic	1323	75	12	High-dimension, high tuples
Waveform	5000	40	3	High-dimension, high tuples
Pen Digits	6970	16	10	Low-dimension, high tuples
German	1000	24	2	Low-dimension, high tuples
Glass	165	9	6	Low-dimension, low tuples
Diabetes	569	8	2	Low-dimension, low tuples

Table 2. Evaluation of K-means+kNN classifier on various datasets

Dataset	Classification Accuracy		Execution time(sec) for Classification	
	kNN(k)	K-means + kNN(k,K)	kNN	K-means+kNN
GCM	**54.28(5)**	54.05(5,4)	57.89	**2.85**
B-cell2	76.47(5)	**76.92(5,10)**	2.39	**1.22**
B-cell3	78.26(5)	**81.82(5,5)**	2.80	**0.25**
Leukemia1	85.71(5)	**88.88(5,2)**	1.12	**0.18**
Leukemia2	90.90(5)	**100(5,2)**	0.95	**0.15**
Tumer	70.83(15)	**80(5,2)**	3.70	**0.5**
B-cell1	90.90(5)	**100(5,5)**	2.35	**0.26**
Colon	85.71(15)	**88(5,5)**	0.74	**0.13**
Bank	**90.83(10)**	90.39(10,9)	19835.62	**34.56**
Pen Digits	**99.04(5)**	72.40(10,5)	163.91	**1.99**
Synthetic	88.64(10)	**93.56(5,9)**	37.77	**0.31**
German	71.30(10)	**73.17(3,9)**	2.72	**0.15**
Waveform	82.77(10)	**83(10,15)**	259.99	**2.12**
Glass	**59.65(10)**	57.69(5,7)	0.12	**0.04**

in bracket. For datasets with low dimension and low tuples, kNN is recommended over blended model K-means+kNN. For dataset with low dimension and high tuples, there is no drastic difference between the conventional kNN and blended model. However, for low tuples and high dimensions, blended model has good accuracy for classification. Results show that for all datasets execution time for proposed blend is quite low than conventional kNN model. Thus there is a trade-off between accuracy and execution time. The complexity of conventional kNN is *O(Nkd)*. However, this blended model has low execution time for classification during phase 2. For a test sample *Xnew*, only one of the clusters *Cnew* is used by kNN for classification. The number of data points in the chosen cluster, |*Cnew*|<< N. Thus the complexity of blended model for classification is *O(|Cnew|kd)<<O(Nkd)*. Thus total data points, *N,* has reduced to just the data points in one of the clusters *Cnew* with no change in k and d. For datasets with less number of data points, the difference in execution time of kNN and K-means+kNN is not very high. But as the number of data points increase, as in *Bank* dataset, the blended model shows a decrease of at least two orders of magnitude in execution time.

Combination of kNN With PCA, kNN With PCA and K-Means

Experimental results of combination of kNN and dimensionality reduction algorithm PCA (Principal Component Analysis) for classification are shown in Table 3. Experiment of dimensionality reduction on clustered data used for kNN is also conducted and the results are shown in Table 3. Here best classification accuracy by chosing optimal value for number of principal components(r), number of clusters (K), and number of nearest neighbors(k) for various datasets, is depicted. Dimensionality reduction of high dimensional data removes redundant features. Classification on the transformed data gives improved accuracy. Hence in almost all high dimensional data PCA+kNN gives better accuracy than conventional

Table 3. Evaluation of various blended models on various datasets

Dataset	Classification Accuracy		
	kNN(k)	**PCA+kNN(r,k)**	**K-means + PCA + kNN (K,r,k)**
Pen Digits	**99.04(5)**	74.04(14,10)	59.64(4,14,10)
Waveform	**82.77(10)**	46.31(6,10)	56.33(4,6,10)
GCM	54.28(5)	**60.87(6,10)**	33.33(4,14000,10)
B-cell2	76.47(5)	**90.9(3800,10)**	25(4,6,10)
B-cell3	78.26(5)	**96.51(6,10)**	50(4,6,10)
Leukemia1	**85.71(5)**	**85.71(6,10)**	50(4,6,10)
Leukemia2	90.90(5)	**98.23(6,10)**	85.71(4,500,10)
Tumer	70.83(15)	**90.05(4000,20)**	83.33(4,500,20)
B-cell1	90.90(5)	**98.5(6,10)**	42.85(4,6,10)
Colon	85.71(15)	**88.88(200,10)**	66.66(4,200,10)
Synthetic	88.64(10)	**99.8(6,10)**	29.18(4,6,10)
German	**71.30(10)**	**71.30(5,10)**	70.41(4,6,50)
Glass	**59.65(10)**	59.09(2,20)	55.17(4,6,20)
Diabetes	**77.72(10)**	77.27(2,20)	66.94(4,2,20)

kNN. However for Waveform dataset with 40 dimensions, kNN gives better accuracy. This is due to the fact that all 40 features in the dataset are important and reducing the dimensions as low as 10 leads to loss of information. For low-dimensional data such as Pendigits, Diabetes, Glass, and German, the blended model PCA+kNN does not give improved accuracy as all the features play an important role in identifying class of the data points. Hence dimensionality reduction leads to loss of information. The maximum improvement obtained in accuracy is 27% for *Tumer* dataset and on an average 3% improvement is obtained in accuracy.

The model K-means+PCA+kNN is not a good blend for classification. The main reason for this is, during K-means entire features are considered. After formation of clusters, proper correlation of features are not obtained in a small partition. So sufficient samples to understand reduce the dimensions in consistent with the labeling is difficult.

Combination of Parzen With K-Means

Parzen window classifier is a non-parametric classifier where the crucial factor is window size. Accuracy of Parzen is plotted by changing the window size as shown in Fig 7A(a). Accuracy of blended model K-means+Parzen by varying K of K-means for a fixed window size, is shown in Fig. 7A(b). Figures 7B(a) and (b) shows the execution time of Parzen and K-means+Parzen respectively.

It is observed that for a given window size, accuracy of Parzen+K-means model remains almost constant. However the execution time is quite less than Parzen classifier. The improved execution time is due to the fact that classification is done on one of the clusters than the entire dataset. Thus K-means+Parzen

Figure 7. For synthetic dataset. (a)Accuracy of Parzen window estimation for classification by varying the parameter window size (b) Accuracy of Blended model K-means+Parzen for classification by varying K of K-means clustering.

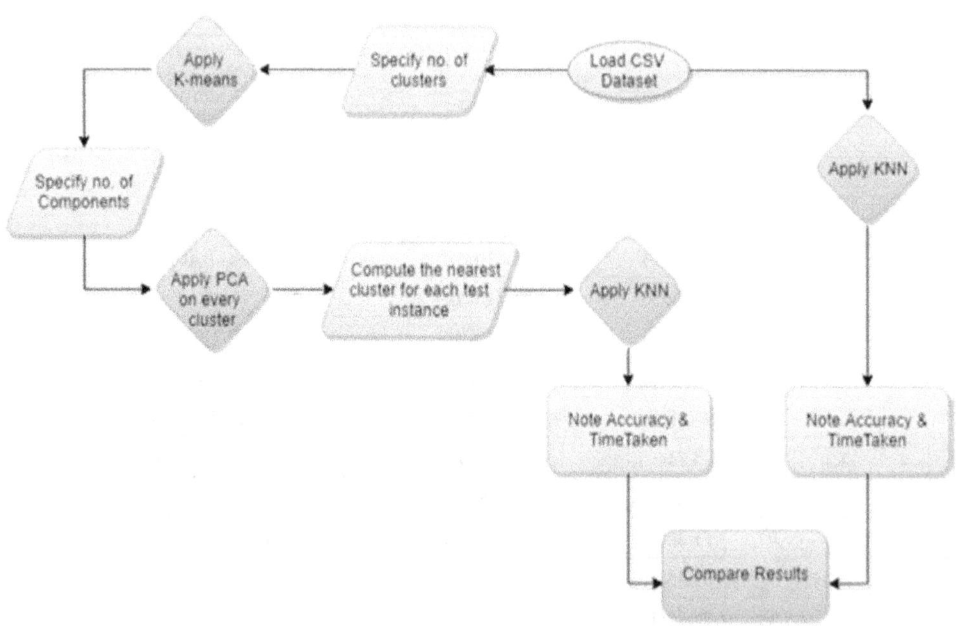

Figure 8. For synthetic dataset. (a)Execution time of Parzen window estimation for classification by varying the parameter window size (b) Execution time of Blended model K-means+Parzen for classification by varying K of K-means clustering.

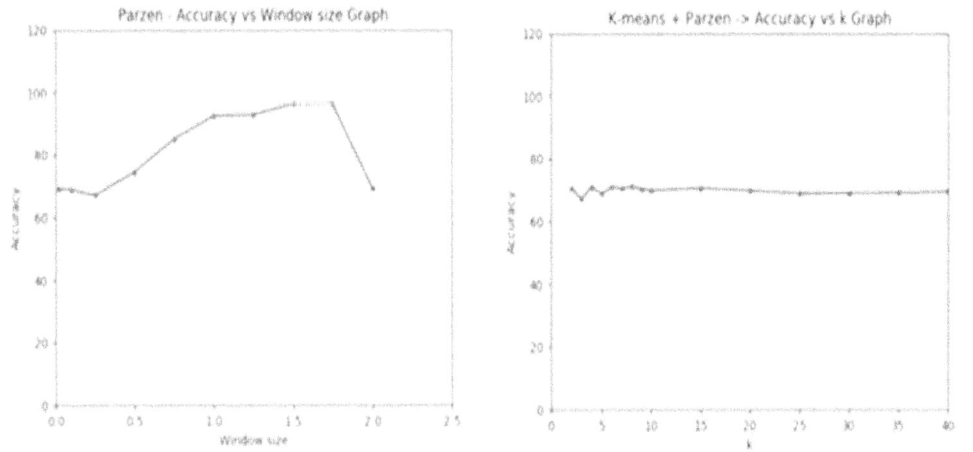

and K-means+kNN are good blended models to capture distributions of data first for proper classification. However, how to choose parameters, k and window size in kNN and Parzen respectively is still required to be explored. The choice of window size determines the efficiency of the estimator.

Accuracy Comparison of kNN, PCA+kNN, K-Means + PCA+ kNN

Different types of datasets are used to compare accuracy of various blended models by varying parameter *k* of kNN. It has been observed that for high dimensional and high tuples data, PCA+kNN is the best model as shown in Figure 8a. As *k* increases, the bias in kNN increases thereby leading to lower accuracy. So even if PCA is applied on the dataset, for very high value of k, kNN suffers from high bias if majority of data points belong to a single class. K-means+PCA+kNN is not a suitable blend for high-dimensional and high-tuples dataset. Once the dataset is clustered, each cluster may have less number of samples. Less samples in each cluster are not sufficient for getting the correlation of the dimensions so as to reduce the dimensionality. Hence PCA after K-means and subsequently kNN does not give good accuracy.

For high dimensional and low tuples data also, PCA+kNN is the best model as shown in Figure 8(b). For high value of *k*, the accuracy decreases due to high bias, similar to Figure 8(a). K-means+PCA+kNN is not a good blend for low tuples and high dimensions due to similar reasons for high tuples and high dimensions.

Figure 8(c) shows the accuracy of low dimensional and low volume data on varying parameter *k*. It is observed that kNN is best model for classification. Dimensionality reduction is not preferable since the number of dimensions is low and hence all of the dimensions are necessary for classifying a data sample. Thus PCA is not mandatory. If the dimensions are reduced, important dimensions may be removed that leads to loss of information thereby decreasing the accuracy. Though K-means prior to PCA can help in knowing the distribution of data, the blended model is not preferable for low dimensional data. K-means+PCA+kNN is a preferred blend over PCA+kNN if the number of tuples as well as dimensions is less.

Figure 9. Accuracy of High dimensional and high volume data. Synthetic dataset has d=75 and N=1323

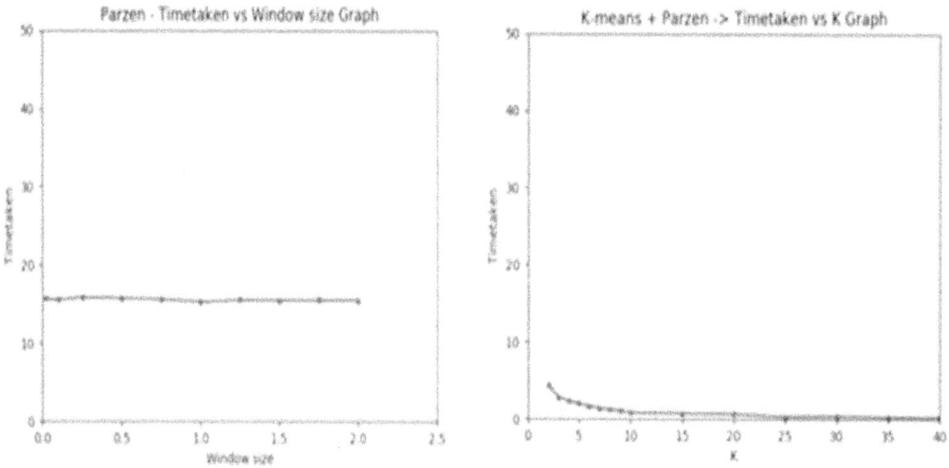

For low dimensional and high volume data too, blended models are not preferable over kNN as shown in Figure 8(d). The blended models give almost same accuracy for higher values of k. This happens since while clustering, in case of low volume dataset, almost all the data points may be considered for finding neighbors. Hence, as the value of *k* increases, the classification accuracy decreases faster than kNN. Thus, PCA+kNN and K-means+PCA+kNN are not preferred models for low dimensional and high volume data. However, kNN is preferred if dimensions are low.

Figure 10. Accuracy of High dimensional and low volume data. GCM dataset has d=16063 and N=114

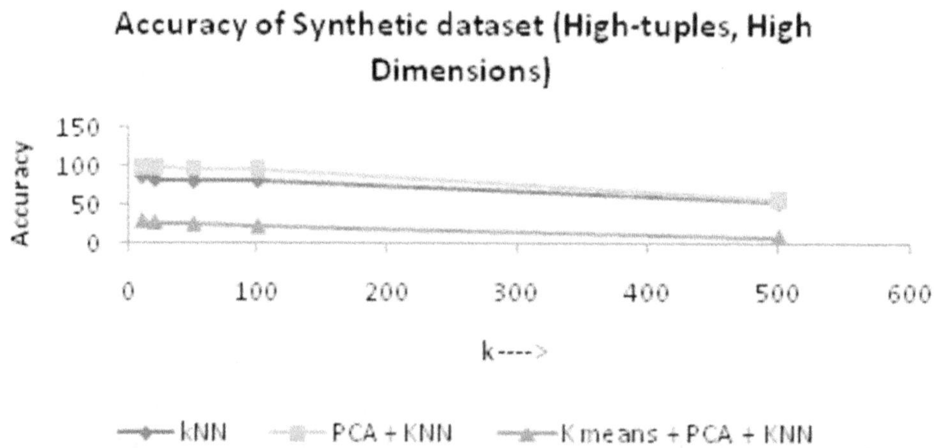

Figure 11. Accuracy of Low dimensional and low volume data. Glass dataset has d=9 and N=165

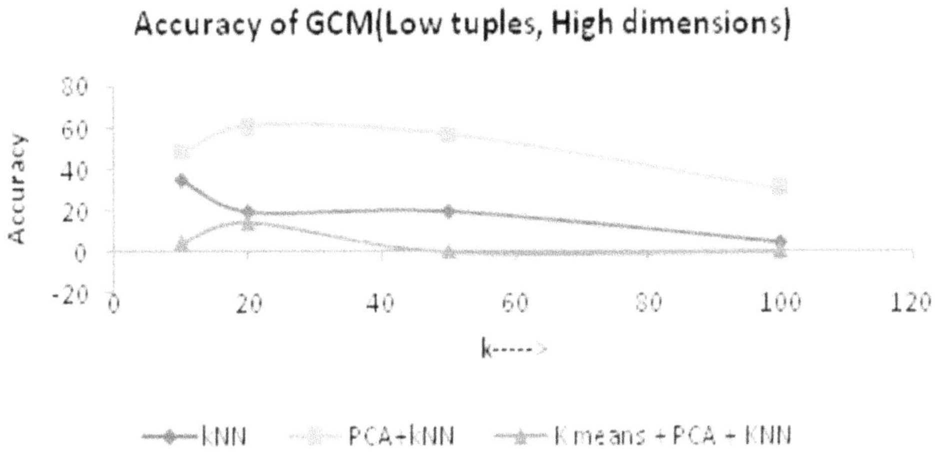

Figure 12. Accuracy of Low dimensional and high volume data. Pendigits dataset has d=16 and N=6970

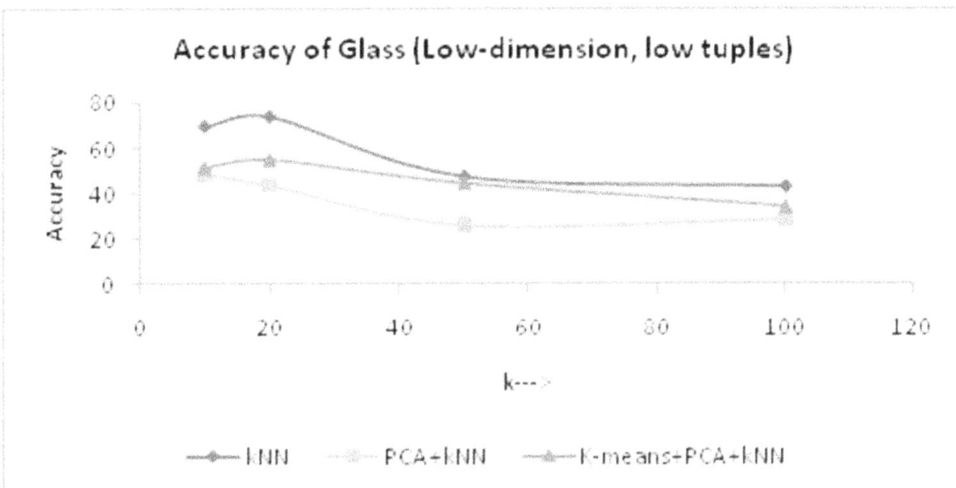

CONCLUSION AND FUTURE DIRECTIONS

This chapter has provided an insight into non-parametric classifiers combined with dimensionality reduction and clustering. For domains such as health care, where the type of data varies frequently, the various models give an idea about what type of combination is suitable. The chapter effectively proposed viable blended models for various types of data that have high or low dimensions as well as large or less number of tuples. Various blended models have been evaluated that combine basic classifiers such as kNN and Parzen window estimator with clustering and dimensionality reduction for better classification accuracy and reduced execution time. It is found that the combination of K-means and kNN removes the need for knowing all the training samples beforehand. A considerable difference in the execution time, as well as an increase in accuracy measure is observed for few datasets with less dimensions and less tuples, by conventional kNN. However for high dimensional data the blended models outperform kNN with a good reduction in execution time. It is noticed that the combination of PCA with kNN reduces the dimension of original data prior to classification. This helps in removing irrelevant attributes and classification is based on only relevant attributes. Hence it is inferred that PCA + kNN gives considerable results for high dimensional data where the time of execution has decreased and accuracy has increased. But, though the blend of K-means + PCA + kNN does not improve accuracy, there has been a considerable decrease in the execution time for high dimensional data sets with fewer tuples. The evaluation of various blended models reveals that K-means and kNN is suitable for low dimensions and huge number of tuples. PCA + kNN is suitable for high dimensional data. K-means + PCA + kNN is not a good mechanism for high dimensional data. Blended models thus depend on the nature of data i.e, number of dimensions, number of tuples, and the type of distributions that generated the data.

Future work aims to explore the ensemble models in a distributed environment where health data is distributed across different sites or organizations. Nowadays, emerging trend is on subspace clustering where the clusters are found in subspaces of data. Whether a non-parametric model is applicable after subspace clustering can be one of the future works. How to embed these models within DBMS (Database Management Systems), where the data actually resides is also one of the crucial works that can be researched upon. A comparison with other ensemble models and theoretical proof of correctness for such blended models are few of the further research works that can be attempted.

ACKNOWLEDGMENT

I thank my colleagues and students in the department of computer science and engineering, who helped me in my endeavor of completing this chapter by giving suggestions and helping in experimentation of various models with different datasets.

REFERENCES

Aggarwal, C. C. (2014). *Data Classification: Algorithms and Applications* (1st ed.). Chapman & Hall/CRC. doi:10.1201/b17320

Anava, O., & Levy, K. Y. (2016). k*-Nearest Neighbors: From Global to Local. *Proceedings of 30th Conference on Neural Information Processing Systems (NIPS).*

Chakraborty, T. (2017). EC3: Combining Clustering and Classification for Ensemble Learning. In *Proceedings of IEEE International Conference on Data Mining (ICDM).* New Orleans, LA: IEEE.

Chen, M., Hao, Y., Hwang, K., Wang, L., & Wang, L. (2017). Disease Prediction by Machine Learning Over Big Data From Healthcare Communities. *IEEE Access: Practical Innovations, Open Solutions, 5,* 8869–8879. doi:10.1109/ACCESS.2017.2694446

Chinmay, C., Gupta, B., Ghosh, S. K., Das, D., & Chakraborty, C. (2016). Telemedicine Supported Chronic Wound Tissue Prediction Using Different Classification Approach. *Journal of Medical Systems, 40*(3), 1–12. PMID:26573639

Cover, T., & Hart, P. (2006). Nearest neighbor pattern classification. *IEEE Transactions on Information Theory*, *13*(1), 21–27. doi:10.1109/TIT.1967.1053964

Cunningham, J. P., & Ghahramani, Z. (2015). Linear dimensionality reduction: Survey, insights, and generalizations. *Journal of Machine Learning Research*, *16*(1), 2859–2900.

Duda, R. O., Stork, D. G., & Hart, P. E. (2001). *Pattern classification* (2nd ed.). Wiley.

Friedman, J. H., Bentley, J. L., & Finkel, R. A. (1977). An algorithm for finding best matches in logarithmic expected time. *ACM Transactions on Mathematical Software*, *3*(3), 209–226. doi:10.1145/355744.355745

Gutjahr, G., Krishna, C. L, & Nedungadi, P. (2018). Optimal Tour Planning for Measles and Rubella Vaccination in Kochi, South India. *Proceedings of International Conference on Advances in Computing, Communications and Informatics (ICACCI)*.

Han, E.-H., Karypis, G., & Kumar, V. (2001). Text Categorization Using Weight Adjusted k-Nearest Neighbor Classification. In *Proceedings of the 5th Pacific-Asia Conference on Knowledge Discovery and Data Mining* (pp. 53-65). Springer-Verlag. 10.1007/3-540-45357-1_9

Islam, M. S., Hasan, M. M., Wang, X., Germack, H. D., & Noor-E-Alam, M. (2018). A Systematic Review on Healthcare Analytics: Application and Theoretical Perspective of Data Mining. *Health Care*, *6*(2), 54. PMID:29882866

Jain, A. K. (2010). Data clustering: 50 years beyond K-means. *Pattern Recognition Letters*, *31*(8), 651–666. doi:10.1016/j.patrec.2009.09.011

Kavilkrue, M., & Boonma, P. (2015). Dimensionality Reduction Algorithms for Improving Efficiency of PromoRank: A Comparison Study. In H. Unger, P. Meesad, & S. Boonkrong (Eds.), *Recent Advances in Information and Communication Technology 2015. Advances in Intelligent Systems and Computing* (Vol. 361). Springer. doi:10.1007/978-3-319-19024-2_3

Kittler, J., Hatef, M., Duin, R. P. W., & Matas, J. (1998). On combining classifiers. *IEEE Transactions on Pattern Analysis and Machine Intelligence*, *20*(3), 226–239. doi:10.1109/34.667881

Koppen, M. (2008). The curse of dimensionality. In *Proceedings of the 5th Online World Conference on Soft Computing in Industrial Applications (WSC5)* (pp. 4-8). Academic Press.

Kriegel, H.-P., Kröger, P., & Zimek, A. (2009). Clustering high-dimensional data: A survey on subspace clustering, pattern-based clustering, and correlation clustering. ACM Trans. Knowl. Discov. Data., 3(1). doi:10.1145/1497577.1497578

Lloyd, S. P. (1982). Least squares quantization in PCM. Information Theory. *IEEE Transactions on Information Theory*, *28*(2), 129–137. doi:10.1109/TIT.1982.1056489

MacQueen, J. (1967). Some methods for classification and analysis of multivariate observations. In *Proceedings of the Fifth Berkeley Symposium on Mathematical Statistics and Probability. Volume 1: Statistics* (pp. 281-297), University of California Press.

Murphy, K. P. (2013). *Machine Learning: a Probabilistic Perspective*. MIT Press.

Nedungadi, P., Iyer, A., Gutjahr, G., Bhaskar, J., & Pillai, A. B. (2018). Data-Driven Methods for Advancing Precision Oncology. *Current Pharmacology Reports*, *4*(2), 145–156. doi:10.100740495-018-0127-4

Niu, K., Zhao, F., & Zhang, S. (2013). A Fast Classification Algorithm for Big Data based on KNN. *Journal of Applied Sciences (Faisalabad)*, *13*(12), 2208–2212. doi:10.3923/jas.2013.2208.2212

Ougiaroglou, S., & Nanopoulos, A. (2007). Adaptive k-Nearest-Neighbor Classification Using a Dynamic Number of Nearest Neighbors. In Y. Ioannidis, B. Novikov, & B. Rachev (Eds.), *Advances in Databases and Information Systems* (pp. 66–82). Springer Berlin Heidelberg. doi:10.1007/978-3-540-75185-4_7

Parzen, E. (1962). On estimation of a probability density function and mode. *Annals of Mathematical Statistics*, *33*(3), 1065–1076. doi:10.1214/aoms/1177704472

Rajaraman & Ullman. (2011). *Mining of Massive Datasets*. New York: Cambridge University Press.

Rashid, T. A., & Abdullah, S. M. (2018). A Hybrid of Artificial Bee Colony, Genetic Algorithm, and Neural Network for Diabetic Mellitus Diagnosing. *ARO-The Scientific Journal of Koya University.*, *6*(1), 55–64. doi:10.14500/aro.10368

Saleh, E., Błaszczyński, J., Moreno, A., Valls, A., Romero-Aroca, P., de la Riva-Fernández, S., & Słowiński, R. (2017). Learning ensemble classifiers for diabetic retinopathy assessment. *Artificial Intelligence in Medicine*, *85*, 50–63. doi:10.1016/j.artmed.2017.09.006 PMID:28993124

Sathya, S., Joshi, S., & Padmavathi, S. (2017). Classification of breast cancer dataset by different classification algorithms. *Proceedings of 4th International Conference on Advanced Computing and Communication Systems*. 10.1109/ICACCS.2017.8014573

Shesternikova, O. P., Agafonov, M. A., Vinokurova, L. V., Pankratova, E. S., & Finn, V. K. (2016). Intelligent system for diabetes prediction in patients with chronic pancreatitis. *Scientific and Technical Information Processing*, *43*(5-6), 315–345. doi:10.3103/S0147688216050051

Song, Y., Huang, J., Zhou, D., Zha, H., & Giles, C. L. (2007). IKNN: Informative K-Nearest Neighbor Pattern Classification. In *Proceedings of the 11th European conference on Principles and Practice of Knowledge Discovery in Databases* (pp. 248-264), Springer Berlin Heidelberg.

Taniar, D. (2008). *Data Mining and Knowledge Discovery Technologies*. Hershey, PA: IGI Global. doi:10.4018/978-1-59904-960-1

Wu, J., Cai, Z., & Gao, Z. (2010). Dynamic K-Nearest-Neighbor with Distance and Attribute Weighted for Classification. In *Proceedings of the International Conference on Electronics and Information Engineering* (vol. 1, pp. 356-360). Kyoto. 10.1109/ICEIE.2010.5559858

Wu, X., & Vipin Kumar, J. (2007). Top 10 algorithms in data mining. *Knowledge and Information Systems*, *14*(1), 1–37. doi:10.100710115-007-0114-2

Xie, Liu, & Xue. (2017). *A survey of dimensionality reduction techniques based on random projection*. CoRR abs/1706.04371.

ENDNOTES

1 https://www.kdnuggets.com/2017/04/must-know-curse-dimensionality.html

2 Anand Rajaraman and Jeffrey David Ullman. 2011. *Mining of Massive Datasets*. Cambridge University Press, New York, NY, USA.

3 Anand Rajaraman and Jeffrey David Ullman. 2011. *Mining of Massive Datasets*. Cambridge University Press, New York, NY, USA.

4 http://archive.ics.uci.edu/ml/index.php

Chapter 4
Developing Security Solutions for Telemedicine Applications:
Medical Image Encryption and Watermarking

Pavithra V.
Thiagarajar College of Engineering, India

Jeyamala Chandrasekaran
https://orcid.org/0000-0001-5233-4393
Thiagarajar College of Engineering, India

ABSTRACT

Telemedicine is defined as the means of providing healthcare for people from a distance by the use of telecommunication and information technology. This technology is mainly useful in overcoming the obstacles of distance and provide enhancement in the access of medical services that would not be easily available in different rural areas. Telemedicine security includes issues such as confidentiality, integrity, and authentication that are also present in other systems involving information and data. Maintaining integrity of data stored and used is a huge problem for medical applications because it contains more sensitive medical records of patients which can cause severe ill effects on slight modification. In order to resolve the confidentiality and integrity issues of telemedicine applications, medical image encryption and watermarking comes into play. The security issues in telemedicine applications is to be given higher importance and thus choosing a reliable and effective approach or framework is more essential.

DOI: 10.4018/978-1-7998-0261-7.ch004

INTRODUCTION

Telemedicine is essentially the remote diagnosis and treatment of patients by means of telecommunications technology This technology is mainly useful in overcoming the obstacles of distance and provide an enhancement in the access to medical services that would not be easily available in different rural areas. This would be most helpful to safeguard lives in emergency and critical situations. Telemedicine allows the interpretation of medical data, medical images and other information related to patients between the patients and the doctors or other hospital staffs. Telemedicine can be beneficial to human beings in places which are isolated and remote areas where instant care from doctors is not possible. The process of remote monitoring of patients using technology can lower the need for outpatient visits and helps in enabling remote verification of prescriptions and administration of drugs.

However, telemedicine applications are highly prone to cyber security attacks that cause serious effects on the confidentiality, integrity and authentication factors. The increasing adoption and usage of internet, smart phones, mobile health care devices and wearable health technology have significantly impacted the growth of telemedicine over the years. Telemedicine involves large volume of storage and exchange of electronic health records among physicians, patients and health care professionals for better health services. Health records involve extensive usage of multimedia especially images, which are generated from various imaging technologies like conventional X-rays, ultrasound imaging, digital mammography, Computed Axial Tomography (CT), Positron Emission Tomography (PET) and Magnetic Resonance Imaging (MRI). These medical images are highly sensitive and are to be operated in a resource constrained environment characterized by lower band width, limited processing power and limited memory. The strong privacy requirements of medical images with the operating constraints demand strong security algorithms with optimal processing requirements.

Challenges and Security Issues in Telemedicine

There are significantly more privacy and security concerns in tele health applications that can cause adverse effects on the patient's clinical treatment. Some privacy risks include the failure of sensors and telehealth devices that fail to collect and transmit complete information and a lack of control over the patient's data. Maintaining integrity and privacy of data (Qasim, Mezinane, & Aspin, 2018) is a major concern when it comes to securing telemedicine applications where large amounts of patient's health data are collected and transmitted over the telecommunication system.

Telemedicine applications are highly prone to cybersecurity attacks that cause serious effects on the confidentiality, integrity and authentication factors. Medical records of patients contain confidential and sensitive information which should not be accessed by unauthorized persons in order to maintain confidentiality, integrity, and privacy. Higher care should be taken such that the medical reports are readily available at any time for authorized access. A good and usable framework for telemedicine demands the following security requirements:

- **Confidentiality**: Confidentiality is the process of keeping the patient's personal health information private unless the permission is provided by the patient to release. It should be maintained by the users (patients, healthcare professionals) and service provider. The users store the data in the encrypted form to maintain the confidentiality. While storing and retrieving the data key management issues should be addressed.

- **Integrity**: Integrity is the process of ensuring that the medical records captured or provided is the original representation of the information and has not been modified. Since many participants (patients, health professionals, specialists from various hospitals) are involved in telemedicine, any modification can occur due to the participants intentionally or unintentionally.
- **Access Control**: The unauthorized access to medical records can be prevented with the help of access control policies. Many organizations allow the users who have previously registered with their valid credentials only to access the resources. The access control policies defined varies for the patients and healthcare professionals.
- **Data Ownership**: Most of the unauthorized users get access to the medical images due to the missing of the owner's identity in the encrypted medical images. If the embedding of the owner's seal or identity is done in the encrypted images through encryption or watermarking methods, it is difficult for the attackers to gain access.
- **Privacy**: Privacy refers to the right of patients to determine when, how and to what extent their health information is shared with others. It involves maintaining confidentiality and sharing identifying data, only with healthcare providers and related professionals.
- **Authentication**: The medical records should be accessed only by the authorized patients and doctors. The credentials provided by the users must match with the stored credentials of the users in the authentication process. If the credential details are leaked out, there occurs a possibility for the unauthorized users to access the data.

The article discusses about the state of the art security solutions for confidentiality integrity and authentication service. To resolve the confidentiality and integrity issues of telemedicine applications, medical image encryption (Nematzadeh, Enayatifar, Motameni, Guimareaes & Coelho, 2018) and Watermarking comes into play.

Survey on Security Solutions for Confidentiality

Image encryption (Nematzadeh et al., 2018) s considered as one of the most important fields of cryptography which should be done with algorithms that requires less time and less cost. By the process of encrypting an image, it is essential to apply a symmetric or asymmetric encryption algorithm for the input image to get converted into a cipher image using symmetric or asymmetric keys. Symmetric ciphers use only one key for encryption and decryption process while asymmetric ciphers use different keys for encryption and decryption.

To address the confidentiality issues in telemedicine applications encryption technique is used. Medical image encryption can be performed using various algorithms using different parameters. Encryption of medical images can be done by high-speed scrambling, bitwise xor diffusion, chaotic (Kanso & Ghebleh, 2015) and edge maps and so on. The performance of the algorithm which was used to encrypt the medical image can be analyzed using measures such as peak signal to noise ratio, bit error rate, fidelity and mean square error.

The main purpose of medical image encryption is for the

- Secure transmission of medical records of patients
- Ensuring confidentiality and integrity
- Avoiding changes in medical images that may lead to a false diagnosis
- Persist from cybersecurity attacks and threats.

By the process of encrypting an image, it is essential to apply a symmetric or asymmetric encryption algorithm for the input image to get converted into a cipher image using symmetric or asymmetric keys. Symmetric ciphers use one key for encryption and decryption process while asymmetric ciphers use different keys for encryption and decryption.

Medical image encryption can be performed using various algorithms using different parameters. Encryption of medical images can be done by high-speed scrambling, bitwise xor diffusion, chaotic and edge maps (Cao, Zhou, Chen, & Xia, 2017) and so on. The performance of the algorithm which was used to encrypt the medical images can be analyzed using measures such as peak signal-to-noise-ratio, bit error rate, fidelity and mean square error.

Medical Image Encryption Evaluation Metrics

Security of medical image encryption is analyzed using the following:

A. Peak Signal-to-Noise-Ratio (PSNR)

PSNR (Figure 1) can be defined using the Mean Squared Error(MSE) (Figure 2) which is the mean value or average of the square of errors. PSNR is the ratio between the maximum power to the corrupted value of a signal or image. Figure 1 represents the PSNR and Figure 2 represents the MSE formula for calculating the corresponding values. Where M and N represented in Figure 1 and Figure 2 are the dimensions of the image used. Here I and I' represents the Intensity of the original image and the encrypted image.

B. Mean, Variance and Standard Deviation

Mean (Figure 3) is the average value for the given data values. In the case of medical images, the mean value of the image results is taken into consideration. Here n is the total number of the dataset used and xi is the sum of all the data values. Figure 3 represents the formula for calculating the mean of given data values.

Variance (Figure 4) is the difference between all the data in the data set and their means. Here X denotes the data values and μ denotes the mean value of the data points. Figure 4 represents the formula for calculating the variance of given data values.

Standard Deviation (Figure 5) is the square root of the variance. It is used to measure the amount of deviation of the data from the mean value. Figure 5 represents the formula for calculating the standard deviation of given data values.

Figure 1. PSNR Formula

$$PSNR = 10 * \lg(255^2 / MSE)$$

Figure 2. MSE Formula

$$MSE = 1 / M * N\sum_{i=1}^{N}\sum_{j=1}^{M}[I(i,j) - I'(i,j)]^2$$

Figure 3. Mean Formula

$$x' = 1 / n * (\Sigma xi)$$

Figure 4. Variance Formula

$$\sigma^2 = \sum X^2 / N - \mu^2$$

Figure 5. Standard Deviation Formula

$$\sigma = \sqrt{\sum f(x - x')^2 / \sum f}$$

C. Bit error rate

The bit error rate can be explained as the rate at which the transmission error occurs.

D. Structural Similarity Index (SSIM)

Structural similarity index (Figure 6) is a measure for measuring the quality of the image and measures the degradation in the image quality. Here μ and μ(w) represent the mean value and σ denotes the standard deviation value of the dataset. C1 and C2 are constants. Figure 6 represents the formula for calculating the structural similarity index of given data values.

E. Information Entropy

Information entropy (Figure 7) is the statistical measure of randomness associated with an image. The probability of making predictions from the cipher image decreases with the increase in randomness. The entropy of plain and cipher medical image samples H(m) are calculated as can be seen from Figure 7 where P(mi) represented in Figure 7 re.ers to the probability of occurrence of particular intensity. The entropy of a truly random source emitting 2N symbols is H(m) = N and hence for a cipher image with 256 grey levels, the entropy should ideally be H(m) = 8. There exists certain degree of predictability if the output of a cipher emits symbols with lower entropy.

F. Differential Analysis

The immunity of an image cryptosystem towards differential attack is measured by Number of Pixel Change Rate (NPCR) and Unified Average Changing Intensity (UACI) (Figure 8), which are calculated as in Figure 8 where R" and C" represented in Figure 8 are the width and height of the medical image, c1 and c2 are two encrypted images with slightly different keys. D(i,j) is a bipolar array with the same size as that of c1 and c2. If c1(i,j) and c2(i,j) are identical, then D(i,j) is set to 0, else set to 1.

Figure 6. SSIM Formula

$$SSIM(I, I_w) = \frac{(2\mu\mu_w + C_1)(2\sigma(I, I_w) + C_2)}{(\mu^2 + \mu^2 w + C_1)(\sigma(I)^2 + \sigma(I_w)^2 + C_2)}$$

Figure 7. Information Entropy Formula

$$H(m) = -\sum_{i=1}^{n} P(m_i)\log_2 P(m_i)$$

Figure 8. NPCR and UACI Formula

$$NPCR = \frac{\Sigma_{i,j} D(i,j)}{R'' \times C''} \times 100$$

$$UACI = \frac{1}{R'' \times C''} \sum_{i,j} \frac{\left| c1(i,j) - c2(i,j) \right|}{255} x100$$

Medical Image Encryption Techniques

Using Edge Maps

In the event of using edge maps (Cao, Zhou, Chen, & Xia, 2017), three different processes are involved. They are bit plane decomposition, generation of random sequence and permutation process. The usage of edge maps is considered advantageous because any type of source image can be used, the choice of usage of bit plane decomposition method is flexible and the number of permutations is also flexible. Furthermore, security benefits are also higher in edge maps considered to other encryption technologies used.

Adaptive Medical Image Encryption

This makes use of multiple chaotic mapping to overcome the defects of the existing chaotic networks. Chaotic logistic maps (Chen & Hu, 2017) are used to generate a sequence of subkeys and the image is encrypted using those subkeys generated by logistic maps. Then subkey generation is done using chaotic maps and those keys are used to encrypt the region of interest in the medical image.

The receiver can use the same subkeys to decrypt the digital medical image and the encryption method is evaluated using loss, peak signal to noise ratio, cross-correlation and so on.

Improved ElGamal Encryption

Simple ElGamal encryption (Laiphrakpam & Khumanthem, 2017) involves the process of encoding the plain message into the coordinates of the elliptic curve before the process of encryption takes place. In the process of improved ElGamal encryption, the problem of data expansion is solved, and the time taken for the entire encryption process is also reduced. The performance of the method can be measured using various statistical and analytical methods.

Scrambling and Diffusion

Scrambling (Nematzadeh et al., 2018) is a method of data encryption and authentication mechanism that is used to protect the medical image or any information from being stolen, distributed and modification. This is one of the copy protection methods that are widely used. In general, scrambling changes the understandable format of text to non-understandable format to avoid illegal viewing of confidential data. Scrambling process is now automated using scramblers which are highly used in telecommunication systems.

This scrambler replaces some sequence of data into other sequences and as a result, the sequence remains scrambled and non-understandable. Scrambling is mainly used for two reasons:

- To ensure recovery of confidential data
- To ensure that no data is modified or lost during transmission.

Diffusion is the process where a single bit change can lead to serious changes in the input text. A single bit change in the plaintext should possibly change half of the bits in the ciphertext that is generated and similarly, a one-bit change in the ciphertext should change one half of the plaintext.

Diffusion can be done using bitwise xor and modulo arithmetic. While bitwise xor provides higher efficiency in case of hardware platforms, modulo arithmetic provides faster execution speed in case of software platforms.

Diffusion (Nematzadeh et al., 2018) often refers to the property of redundancy that the change of plaintext can change the ciphertext. Transposition is an important technique of diffusion where there is a dependency between input and output bits. In a good diffusion process, flipping of one bit in the input should essentially change half of the bits in the resulting ciphertext.

Related Works

This paper provides a better encryption scheme for the process of protecting medical images. This method has better efficiency and robustness in comparison to other methods based on the experimental results. In the first step, some amount of random data are inserted into the ends of the image. The second step focuses on two rounds of scrambling which has higher speed and pixel adaptive diffusion is performed in order to shuffle the data randomly inside the image. In this, they have proposed an encryption scheme that can be applied to any source image without any standard format. Two different types of practices are implemented to perform the diffusion process namely bitwise XOR and modulo arithmetic. While bitwise XOR has higher efficiency in case of hardware platforms, the modulo arithmetic diffusion process can achieve higher speed and higher security in case of software platforms. The problem of data loss interference is also addressed in this paper (Nematzadeh et al., 2018).

Digital Imaging and Communications in Medicine(DICOM) is a common standard that is mostly used for representing medical images of patients such as x-ray, MRI, and endoscopy. This paper mainly focuses on enhancing the security measures over transmission since the medical record of patients has greater importance in telehealth applications. This method combines the process of both encryption and watermarking which enhances the process of authentication and safer transmission of data thus enhancing the security in telecommunication systems. In this, the author has made use of a fuzzy chaotic map for the process of encryption and for the process of watermarking Discrete Wavelet Transform (DWT) is used. This method has also resolved the problems with Arnold transform which is known to be the most utilized mechanisms in encryption and ciphering of medical images. Performance measurement has been evaluated for better enhancement. This work can be further extended with the use of neural networks to provide much more security to the storage and transmission of medical images (Qasim, Mezinane, & Aspin, 2018).

In this paper, they have presented the design of the double hump logistic map that is generalized, and they have used it as a pseudo-random number generator. The parameter of generalization provides much control of the user over the chaotic logistic maps. Also, it has the benefit of obtaining a special map on the zooming effect of the medical image that is obtained by the process of generalization parameter value manipulation. The generalized map behaves dynamically, and all the activities are analyzed including the points that are fixed and the ranges that are stable. The encryption algorithm is based on the pseudo-random number generation using the dynamic hump logistic map that is generalized thus providing secure storage and transmission of medical data. Analysis of security measures is done based on the two parameters namely key sensitivity, analysis of keyspace, analysis of histograms and correlation coefficient. The robustness of the system has also been projected in this paper by avoiding the noise attacks along with the national institute of standards and technology thus making sure of the system efficiency. Also, the comparison of the proposed work and existing work has also been tabulated (Cao, Zhou, Chen, & Xia, 2017).

Medical image data are the most significant data in the medical systems. The analysis methods that are used for the medical images are getting modernized day by day with new medical image devices and different unique and distinct medical image processing mechanisms. The paper presents an encryption method for medical images based on a genetic map algorithm and map lattices. First, the proposed method employs coupled map lattices to generate different cipher images that are secured and then it makes use of a modified genetic algorithm to increase the entropy of the encrypted and ciphered medical images and also to decrease the computational time that is required for the complete encryption and decryption process. The experimental results depict that the proposed method not only does good encryption but also is capable of being robust and resistant to various cybersecurity attacks. The results also show that the proposed methods perform better than other methods that exist and the better results are highlighted in each case. Finally, the proposed method also achieves outstanding results in decreasing the time for the execution of medical image encryption (Nematzadeh et al., 2018).

This paper proposes an encryption scheme for the protection of medical images in modern clinical diagnosis. The patient's health record and other confidential information are stored and transmitted for communication over public networks. Confidentiality need for the protection of those medical images is increasing. This paper describes an adaptive medical image encryption scheme that is based on chaotic maps to overcome the issues in the existing chaotic encryption algorithm used for the encryption of medical images. In the first step logistic chaos mapping is used to perform high-speed scrambling and then further the scrambled image is divided into two sub-blocks. Then by using a hyperchaotic system the sub-blocks are encrypted adaptively thus completing the encryption of thesesub-blocks. The performance measures that are used are correlation coefficient and information entropy thus giving the experimental results making the proposed algorithm a better efficient one (Chen & Hu, 2017).

In this paper, the author proposes a novel and efficient encryption scheme that is chaos based that is much suitable for the encryption process of medical images. This includes two processes namely shuffling and masking process. All the phases are computed based on blocks and they have made use of chaotic maps to implement the process of shuffling and masking the input to the image. To improve efficiency and security, the author has made use of a pseudo-random matrix that is of the same size as of the input medical image. Blocks of the pseudorandom image can undergo permutations before the shuffling process based on the outputs of the chaotic maps. This method also applies the execution of mixing the different blocks of an image to prevent from different attacks. Also, results depict that the proposed scheme provides a higher performance rate and also shows that the robustness of the system is higher and persistent against cryptanalysis attacks thus providing confidentiality, integrity, and authenticity. The mixing of blocks is the reason for the excellent performance of the proposed scheme (Kanso & Ghebleh, 2015).

Integrity and Authentication Survey

This paper provides a survey on the security of the medical record of patients and medical images. Since there are chances of the medical image being manipulated intentionally or unintentionally from outside as medical images involve processing techniques such as viewing, extracting and transmission using telecommunication systems. This method focuses the survey on the imaging standard known as picture archiving and communication systems which are intended to provide higher security. Digital watermarking is one of the best approaches that mainly ensures the authenticity and integrity of medical images that are archived and transmitted over the public network. This also provides an evident scene by the process of analysis of robustness and efficiency of the transmission system. This survey also works on the study of different security levels that need to be implemented along with the picture archiving and communication system and thus clarifies the need and requirement for medical image watermarking. This survey also mainly focuses on the purpose of digital watermarking which need to be applied to medical images (Qasim, Mezinane, & Aspin, 2018).

In this paper, they have proposed medical image encryption that is based on the edge maps that is derived from the source image. The algorithm comprises of three main parts: decomposition of the bit-plane, random sequence generation and the process of permutation. The major advantages with this methodology are that the source image need not follow any standard format and any type of image can be used. Other advantages include different edge maps generation could be different for distinct edge detectors and unique thresholds, the selection of the method for performing bit-plane decomposition is flexible and the number of permutations to be performed can also be adjusted and is flexible. The algorithm proposed generated a large key space and a large sensitive key in order to provide a higher level of security to the medical images. This method is known to be widely applied than other fuzzy logic methods. Experimental results also depict that the proposed method has higher resistance and robustness against various security attacks and other methods (Cao, Zhou, Chen, & Xia, 2017).

Elliptic curve based ElGamal encryption technique mainly requires the process of encoding the plain message into the original image and this paper uses the koblitz encoding technique before performing the process of encryption. This paper presents an advanced image encryption scheme based on advanced ElGamal encryption technique. A new method that has been implemented in this paper is that there is no need for separate calculations for the process of encoding the plain message to the elliptic curve. This algorithm is just an improved version of the existing ElGamal encryption technique in which the problem of data expansion is resolved. The execution speed has also been increased to reduce the time complexity of the encryption and decryption process. The performance of the proposed system has been measured using various security analyzers and statistical analysis. The new finding made is that the process of base operation helps in encrypting multiple pixel values at once thus enhancing the execution speed of the process (Laiphrakpam & Khumanthem, 2017).

This paper presents a joint watermarking and lossless compression of the medical image in order to maintain the originality of the medical image and lossless compression is achieved by the process of the bitwise substitution modulation method. This also enables watermarking based security solution without any loss in the image and without decompressing the image. This also makes it possible to verify the authenticity of the medical image from the bit stream generated. An original medical image of the patient is subjected to watermarking or JPEG lossless compression as the output of which compresses watermarked bitstream is generated. In the end, the compressed image can be decompressed using the same algorithm that was used for compression and using the decryption key the original image and message can be extracted without causing integrity and authenticity issues. At the stage of the verificationstage, the message is extracted from the bitstream by identifying the bit sequences that are present within the compressed image (Haddad, Coatrieux, Cozic & Bouslimi, 2017).

This paper presents a selective encryption scheme for the secured transmission of medical images which is based on the process of JPEG based compression algorithm. The magnanimous development of the telecommunication is due to the wide usage and the data involved in it. This work mainly focuses on the partial or selective encryption process which is based on the discrete cosine transform which reduces the processing and execution time for the process. The experimental results depict that the proposed scheme is secured, faster and efficient in terms of robustness and security. Since the digital medical images have gigantic sizes they are compressed in order to improve the storage capacity and to ensure the easy transmission of data. First, an approach is applied to compress the original image to a smaller size for increasing the space and then the output which is a compressed image is finally encrypted with any independent cryptographic algorithm such as advanced encryption standard and data encryption standard and so on. The results clearly depict that the symmetric and asymmetric cryptographic systems combined with the compression process can highly ensure secure transfer of medical images (Abdmouleh, Khalfallah, & Bouhlel, 2017).

In this paper, the author has proposed a novel based encryption scheme which makes use of the region of interest-based data hiding scheme in order to achieve higher security of medical images. As the first step, the medical image of the patient is divided into a region of interest (ROI) and region of non-interest(RONI) and then encryption of both the regions are done using the encryption key generated. A data hider is used to concatenate the least significant bit of the encrypted region of interest and the digital record of patients. Finally embedding the concatenated data into the original medical image is done through the least significant bit (LSB) substitution method. When the receiver receives the encrypted medical image along with the concatenated data, it is possible for the receiver to extract the data that is embedded using the key which was used for hiding the data. If the receiver possesses the encryption key, it is possible for the receiver to get a medical image that is like the original image by decrypting the encrypted image. If the receiver has both the data hiding key and encryption key, the embedded data, as well as the original medical image, can be obtained without any data loss and error. It is also possible to recover the region of interest and region of non-interest separately without any loss after the process of extracting the embedded data gets completed (Liu, Qu, & Xin, 2016).

This paper proposes a cryptographic watermarking system that is meant for checking the integrity of the medical images and also enables tracking of those medical images. Tracking enables the process of identifying the origin of the process that seems to be illegal. This paper proposes a double watermarking system approach which involves joint watermarking decryption and modulation of quantization index. When the medical image is sent a watermark is sent as a proof of reliability before the encrypted image is sent. This approach eliminates the issues of interference between two adjacent watermarks that interferes horizontally and vertically. Experimental results depicted in the paper assure that the efficiency of the system is highly improved and also traceability can be used to identify the origin of an illegal process. The receiver is provided access to both the reliability and traceability proofs. This method was proposed to highly guarantee the confidentiality of the image through the process of encryption and reliability through traceability of the origin (Bouslimi & Coatrieux, 2016).

In this paper, an encryption scheme is introduced in which the cosine number transform is used. Since the cosine number transform is used along with algebraic structures only modular arithmetic can be used. Cosine number transform is a tool in mathematics that is used for modular arithmetic applications. If the property of modular arithmetic is used the round off errors can be resolved. This also avoids the round off errors and allows the recovered image to be identical to the original image after the encryption and decryption process. This method proposed also ensures that it can avoid all the important cryptographic attacks. The method that has been introduced divides the image into blocks in which overlapping exists vertically and horizontally with the other blocks that are adjacent to each other. Then the sub-blocks are taken into consideration and computation of a two-dimensional cosine number transform takes place. The number of times the process takes place depends on the secret key and this can be also encoded as the bit sequence. Encryption is completed after the original medical image of the patient is processed twice and the decryption process involves the same process in the reverse order. This method that has been proposed is seen to be flexible since the number of rounds depends on the secret key generated and the number of computations is less when compared to other encoding schemes (Lima, Madeiro & Sales, 2015).

This paper proposes a method of exploiting Joint photography experts group method to enhance the security and integrity of the medical image since the need for the protection of medical images has been increasing day by day to resist those confidential data against different kind of attacks and also to ensure that transmission takes place in a secured manner. This method aims to achieve the privacy goals of cryptography including authentication, confidentiality,and integrity. In this case, encryption is applied to the output of the JPEG discrete cosine transform encoding process. Here the parsing of JPEG bitstream takes place by encrypting both the AC and DC coefficients in an 8*8 block image. This method also provides a lower complexity of time and space, a compression method that is efficient and enhances the integrity of the medical image thus providing robustness to the entire system. The experimental results depict that the method that has been proposed has reached a higher level of robustness having 60.4 dB of peak signal to noise ratio and the bit error rate of 0.006% on an average. The original image is fed into the original block of the luminous component and then into the quantization matrix to achieve higher

Table 1. Results comparison

Author	Type of Image	Size of Image	Technique Used	Evaluation Metrics			Values		
Zhongyun Hua, [1]	DICOM	8 bits, 16 bits, 24 bits, 256 * 256	Scrambling and Diffusion	PSNR	MSE	Information Entropy	35.4874	8	
C. Lakshmi, [2]	DICOM	8 bits, 400 * 400	Watermarking	PSNR	MSE	SSIM	88.1	0.0001	0.9999
Samar M. Ismail, [3]	PNG and JPG	16 bits	Double humped logistic map	Correlation Coefficient	Entropy	NPCR	0.85	7.9885	75.6256
Hossein Nematzadeh,	DICOM	8 bits	Modified genetic algorithm	NPCR	UACI	-	0.990817	0.331845	-
Asaad F. Qasim	DICOM	8 bits	Survey on Watermarking	-	-	-	-	-	-
Weijia Cao	DICOM	16 bits	Edge Maps	NPCR	UACI	-	-	-	-
Dolendro Singh Laiphrakpam	DICOM	8 bits	ElGamal encryption technique	PSNR	SSIM	Entropy	6.94815	0.006167	7.9993
Xiao Chen	PNG and JPG	-	Chaotic Maps	Correlation Coefficient	NPCR	UACI	0.0171	0.9959	0.3342
S. Haddad	JPEG	8 bits	Watermarking and Lossless compression	-	-	-	-	-	-
Med Karim Abdmouleh	JPEG	8 bits	Compression based encryption of DCT	-	-	-	-	-	-
Yuling Liu	DICOM	16 bits	Reversible data hiding scheme	PSNR	-	-	131.48	-	-
Dalel Bouslimi	DICOM	8 bits	Crypto Watermarking	PSNR	Standard Deviation	-	45.65	0.82	-
J. B. Lima	DICOM	8 bits, 16 bits	Cosine number transform	NPCR	UACI	-	99.6082	33.4682	-
Musab Ghadi	JPEG	8 bits	Bitstream encryption	PSNR	Correlation Coefficient	BER	67.6862	0.99	0.0003
Kanso	DICOM	16 bits	Shuffling and Masking	Correlation Coefficient	-	-	0.9847	-	-

security levels. Then a discrete cosine transform method is employed to obtain 8*8 DCT coefficients which then performs difference coding of DC coefficients and AC coefficients (Ghadi, Laouamer, & Moulahi, 2015).

Comparison of performance for the distinct approaches that have been presented in these paradigms has also been demonstrated in Table1. The objective is to have a better understanding of the results and differences between then existing methodologies. In common, it is very much essential to preserve the quality of the medical images without any damage or changes. So, for evaluating the image with those constraints, several metrics have been used. In any medical encryption scheme, the first aim should be to measure the standard of images whereas the second aim should be to maintain and asses the accuracy of the encrypted medical images.

State-of-the-Art Solutions for Integrity and Authentication Service

Digital Watermarking

Also, ensuring trust within the workflows of medical images is much required. Digital Watermarking of medical images has become a highly effective means for achieving integrity and authenticity in medical images. Authentication is the means of verifying the root source of the information and ensuring that the treatment is delivered to the right patients at the right time. Integrity ensures that confidential information has not been altered without proper authorization mechanisms.

Most of the information systems and hospital managements maintain systems to store medical information and medical images such as X-ray, Magnetic Resonance Image (MRI), and Computerized Tomography (CT) which are mostly DICOM (Qasim, Mezinane, & Aspin, 2018) (Digital Imaging and Communications in Medicine) images. Initially, all the medical images are collected in a hospital and stored in the PACS (Picture Archiving and Communication Systems). Digital Watermarking requires some parameters including fidelity, robustness, data payload, security, perceptibility, imperceptibility, and reversibility.

Fidelity is a measure that depicts the similarity between the original image and the encrypted image to ensure that the watermarking (Ghadi, Laouamer, & Moulahi, 2015) is made invisible to the human view so that no distortion occurs. Robustness defines the ability of the image and the information system that remains to be resistant against several cryptographic attacks. Data payload gives information about the number of bits that can be modified without affecting the quality of medical images. Perceptibility defines the distortion in the image that has occurred due to the embedding of data. Imperceptibility which is commonly referred to as fidelity or invisibility is the most essential requirement of medical images. This ensures that the original image and watermarked image are similar in perception and can be done with higher robustness and security.

The predominant processes in Digital Watermarking (Bouslimi & Coatrieux, 2016) include watermark generation, watermark hiding, and watermark extraction. Watermark generation is where the original data and the message is given as input and a watermark is received as output. The watermark has specific properties based on the objectives designed. Patients can ensure the integrity and authenticity of the medical image using its features. Watermark hiding is used done by the sender. In this process, a watermark is embedded into the original data or image using some algorithm and a secret key is generated to obtain the watermarked image. Original data, secret key,anda watermark generated in the previous process are given as input to obtain watermarked data. In watermark extraction, the watermarked data, original data and secret key are given as inputs to generate the watermark that was hidden within the original medical images.

To resolve authenticity issues (Qasim, Mezinane, & Aspin, 2018), user authentication is other means of ensuring a higher level of security. Any doctor or hospital staff or patients accessing the medical records of patients or their own medical records need to be provided with a user name and password and even multi-factor authentication to prevent unauthorized access

All the medical image sent inside and outside of the secured medical system can be modified since the images are transmitted over the public networks. Many organizations make use of Digital Imaging and Communications in Medicine (DICOM) standard whereas several organizations make use of Picture Archiving and Communication Systems (PACS) for enhancing the security aspect of medical images. However, since the transmission of electronic health records and medical images between different health institutions and care providers is common, it is essential to ensure trust between those service providers (Pianykh, 2009). Medical image Watermarking seems to be an effective approach which mainly ensures the authenticity and integrity of the medical images. Authenticity is where an approach of identity management is implemented to verify that the medical records match to the exact person and Integrity is required to ensure that the data or information has not been viewed or altered without proper authentication and authorization.

Need for Watermarking in Medical Images

The major requirement in medical images is that it requires the implementation of ethics and rules that the doctors and patients must follow. In case of securing the medical images, three factors come into play: confidentiality, reliability, and availability. Confidentiality mainly ensures that only authenticated and authorized persons can access and modify the information. Reliability is sub-divided into 2 parts namely integrity and authentication. Integrity is where verification is done to verify that no data has been modified and authentication is where verification is done for the process of ensuring that the data belongs to the respective patient and the data comes from the reliable source.

Availability is where it is made sure that an authorized person can access the information whenever he/she needs it. Confidentiality in case of medical data can be achieved by some mechanism such as encryption, access control, Intrusion detection systems, and firewalls. Integrity can also be achieved by encrypting the pixels of the medical image which provides a higher level of security when transferred over the public network. Confidentiality ensures whether the confidentiality or integrity mechanism has been breached (Fontani, De Rosa, Caldelli, Filippini, Piva & Consolvo, 2010).

To achieve higher levels of security, integrity and authenticity need to be ensured within the data. This can be done using two techniques namely metadata and digital watermarking. Metadata usually is defined as the data about the data. But in the case of medical images, metadata refers to the data along with the images. The digital signature of the medical image is placed in the header of the metadata. Digital signatures are used to avoid manipulation in patient data which would lead to the false diagnosis of patients (Liew, Zain & Tamper, 2011). The metadata also ensures confidentiality by using the DICOM header to encrypt the entire medical image. Since most of the existing metadata techniques do not provide a higher level of robustness between the medical image and the corresponding metadata, there are chances of manipulating the metadata leading to the change in the medical image data. These cons can be avoided using digital watermarking. Digital Watermarking is where a data known as the watermark is hidden inside the digital medical image with an added advantage that the watermark can be extracted to highly ensure the integrity of the medical image. Watermarking in images is an old technique for ensuring integrity and authenticity but in the years later authentication has become one of the major requirements when it comes to digital watermarking.

When it comes to analyzing the requirements that are required for the efficient implementation of digital watermarking the following considerations are required namely fidelity, robustness, data payload, security, computational complexity, perceptibility, imperceptibility, reversibility, and reliability. Fidelity measures the similarity between the original image and the watermarked medical image. Fidelity is one of the most important aspects of the digital watermarking system. The watermark should always remain invisible to the human view to provide and ensure higher security levels. Robustness mainly defines the resistance of the medical images against several attacks in the public networks since most of the medical data are transmitted over those networks. Some attacks in the public network include cryptographic attacks, sniffing and manipulation attacks Memon, Chaudhry, Ahmad & Keerio, 2011).

Data payload count the number of bits that can be hidden such that no change to the quality of the image happens. It also measures the number of bits that can be hidden within the image so that the extraction of the watermarked bits at the other end becomes easier (Dehkordi, Esfahani & Avanaki, 2011). The number of hidden bits is decided based on the size of the image. As the size of the image increases, the number of bits to be hidden also increases i.e. the size of the image is directly proportional to the number of hidden bits. Security is a major factor that defines the resistance capacity of the medical image against attacks that are intentional and non-intentional. Also, the digital watermark generated is said to be secure if and only if the authorized users can extract and modify the watermark thus prohibiting the unauthorized users from even accessing it.

Computational Complexity calculates the time required for the embedding and extraction process of medical images. For the higher performance of the medical application, it is required to maintain higher values of computational complexity. Imperceptibility is a factor where the original medical image and watermarked medical image must be similar only in the case of perception. This can be achieved by either reducing the robustness, capacity or both. Reversibility is a major factor since a minor distortion to the medical image can cause false diagnosis and severe ill effects to the patients. This is the process where the image and the watermark can be embedded and extracted such that any distortion does not make any changes to the image and the watermark embedded in the medical image (Richardson, Frank, & Stern, 1995).

Watermarking System and Its Principal Components

The watermarking system mainly consists of three main components which ensure the effective working of the watermarking system. These include three processes namely generation of watermarks, hiding the watermarks and finally extracting the watermarks.

Watermark generation is the process where watermarks are created based on the application and its functions. In case of a simple application, watermark generation is only about the image and its functions but when it applies for a higher end application, the properties are also taken into consideration which makes the process tedious. Watermark hiding is done at the sender level where the generated watermark is hidden inside the image using some algorithm and a key is generated which could be used for the extraction process at the receiver end. Watermark extraction is done by using the same algorithm used for hiding but in a reverse manner and the secret key is useful for extracting the original data without any disruption or modification (Dehkordi, Esfahani & Avanaki, 2011).

When it comes to classifying the watermarking methods, they are mainly subdivided based on some properties that are being used. Based on the type of document, we have 4 types of watermarking techniques namely audio files watermarking, video files watermarking, text files watermarking and image files watermarking. Similarly, based on the domain in which the watermark is hidden we have 2 types namely spatial hiding scheme and transform hiding scheme. Also, based on the reversibility property watermarking can either be reversible or irreversible. Watermarking can also be classified based on the human view namely visible watermarking, invisible watermarking and combination of both (Wenvin & Shih, 2011).

Watermarking Methods

Based on the properties of the image, we had several types of watermarking schemes. In watermarking methods, we have 3 methods namely traditional methods, watermarking methods based on the region-of-interest and region-of-non-interest and watermarking based on the reversibility techniques. In traditional watermarking methods, the watermark is embedded in the whole image by replacing some data such as least significant bits or some other data which would lead to compression with data loss. Since it is very important to maintain the originality of the medical image in any case, traditional classical methods fail to meet those requirements. Also, the watermark should be reversible and if the watermark remains irreversible it is mostly subjected to examination (Wenvin & Shih, 2011).

The watermarking method which involves separation of Region of Interest and Region of Non-Interest which gives priority to the region which needs to be highly concentrated in medical diagnosis. The region of Non-Interest usually describes the background part of the medical image but there are also chances of having some regions which require slight concentration. In these cases, watermarking is very robust and fragile based on the type of application in which it is being used. The major disadvantage with the process is that the watermark if hidden or embedded behind the Region of Interest of the medical image can also lead to a false diagnosis of patients. But if watermarking needs to be embedded in the Region of Non-Interest then it is limited to size. The size of the watermark purely depends on the size of the Region of Non-Interest and the Region of Interest is mostly prone to several malicious attacks (Dehkordi, Esfahani & Avanaki, 2011).

In watermarking methods that are reversible, the watermark can be generated and embedded at the sender side whereas the watermark can be extracted at the receiver end. It is clearly known that any type of watermarking can cause degradation to the quality of the image even though a robust watermarking method is employed (Cheng, Chen, & Tsai, 2013). Since modification in the image can lead to severe effects in case of medical, military and other trivial applications, this type of reversible watermarking scheme has been introduced where embedding of the watermark and extraction of the original image is possible. When reversible watermarking techniques are used for authentication systems, it highly protects the integrity of the medical image and the property of reversibility of the watermark technique highly protects it from several malicious attacks. Better clarity of watermarking techniques can be achieved by explaining the classified parts of watermarking techniques namely watermarking based on compressing the image, watermarking based on the modification of the histogram, watermarking based on expansion and finally watermarking based on quantization technique. In compression-based technique, some additional information needs to be embedded along with the watermark to ensure the integrity at the receiver side. In the process, as an initialstep, the image is modified into a domain transform using wavelet transform equations. In the second step, the transformed image is divided into blocks then the watermarking process is carried out for each block and finally, all the blocks are integrated to obtain the original image (Fontani et al., 2010).

Histogram related watermarking is mainly implemented to ensure the robustness of the medical image against various attacks during the processing of the entire image. In this technique, histogram replaces the embedding part thus introducing higher robustness levels. This technique can also be implemented by dividing it into blocks where these blocks having higher resistance against attacks and this is only implemented where robustness is of higher importance. The only disadvantage is that it does not prove to perform high in cases of data hiding mechanisms. Watermarking method based on quantization is-like compression-based watermarking but the only thing that differs is that this can be executed both in spatial and transform domains.

The watermarking method based on expansion was introduced as an improvement for the reversible watermarking technique. In this technique, one bit of the watermarked data is embedded to the difference in the least significant bit of two values in the pixels of the image (Cheng, Chen, & Tsai, 2013). The major disadvantages that the capacity of the hiding scheme is very much less, and the embedding capacity is also reduced.

CONCLUSION

The need for the protection of medical image is not only to ensure confidentiality and to resolve confidentiality issues but also to prevent the medical images from modification which can be done by both authorized and unauthorized users. Thus, there is a method for ensuring security in terms of all the data including medical images. Medical image encryption has been a well-known approach that ensures data and image confidentiality in medical paradigms. In this paper we have presented a detailed review of medical image encryption techniques (Table1) and discussed several information accompanying to it. Several methodologies have been proposed indifferent papers considering both in spatial and frequency domains. Also, data hiding using Region of interest and Region of non-interest (Liu, Qu, & Xin, 2016) segmentation was also present. Medical care requires best quality of image and do not accept any modification made to the images. So, the process of medical image encryption needs to be resistant against any type of attacks over the network.

From the critical survey of literature, it could be inferred that majority of the research focus for medical image encryption is based on chaotic maps. The randomness and sensitivity to initial conditions of chaotic maps makes it suitable to address the cryptographic requirements such as confusion and diffusion. However, Lower dimensional chaotic maps suffer from the limitation of low cycle lengths. High dimensional chaotic maps have larger key space, at the cost of large number of computations. Many of the chaotic algorithms for medical image encryption operate at an encryption speed of 10-50 Kbps. Standard non chaotic algorithms such as AES operate at an encryption rate of 50-200 Mbps in a 1 GHz Pentium processor.

The second limitation of chaotic maps is that they operate with floating point numbers. Manipulations of floating point numbers are not as efficient as integer operations. For instance, a 64 bit Intel processor, the clock cycles used for floating point arithmetic is 6 times more than the integer point arithmetic.

The high sensitivity to initial conditions of chaotic maps is a great asset for cryptographic applications. However, it remains as a practical weakness, when encryption and decryption are to be carried out in different computing devices. This may lead to a situation, where message encoded by one processor is not correctly decoded by a different processor. For successful implementation of chaos based cryptography, encryption and decryption are to be carried out in identical processors and in identical software implementations. Rounding algorithms used in software implementations are to be identical to avoid errors in decoding.

The above mentioned limitations have necessitated the need for enhancement of existing medical image encryption algorithms to support operating requirements in constrained environments. In the process of implementing the medical image encryption method, it is much essential to use an effective and suitable algorithm and approach. Thus, medical image evaluating expert systems to monitor the distinguishing features between the original image and encrypted image can be considered as a promising direction of research.

In this chapter, we also made a brief review on the watermarking methodologies and the need of watermarking. For the future scope, multi-level watermarking can play its roles since it extends the simple watermarking to multiple levels with different variants. Also, reversibility and security of the watermarked images can also be taken into consideration with additional steganalysis.

REFERENCES

Abdmouleh, M. K., Khalfallah, A., & Bouhlel, M. S. (2017). A Novel Selective Encryption Scheme for Medical Images Transmission based-on JPEG Compression Algorithm. *Procedia Computer Science*, *112*, 369–376. doi:10.1016/j.procs.2017.08.026

Ali, M., Ahn, C. W., & Pant, M. (2014). A robust image watermarking technique using SVD and differential evolution in the DCT domain. *Optik-Int. J. Light Electron Opt*, *125*(1), 428–434. doi:10.1016/j.ijleo.2013.06.082

Bouslimi, D., & Coatrieux, G. (2016). A crypto-watermarking system for ensuring reliability control and traceability of medical images. *Signal Processing Image Communication*, *47*, 160–169. doi:10.1016/j.image.2016.05.021

Cao, W., Zhou, Y., Philip Chen, C. L., & Xia, L. (2017). Medical image encryption using edge maps. *Signal Processing*, *132*, 96–109. doi:10.1016/j.sigpro.2016.10.003

Chakraborty, C. (2011). Mobile Telemedicine Systems for Remote Patient's Chronic Wound Monitoring. In M-Health Innovations for Patient-Centered Care. IGI Global.

Chakraborty, C. (2013). Review on Telemedicine-Based WBAN Framework for Patient 26Monitoring. *Int. Journal of Telemedicine and e-Health*, *19*(8), 619–626.

Chakraborty, C. (2019). Performance Analysis of Compression Techniques for Chronic Wound Image Transmission under Smartphone-Enabled Tele-wound Network. *Int. Journal of E-Health and Medical Communications, 10*(2), 1–15.

Chang, J. D., Chen, B. H., & Tsai, C. S. (2013). LBP-based fragile watermarking scheme for image tamper detection and recovery. *Next-Generation Electronics (ISNE), 2013 IEEE International Symposium on*, 173–176.

Chen, X., & Hu, C.-J. (2017). Adaptive medical image encryption algorithm based on multiple chaotic mapping. *Saudi Journal of Biological Sciences, 24*(8), 1821–1827. doi:10.1016/j.sjbs.2017.11.023 PMID:29551931

Dehkordi, A. B., Esfahani, S. N., & Avanaki, A. N. (2011). Robust LSB watermarking optimized for local structural similarity. *2011 19th Iranian Conference on Electrical Engineering*, 1–6.

Ghadi, M., Laouamer, L., & Moulahi, T. (2015). Enhancing digital image integrity by exploiting JPEG bitstream attributes. *Journal of Innovation in Digital Ecosystems, 2*(1-2), 20–31. doi:10.1016/j.jides.2015.10.003

Haddad, S., Coatrieux, G., Cozic, M., & Bouslimi, D. (2017). Joint watermarking and lossless JPEG-LS compression for medical image security. *Proceedings of the International Conference on Watermarking and Image Processing - ICWIP 2017*. 10.1145/3150978.3150985

Hua, Z., Yi, S., & Zhou, Y. (2018). Medical image encryption using high-speed scrambling and pixel adaptive diffusion. *Signal Processing, 144*, 134–144. doi:10.1016/j.sigpro.2017.10.004

Kanso, A., & Ghebleh, M. (2015). An efficient and robust image encryption scheme for medical applications. *Communications in Nonlinear Science and Numerical Simulation, 24*(1-3), 98–116. doi:10.1016/j.cnsns.2014.12.005

Kaur, M., & Kaur, R. (2012). Reversible watermarking of medical images: Authentication and recovery-a survey. *J. Inf. Oper. Manag, 3*, 241.

Laiphrakpam, D. S., & Khumanthem, M. S. (2017). Medical image encryption based on an improved ElGamal encryption technique. *Optik - International Journal for Light and Electron Optics, 147*, 88–102.

Lakshmi, C., Thenmozhi, K., Rayappan, J. B. B., & Amirtharajan, R. (2018). Encryption and watermark-treated medical image against hacking disease—An immune convention in spatial and frequency domains. *Computer Methods and Programs in Biomedicine, 159*, 11–21. doi:10.1016/j.cmpb.2018.02.021 PMID:29650305

Liew, S. C., & Zain, J. M. (2011). Tamper localization and lossless recovery watermarking scheme. In Software Engineering and Computer Systems. Springer. doi:10.1007/978-3-642-22170-5_48

Lima, J. B., Madeiro, F., & Sales, F. J. R. (2015). Encryption of medical images based on the cosine number transform. *Signal Processing Image Communication, 35*, 1–8. doi:10.1016/j.image.2015.03.005

Liu, Y., Qu, X., & Xin, G. (2016). An ROI-based reversible data hiding scheme in encrypted medical images. *Journal of Visual Communication and Image Representation, 39*, 51–57. doi:10.1016/j.jvcir.2016.05.008

Memon, N. A., Chaudhry, A., Ahmad, M., & Keerio, Z. A. (2011). Hybrid watermarking of medical images for ROI authentication and recovery. *International Journal of Computer Mathematics*, *88*(10), 2057–2071. doi:10.1080/00207160.2010.543677

Nematzadeh, H., Enayatifar, R., Motameni, H., Guimarães, F. G., & Coelho, V. N. (2018). Medical image encryption using a hybrid model of modified genetic algorithm and coupled map lattices. *Optics and Lasers in Engineering*, *110*, 24–32. doi:10.1016/j.optlaseng.2018.05.009

Ni, Z., Shi, Y. Q., Ansari, N., & Su, W. (2006). Reversible data hiding. *IEEE Transactions on Circuits and Systems for Video Technology*, *16*(3), 354–362. doi:10.1109/TCSVT.2006.869964

Qasim, A. F., Meziane, F., & Aspin, R. (2018). Digital watermarking: Applicability for developing trust in medical imaging workflows state of the art review. *Computer Science Review*, *27*, 45–60. doi:10.1016/j.cosrev.2017.11.003

Richardson, M. L., Frank, M. S., & Stern, E. J. (1995). Digital image manipulation: What constitutes an acceptable alteration of a radiologic image? *AJR. American Journal of Roentgenology*, *164*(1), 228–229. doi:10.2214/ajr.164.1.7998545 PMID:7998545

Wenyin, Z., & Shih, F. Y. (2011). Semi-fragile spatial watermarking based on local binary pattern operators. *Optics Communications*, *284*(16-17), 3904–3912. doi:10.1016/j.optcom.2011.04.004

Chapter 5
Smart Healthcare Monitoring System for War-End Soldiers Using CNN

Preethi S.
https://orcid.org/0000-0002-4817-9471
Dr. N. G. P. Institute of Technology, India

Prasannadevi V.
Dr. N .G. P. Institute of Technology, India

Arunadevi B.
Dr. N. G. P. Institute of Technology, India

ABSTRACT

Health monitoring plays a vital role to overcome the health issues of the patients. According to research, approximately 2000 people die due to carelessness of monitoring their health. Wearable monitoring systems record the activities of daily life. A 24-hour wearable monitoring system was developed and changes were identified. This project is designed for helping the soldiers to maintain their health conditions and to identify their health issues at war's end. Different health parameters are monitored using sensors, and the data are transmitted through GSM to the receiver, and the received data are analyzed using convolutional neural networks, which is performed in cloud IoT. If any abnormalities are found during the analyzing process, the message is sent to military personnel and the doctor at the camp so that they could take necessary actions to recover the ill soldier from the war field and provide emergency assistance on time. The location of the soldier is also shared using the input from GPS modem in the smart jacket.

DOI: 10.4018/978-1-7998-0261-7.ch005

INTRODUCTION

A well-maintained defense system has been set up in our country to protect the country from the external invasion and the internal disturbances. The three pillars of defense system are Army, Navy and Air force. Indian army is the land-based unit, while Indian Airforce deals in air defense and the Indian Navy is the naval unit. In world, our Indian army is the second largest with about 1.23 million personnel on active rolls and another 9.6 lakhs in reserves. The main responsibility of Indian army is to protect the country against land-based attacks. It also joins hands with other agencies in dealing with terrorism, tackling emergencies in the country and also rescuing people in case of natural calamities like floods, earthquake, etc.

In today's word, science and technology are growing rapidly with new inventions, innovations and with advance level of their implementations. These immerging advance technologies are firmly adopted by defense services to provide some safety systems to our soldiers. There are many parameters by which defense services can provide safety to the soldiers. The nation's security is monitored and kept by the army, navy, and air-force. Indian soldiers sacrifice their lives for their country. There are many concerns regarding the safety of the soldier. Due to lack of connectivity, Soldiers entering the enemy lines often lose their lives, it is very important for the army base station to known the location as well as the health status of all soldiers. A leak of proper health backup and connectivity between the soldiers on the war-fields and the officials at the army base stations, many soldiers lost in war fields. All must be concerned about the safety of the soldiers, so decided to build a project which will efficiently keep a check on the health status of the soldier, and his precise location to equip him with necessary medical treatments as soon as possible. A soldier's tracking is done by using GPS and Wi-Fi module, which is used to provide a wireless communication system. IoT based healthcare project help the people to check their historical health data. Here, the monitoring various parameters of the patient will be done using the Internet of Things. Theperiod parameters of the patient's health are sent to cloud exploitation net property. And these parameters were sent to a remote internet location so that the user can view the details from anywhere in the world (Rejab, Nouira & Trabelsi, 2012). In IoT based systems, the details of patient health can be seen by many users. The IoT patient monitoring system has three sensors; temperature sensor, heartbeat sensor, and humidity sensor. This project is very useful since the doctor can monitor the patient just by visiting the website or URL. The Arduino UNO board continuously reads the input from the above sensors. Then it sends these data to the cloud by sending it to a particular URL/IP address.

In (Amor & James, 2015), structural health monitoring, physical or mathematical model are useful for analysis, thus in real-time applications, some type of nonlinearities was performed that lead to expensive model. In this case, the Convolution Neural Networks (CNN) has become popular in real-world applications as it uses the concept of deep learning (Xna & Lee, 2013). CNN is used in areas such as computer vision, speech recognition, biomedical system, and language processing. A a wearable monitoring system records the activities of daily life. A twenty-four-hour a wearable and ambient monitoring system was developed and the opportunities and changes were identified (Shhelhamer, Long & Darrell, 2017). The sensing nodes and a wireless device were replaced to implement the object detection system, visual object identification and tracking along with the exclusive of thousands of meters of electric cable were developed using a wireless sensing network. In the field of healthcare monitoring operation and home security approaches the potential of object detection is done by using the camera-based network, hence by using a camera as a sensing element. Most of the health care systems were based on the Electronic

Medical Record (EMR) which gives the collection of longitudinal data according to patient health. It significantly increases the clinical data and impact discovering new disease patterns and also provides personalized patient care by processing quantities of data automatically. It is becoming challenge.

Real-time health care monitoring system allows the mobile patients to receive the health conditions anytime and anywhere, by the development of a wearable sensing device which is more comfortable (Amor, Hattersley, barber & James, 2015). Recently in a wearable sensing device, the concept of coupling capacitance develops the skin-electrode interface impedance and the non-contact electrodes. The patients are strongly motivated by the use of a wearable monitors to perform predictive monitoring. The cost of a wireless sensor network is low and contains short deployment time with typically higher number of sensors over a limited bandwidth and unreliable connection. The data rates of A wireless Sensor Network (WSN) are higher than the conventional WSN (Gomez, 2016). In WSN, the SHM sensors are being used at various locations throughout a structure. Thus, the sensor collects information and forwards it as a packet. The sensors are to be installed at various locations in order to correctly capture the response and the data are collected at an adequate period. The objective of this system is to provide the early warning about the health condition that is to be taken into account in order to improve the patient's outcomes; it reduces the workload of clinicians and health care workers. The proposed system consists of various sensors connected to a mini computer and then the data is transferred through cloud platform to the military unit at the base station. In the military base station, the databases are created using a convolutional neural network. This network is created with high precision such that the network will be able to communicate a correct solution to the commander and the doctor at the military unit.

LITERATURE SURVEY

The innovative ideas and concepts which helped for the proposal of this Healthcare Monitoring were taken from the following papers and journals. This has helped in gaining information regarding the works and procedures of the existing systems. Encapsulating the advantages and disadvantages of various existing systems henceforth helped in modifying the project.

Wireless Sensor Networks (WSN)

Sensing module which is mainly composed of heart sound sensor and control module realizes raw data collection and the transmission of heart sound signals (Ren, Jin, Chen, Ghayyat & Chen, 2018). The signal is transmitted to an Android phone via Bluetooth 4.0 module Figure 1. Compared with other-wireless technologies, like Zigbee and Wi-Fi, Bluetooth 4.0 has many advantages. The most appealing features are low energy and fairly simple to use. Unlike Wi-Fi which is more complex and requires configuration of software and hardware, Bluetooth can be used to connect multi-peripheral devices at a time. As for the data transfer speed, Bluetooth 4.0 is enough for the transfer of physiological signals. Although the mesh network of Zigbee allows devices to work in the complex system, Zigbee does not support by Android or iOS.

The data acquisition module is controlled by the CC2540 unit, which contains a CC2540 system-on-chip, an external antenna, and other auxiliary components. In this system, the sensing module acts as the peripheral station and the local home gateway as the central station. The local home gateway

Figure 1.

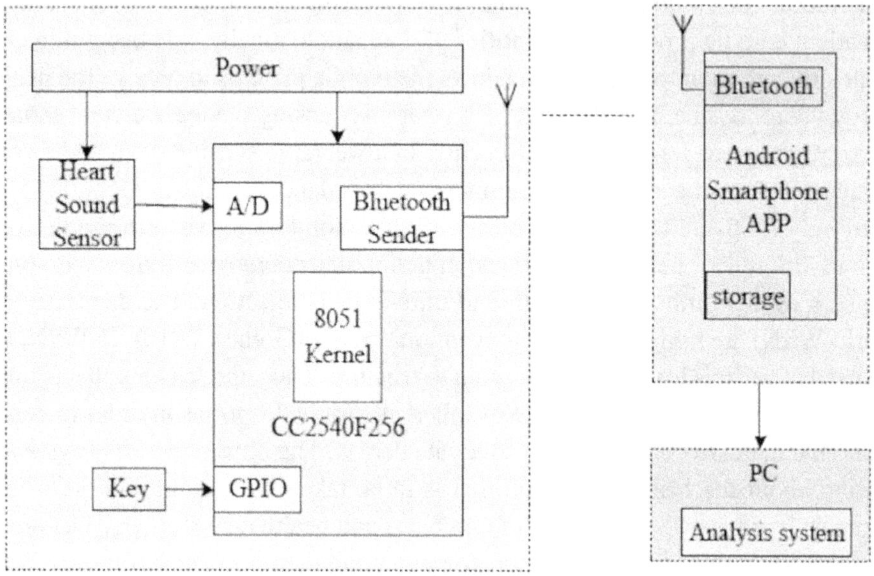

system takes the role of Generic Attribute Profile server and executes the service which contains seven Characteristics. The system uses the seventh characteristic CHAR7 to complete the data transmission, which is a periodic notification mode. When the server data changes, the client obtains CHAR7 notification instead of reading the data. According to the CC2540 transmission format, the length of the payload is 20-byte. Therefore, the heart sound should be collected for ten times, and then transmit them to a Smartphone through the notification of CHAR7. The signal transmission quality in different communication range was tested. The results showed that the PLR was zero when the communication range is less than 10 meters.

Structure Healthcare Monitoring

In WSNs for Structure Healthcare Monitoring (SHM) sensors area unit deployed at numerous sensors collect data regarding their close like acceleration, close vibration, load and stress at sampling frequencies upwards of a hundred rate (Noel & Abdaoui, 2017). Hence, the sensing and sampling rates and the quantity of collected information area unit abundant more than those in alternative applications in WSNs; and as a result, WSNs for SHM introduces challenges in network design. Sensor nodes transmit the detected information to the sink either directly or by forwarding every other's packets, Data aggregation and processing is necessary for the detection and localization of structural damage and can occur in different locations depending on the network topology. Typically, harm detection needs the comparison of the structure's gift modal options to those related to the structure's unmutilated state. Modal options of a structure area unit in the main portrayed by the mode shapes – the natural vibration pattern for a given structure. A diagram outlining the process of SHM using WSNs is displayed in Figure 2. The base station then processes the info and chooses the structure's overall health. This system is one of the largest WSN-based SHM systems to date with a total of 64 sensor nodes deployed on the bridge. The sensors

Figure 2.

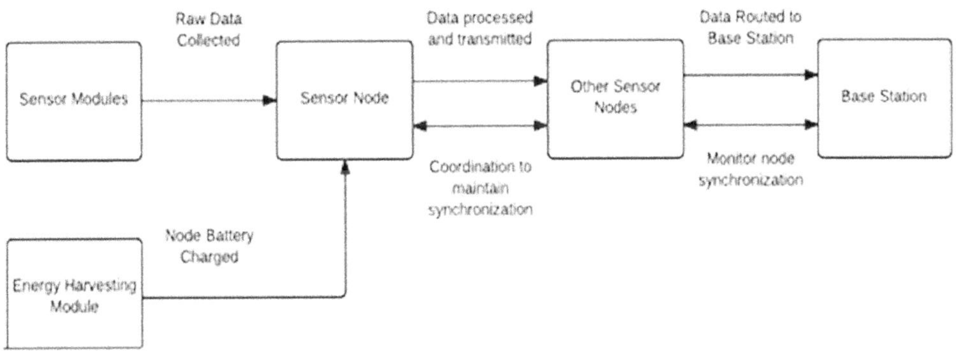

during this network collect close acceleration knowledge and use the quick Fourier rework (FFT) and also the resultant Power Spectral Density (PSD) to see the structure's mode form. This focuses more on the telecommunications component of WSNs for SHM than existing surveys.

Vital Signs Compression and Energy Efficient

A High-level description of the system is illustrated in Figure3,where it consists of the following three major sub-systems/components:

- **Edge Network**: multiple users equipped with PDAs to acquire vital signs using a wearable device (Said, Mohamed, Elfouly & Dennis, 2018). The PDA handles communication with the wearable device, collects, pre-processes and transmits data to the MHC sub-system via the network infrastructure. Pre-processing consists of a compression algorithm that maps the original data to another representation. We propose to use a multiple modalities deep learning compression approach that exploits the availability of multiple modality data and captures the inter-modality correlations to provide an adaptive compression technique. Specifically, here propose SAE-based compression schemes that compress acquired medical data before the transmission to the MHC taking into consideration the network's state and application-level Quality of Service (QoS).
- **Network Infrastructure**: it allows the PDA to communicate with the MHC subsystem. The PDA is battery operated; thus, optimizing its transmission energy is essential. In this work, we formulate an optimization problem for multiple users to minimize energy consumption. We minimize a cost function that models the energy consumed by the different entities in the system, and their allocated resources based on the wireless channel state of each user. Furthermore, our model allows selecting an appropriate compression configuration given the current network dynamics.
- **mHealth Cloud (MHC):** a medical server that receives the compressed data from patients, decompresses and stores them for further analysis by the medical staff.

Figure 3.

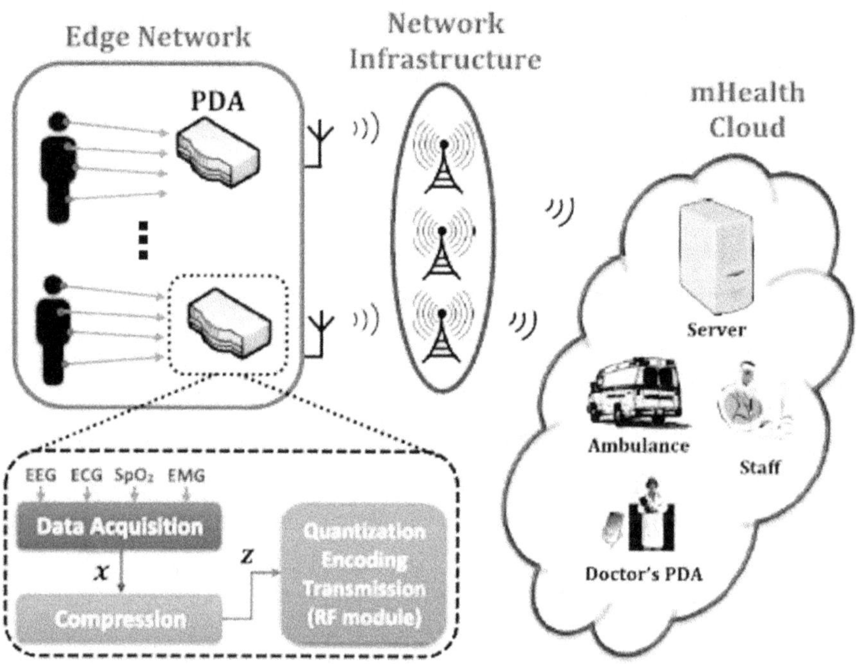

Security Monitoring System via a Wireless Sensing Network

A wireless visual sensing network integrates a variety of camera to gather time-series eventualities, characterize, and establish intrusion targets (Zhu, Bojian, Li, Gu & Yang, 2018). Thereby, corresponding defense actions will be taken in a timely mane. In this study, we tend to so concentrate on the event of security observance system supported image process approaches, through that we will acquire some universal ways to hold out a surveillance system. A a wireless camera sensing network is intended and engineered up in our system. The hardware frame diagram of the security monitoring system is shown in Figure 4. A variety of eventualities similarly as their location data area unit collected from the camera nodes. As such, the AMN14112 camera detector, which is ready to sleuth objects among a spread of 10m, is deployed within the network. Each sensing node is difficult wired to a communication unit at intervals a predefined space. For the aim of communication, the Wi-Fi-based a wireless transmission modules area unit used. which exchanges information based on a wireless sensor networks. Thewireless routers are applied to transmitting the sensing signals from the sensors due to its cost-effectiveness in long-distance utilization. Therefore, the main function of the WIFI network is for delivering captured images from the cameras to the host computer via cooperation.

Figure 4.

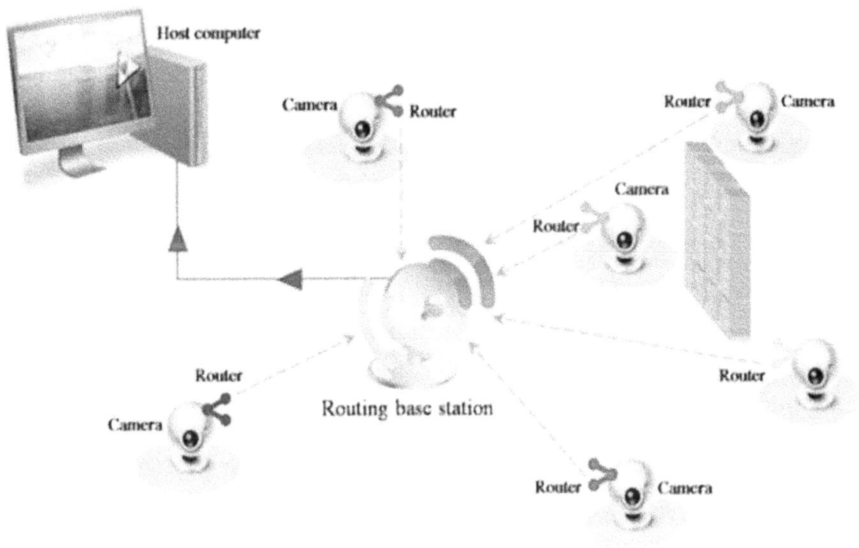

Wearable Health Devices

Wearable Health Devices (WHDs) are an emerging technology that enables continuous ambulatory monitoring of human vital signs during daily life (during work, at home, during sports activities, etc,.) are in a clinical environment, with the advantage of minimizing discomfort and interference with normal human activities (Ou & Li, 2010). WHDs are part of personal health systems, a concept introduced to place the individual citizen in the center of healthcare delivery process, managing its health and interacting with care providers a concept that is commonly referred to as "patient empowerment". These devices created synergy between multiple science domains such as biomedical technologies, micro, and nanotechnologies, materials engineering, electronic engineering and information and communication technologies. In (Olivero, Tosi & Perrone, 2018), we use of WHDs allows the ambulatory acquisition of vital signs and health status monitoring over extended periods and outside clinical environments. This feature allows acquiring vital data during different daily activities, ensuring better support in medical diagnosis and helping in better and faster recovery from medical intervention or bodily injury. WHDs are also very useful in support activities/fitness to monitor athlete's performance or even in first responders or military personnel to evaluate and monitor their body response in different hazardous situations and to better manage their effort and occupational health. These devices can be for both medical and /or activities/fitness/wellness purposes, always targeting the human body monitoring. In (Hao, 2015), Taking this into an account, the best terminology is "health", leading to WHDs. WHDs denomination can be more specifically referring to which areas they are applied to. Independently of WHDs purpose, there are four main requirements on their design: low power consumption, reliability and security, comfort, and ergonomics. Accordingly, the wearable devices market is currently having worldwide revenue of around $26 billion and is expected to reach almost $34 billion in 2019. Regarding healthcare and medical environments, it is expected to grow almost to $15 billion worldwide value in 2019. A wearable device is now at the heart of just about every discussion related to the Internet of Things (IoT), and the full range of new capabilities pervasive connectivity can bring (Shaladi, Alatshan & Yang, 2015). In this perspective, the design and development of A wearablehealth-Monitoring Systems (WHMS) have received lots of attention from the scientific community and industry during the last years. These low-cost systems are made up of various small physiological sensors, transmission modules, and processors. As a result, they are well-suited to a wearable and unobtrusive mental and physical health status monitoring solutions and do not impose limits on time or location. Even though independent sensor information is conducive to revealing the working state of the system to some extent, a comprehensive multi-parameter sensing model is more effective for analysis and evaluation of potential operational risks. To the best of our knowledge, multi-sensor fusion is one of the most suitable technologies to use when dealing with data from disparate sources (Saxena & Saad, 2017). Since the last decade, an aging population and the emergence of chronic diseases lead to a bigger interest in a wearable physiological measurement device. The effort in these developments is resulting in a small wearable device, with the benefits of a lower cost and higher mobility while the data is being collected. The different wearable devices that could be used for health monitoring are listed below in Table 1.

Wrist Wearable Unit (WWU)

WWU is being developed as a part of USEFIL (Unobtrusive Smart Environments for Independent Living) system (WHO, 2012). The requirements for the WWU in the USEFIL system are 1. gather data on the PA (physical activity) of the user, 2. communicate automatically with the USEFIL system 3. Customized

Table 1. Different Wearable Devices: Properties, Capabilities & Application

Type	Properties	Capabilities	Application
Smart Watches	1.Low operating power 2.User-friendly interface	1.Payment 2.Communication	1.Education 2.Business, Administration
Smart eyewear	1.Sends sound directly to the ear 2.Controlled by touching the screen, voice command, etc.,	1.Visualization. 2.Task coordination 3.Language Interpretation	1.Surgery 2.Logistics 3.Infotainment
Fitness Tracker	1.High accuracy 2.Waterproof 3.Lightweight 4. A wireless communication.	1.Physiological wellness. 2.Navigation 3.Heart rate monitor	1.Fitness 2.Health care 3. Professional sport 4.Outdoor/Indoor sport
Smart Clothing	1.Data are obtained by body sensors and actuators 2.No visual interaction with the user via display/screen	1.Heart rate, Daily activities, temperature and body position tracking 2.Heating/cooling the body automatic payment	1.Medicine 2.Military 3.Logistics 4.Professional sport-fitness
Wearable Camera	1.Smaller dimensions. 2.Night vision	1.Live streaming 2.Fitness/Activity tracking	1.Defense 2.Fitness 3.Industry 4.Education
wearable medical devices	1.Pain management 2.Physiological tracking 3.Glucose monitoring 4.Sleep monitoring 5.Brain Activity monitoring	1.Dermatology 2.Rehabilitation 3.NeuroScience 4.Chronic diseases: diabetes 5.Surgery 6.Cardiovascular diseases	1.Fitness 2.Cardiovascular medicine 3.Surgery 4.Oncology 5.Dermatology 6.Respirology

algorithm for data processing (Humphereys, 2012). An analysis of the market reveals that for the health and activity monitoring area, there is a lot number of devices available. They fall into three categories; sensor platforms, health and lifestyle devices, and smart-watches. Of these, the key criteria for USEFIL are smartwatches. Sensor platforms, such as the Altigraph typically do not have the communication or algorithmic flexibility required and health and lifestyle devices, such as the Fitbit are typically locked to proprietary algorithms and data interfaces. To meet the system requirements, an off-the-shelf Android-based smart-watch, the Android Z1 was invented.

The Z1 weighs 160 g and the dimensions of the device are 64 mm × 42 mm × 14.5 mm, with a 50.8 mm capacitive touch screen of 320 × 240-pixel resolution. The base chip is a MT6516 which runs a 416 MHz processor with 256 MB RAM and 8 GB internal memory. The Z1 has full Bluetooth, WIFI and GSM connectivity's as well as GPS and accelerometer sensors. The accelerometer is tri-axis with a range of ± 2 g. The device is limited by its 800 mAh battery, which lets the device record data from the accelerometer of the device, continuously, for ~5 h. The USEFIL system provides several services and applications to assist independent living. One key service is a high-level decision support system (DSS) that will combine the sensor inputs of the USEFIL system and provide suggestions that benefit the healthcare of the user. The WWU acts as a key sensor in this part of the system and provides information on the PA of the user. The WWU pulls data from the accelerometers and runs a suite of algorithms on the data to extract the activity parameters. These parameters are sent back into the USEFIL system through the WWUs Wi-Fi connection and integrated into the USEFIL System DSS. As PA is related to the health of the person, assessing PA levels continuously is essential to recognize the change in health status (Prince, Adamo, Hamel, Hardt, Gorber & Treemblay, 2008). Also, to meet the amount of moderate and vigorous PA for older adults, recommended by the World Health Organization (WHO) (2013), a quantitative or direct measure for activity level is preferred in comparison to self-reported measures (Murphy, 2009). Accelerometers are widely used to monitor PA and the general considerations for choosing an accelerometer for use in studies with older adults given by Murphy (Najafi, Aminian, Loew, Blanc, & Robert, 2002) include the lifestyle PA and step count. Although, the placement of accelerometers is usually chosen based on the application, for example, whole-body movements (chest, sternum, underarm or waist), leg movement (shin, ankle) and Parkinsonian tremor (wrist), for long-term unobtrusive monitoring, as in USEFIL, a simple system using only one sensor attached to the wrist is generally preferred, especially for older people (Nangalia, Prytherch & Smith, 2010). This was reflected in the responses obtained in early focus groups – potential users had a definite preference towards the wrist-mounted devices. PA monitoring to extract various PA parameters using accelerometers is an active area of research. Previous research on activity levels has shown that, as activity intensity increases, the root-mean-square (RMS) of the acceleration signal increases, meaning that the use of RMS score for a measure of activity is valid (Amor, 2011). In (Easton, Philip & Aleksandravicius, 2013), it is shown that the vector magnitude of the tri-axis accelerometers correlates with calorific energy expenditure for a range of activities. In research, Step counts are mostly used to relate activity to the health state, promote a healthy lifestyle (Bravata, Sundaram & Gienger, 2007) and also to show that PA can affect health outcomes, particularly in chronic conditions (Leidy, Kimel, Ajagbe, Kim, Hamilton, & Becker, 2014). Some step count detection algorithms include Pan and Tompkins (1985), originally designed to detect QRS complexes, but more recently applied to step count (Ying, Schintzer, Leonhardt & Schiek, 2007), a peak detection method based on combined dual-axial signals (x and z axes) (Ying, Schintzer, Leonhardt & Schiek, 2007), threshold-based peak detectionand template matching. As mentioned previously, the WWU gathers data from its accelerometers and uses this to perform activity monitoring. In a system such as USEFIL, activity level information combined with step counts can be used to determine activity patterns and daily rhythms. Furthermore, through the detection of PA, it is possible to extrapolate patterns in behavior, such as sleep-wake cycles, which act as key indicators to health status. For example, a person who is ill might spend longer in bed.

Smart Watch

These are computerized devices intended to be worn on the wrist, and the functionality has been expanded which is often related to communication. Most of these models are based on mobile operating systems. Smartwatches can now be used to capture and analyze hand gestures, with the addition of reliable, sensitive inertial sensors on them.

Smart Eyewear

These are used for various applications in Optical Head-Mounted Displays (OHMDs), Heads-Up Displays (HUDs), Virtual Reality(VR). The displays can be monocular or binocular.

Fitness Tracker

It is also known as activity trackers, that are designed to monitor and track outdoor sports activities and measures the fitness-related metrics. These trackers provide health empowerment for users and their adoption can encourage overweight children to exercise more

Smart Clothing

These include a broad list of a wearables, ranging from sportswear and consumers sports apparel, military apparel, and e-textiles. It consists of a range of articles, although it is typically in the form of shirts, socks, yoga pants with secret cameras, helmets, and caps with a wide range of sensors and features. Smart Clothing has the potential to exceed the benefits for firefighters, at construction sites, and for transportation.

Wearable Camera

These wearable cameras have attracted significant interest from consumers. They are well-suited for making first-person videos and photos in a period. It is used to detect and monitor ecological environments.

IoT in Health Monitoring System

Advances in the information and communication technologies have led to the emergence of the Internet of Things (IoT). IoT allows many physical devices to capture transmit data, through the internet, providing more data interoperability methods (Ahanathapillai, Amor, Goodwin & James, 2015). Nowadays IoT plays an important role not only in communication but also in monitoring, recording, storage, and display. Hence the latest trend in the Healthcare communication method using IoT is adapted. Monitored continually, aggregated and effectively analyzed - such information can bring about a massive positive transformation in the field of healthcare. Our matter of concern in this project is to focus on the development and implementation of an effective healthcare monitoring system based on IoT. The proposed system monitors the vital health parameters and transmits the data through a wireless communication, which is further transferred to a network via a Wi-Fi module. The data can be accessed anytime promoting the reception of the current status of the patient. In case any abnormal behavior or any vital signs are recognized, the caretaker, as well as the doctors,are notified immediately through a message service or an audio signaling device (buzzer). To design an efficient remote monitoring system, security plays an important part. Cloud computing and password protected. The Wi-Fi module handles authentication, privacy, and security of patient details by allowing restricted access to the database. Health is an important factor of human life. The health problems should be first diagnosed and then prevented. In traditional approach the healthcare professionals should be on-site to monitor medical parameters of a patient all the time and patient remains admitted in a hospital, wired to biomedical instruments. A new modern healthcare monitoring system introduces a wireless body sensor to monitor their medical parameters at any time in an economic and patient-friendly manner. An IoT method is adapted to access the medical parameters of a patient in a local and remote area. The body sensor network system helps the people by providing a healthcare services such as medical data access and communication with healthcare providers in emergencies through SMS or GPRS.

To move forward, embedding modern Information and Communication Technologies (ICT) in the healthcare system is expected to deliver more effective and efficient healthcare service to patients with chronic disease and the elderly (Saxena & Saad, 2017). In the meantime, several phenomena have been risen, such as Ambient Assisted Living (AAL), ubiquitous healthcare, and IoT for healthcare. Such terms all with each other, while all are co-related. IoT emphasizes the interconnection of all physical and digital items including sensors, smart devices, cyber sensors, and so much more, which allows the automatic and efficient data transmission and shared over the internet. Hence, empowering the utility of IoT in healthcare, with interconnected medial sensors, especially a wearable or implantable, is considered to be able to provide smart accurate and cost-effective personalized healthcare service. The Internet of Things is helping healthcare providers offer new services and solutions through remote health condition monitoring (Jang, 2010). Not to mention, collecting data in real-time helps improve operational efficiency for organizations throughout the healthcare industry:

- Real-time data can be accessed by the Healthcare providers frequently, giving them better visibility into patient health and allowing them to provide timely support and treatment.
- Physicians can monitor the status of a patient's health by allowing them to return home to finish treatment while medical staff continues to monitor their condition remotely.
- In-home services are expanded by the Healthcare companiesusing remote condition monitoring to offer new independent living solutions designed for aging and disabled populations.
- Hence the system provides quality healthcare to all. This paper provides a new novel system for Healthcare Monitoring using IoT.

Hence with the help of various papers and journals, controlling steps for the health monitoring system and the usage of various sensors were inferred.

Classifiers for Smart Health Monitoring

Different types of algorithms and wearable devices are used for smart health care monitoring system implementation.

Decision Tree Algorithm

Decision trees can be visualized as an explicit representation of decisions and decision making. This algorithm could be used for both regression and classifier. When the feature importance is clear, then the relations can be viewed very clearly and this type of decision tree could be used for classification. In a particular group, the mean of the training data sets is considered to be the prediction for that group.

Classification = sum(pk*(pk-1))

where the pk is the proportion of the same inputs present in a particular group. The decision trees lag in overfitting problems. Such trees grow uncontrollably and thus setting a limit for the growth of the tree is a must.

Logistic Model Trees

A Logistic model tree is a good fit example of a supervised learning algorithm. It is a combination of logistic regression and decision tree algorithm. The difference between an ordinary regression tree and the logistic model tree is that the ordinary regression tree will generate a piecewise-constant model whereas the logistic model tree will provide a piecewise linear regression model. In the logistic variant uses the LogitBoost algorithm is used to produce a logistic regression model at every node. The number of iterations in the logistic algorithm is calculated using cross-validation where this facilitates not to overfit the training data.

Random Forest Model

The random forest classifier is a collection of a large number of individual decision trees where the individual trees represent a particular class prediction. The class with a greater number of votes gets the highest priority and could be chosen as the best prediction model. The random forest takes advantage of the sensitivity of the decision trees on which the data is trained on. It allows each tree to randomly sample from the dataset with replacement resulting in different trees.

Meta-Learning

Meta-Learning is a machine learning algorithm thatis trained by large data sets and tested on their ability to learn new tasks. In this process, there are two important terms, the learner which learns the task and the meta-learner which trains the learner. This algorithm plays a vital role in computing several classifiers by implementing the methodology of learning programsto a collection of independent and inherently distributed databases in parallel computation.

Table 2. Comparison of Different Classifiers Performance

Algorithm	Recall	Precision	F- Measure	False alarm Rate
Decision tree algorithm	0.915	0.917	0.910	0.076
Logistic Model Trees	0.906	0.9416	0.920	0.065
Random Forest Model	0.930	0.957	0.942	0.038
Meta-learning	0.9185	0.9314	0.938	0.041
Support Vector Machine	0.925	0.914	0.932	0.042

Support Vector Machine

Support Vector Machine is one of the supervised approaches that learns about the classes from the dataset for classification.SVM divides the data into two classes by projecting the data into higher dimensions. For a patient's data set, there are so many different parameters available like pulse, cholesterol levels, heartbeat rate, temperature, and blood pressure. The SVM prepares the higher dimension characteristics for these measures and divides the data into different classes after identifying the hyperplane. This gives higher reliability in the process of classification such that the data is segmented into a correct form.

The overall performance analysis of these classifier algorithms on the smart health monitoring system is overviewed in the below table 2.

From Table 2, the classifier performance of each classifier is analyzed using the parameters recall, precision, f measure, andfalse alarm rate. From the analysis, it is inferred that the Random forest model has the highestprecision and lowest false alarm rate. Furthermore, a detailed study of the above has helped in overcoming the demerits of the existing system and work for more efficient algorithms.

PROCESS DESCRIPTION

Considering the users and application scenarios, the monitoring system should be portable and simplifies the control of the application. This system includes different types of sensors along with the function of feedback. Thus, the collected data's are uploaded to a cloud platform for further analysis. This cloud platform integrates the data's processing and thus the doctors can get accessed to the cloud platform to get the dataset and the results via the peripheral devices. Moreover, the users can be able to obtain the diagnosed results, and the system realizes the telemedicine eventually.The concept of physiological measurement systems has been a mounting research attention in the last decades, due to the few applications in medicine, sports and security with the growth in the population, as well as the emergence of diseases, there has been a necessity to monitor and analyze the health status of the individuals to avoid the fatal conditions. The wireless health monitoring is encouraged to boost the quality of lifespan. Moreover, unnecessary hospitalization can be avoided, that is used to reduce the cost and increases the quality of care. The total proposed process is explained in the below Figure 5.

- The Health care Monitoring System proposes a novel Smart Jacket for high-quality remote monitoring of military personnel using A wirelessBody Sensor Network.

- The module consists of a body area sensor network that monitors the soldier's health condition continuously and the data is transmitted over a a wireless network to the base military unit.
- In the base military unit, the cloud server consists of the health database collected from the various soldiers (nearly 1000) and trained by the Convolutional Neural Network. This network will test the incoming data and give a result whether the soldier is at risk or normal condition in all aspects.
- If the soldier is found to be under risk the emergency messages are sent to the captain of the camp, and the doctor at the camp along with the position details of the soldier. This will help them to reach the soldier at risk in a short time with proper first aid and medications

HARDWARE DESCRIPTION IN SOLDIER UNIT

A clear view of the hardware requirements of the project is crucial to understand its commissioning and working. The chapter takes a deep analysis of the hardware needing our understanding.

Arduino UNO

The Arduino UNO is a Microchip ATmega328P microcontroller equipped with sets of digital and analog I/O Pins to interface various sensors at a time and process the data. It consists of 14 digital and 6 analog pins that can be used for different operations like pinmode(), digitalwrite(), and digitalread(). These pins are used to interface the different sensors like temperature sensor, heartbeat & pulse rate sensor, ECG sensor, GPS module. The serial In and Serial Out pins are used for serial In/Out operations. The GSM module is connected to this serial Out pin in which the Micro SD Sim Card is inserted for data communication.Figure 6 and Figure 7 depicts the Arduino UNO board and its pin configuration.

Figure 5.

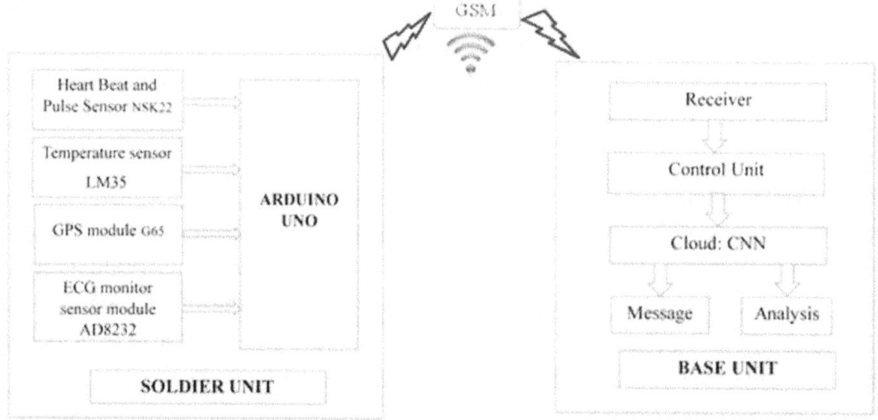

Figure 6.

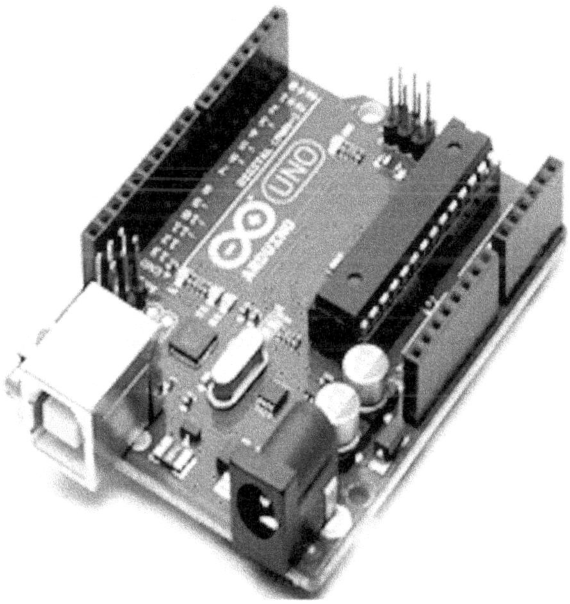

Figure 7.

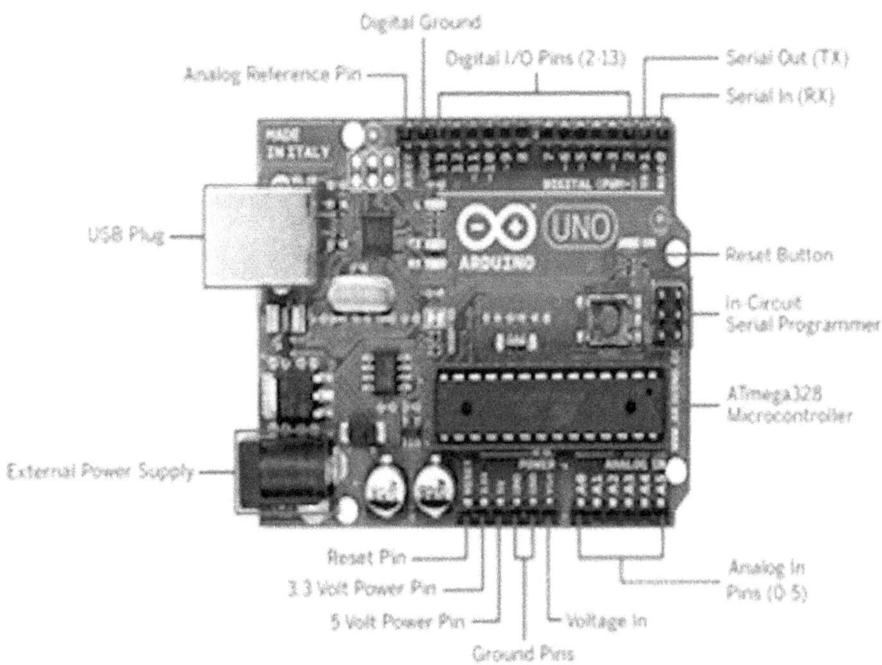

Temperature Sensor LM35

Body temperature is the outcome of the balance between heat loss and heat production in the body. It is divided into two measures; Core Temperature (CT) and Skin Temperature. The skin temperature varies with a wider range than the core temperature. The skin temperature is affected by blood circulation and is related to HR and metabolic rate. The temperature sensor is a thermocouple, made from two dissimilar metals that produce an electrical voltage in direct propagation to change in temperature.

LM35 is a precision IC temperature sensor, used to measure the hotness and coldness of an object. It produces an electrical output (10mv/degree Celsius) proportional to the temperature of the object and is calibrated in degree Celsius. It is a three-terminal device.

Figure 8 refers to a temperature sensor; the circuit will read the temperature of the surrounding environment and relay the temperature to us back in degrees Celsius. The IC will be used to measure the temperature is the LM35 IC. We will integrate this with the Arduino UNO to measure the temperature. The IC has just 3 pins, 2 for the power supply and one for the Analog output. The Analog output is provided by the output pin VOUT that is linearly proportional to the Celsius (Centigrade) temperature. Pin 2 gives an output of 1 millivolt per 0.1°C (10mV per degree).So, to get the degree value in Celsius, all that must be done is to take the voltage output and divide it by 10- this gives out the value degrees in Celsius. Figure 9 gives a description of the working flow of the Temperature sensor when it is interfaced with the Arduino board.

Figure 8.

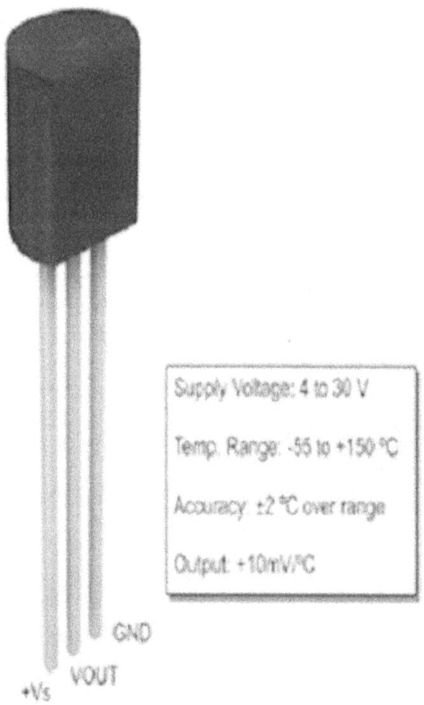

Figure 9.

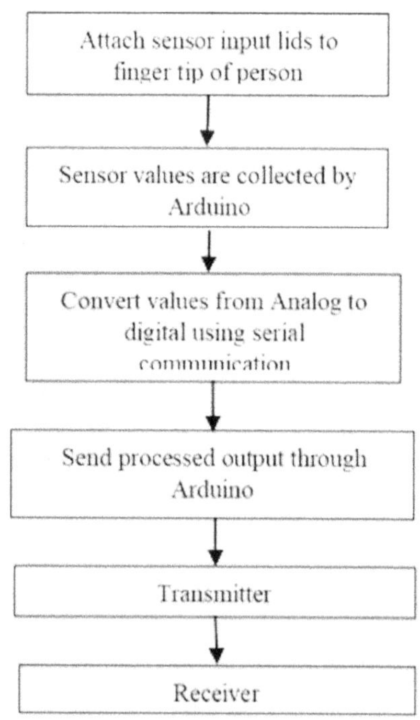

GPS-G65 Method of Operation

The GPS module is used to find out the position and location of the patient using the latitude and longitude received. Then it sends this location to the cloud using the Wi-Fi module. So that the doctors can find out the position of the patient in a case to take some preventive action. A GPS device can receive the information from GPS satellites. Then the geographical position uses to calculate.

Trendily, remote monitoring systems have involved responding to the needs in the healthcare sector, which is an important pillar. The smart system is proposed to monitor a patient's current health condition based on the widely spread technology such as GSM and GPS. The objective of the paper is to provide an effective system model that will track, trace and monitor patient reading to provide major medical service. By using the sensor, the data's will be captured and compared with the threshold. A GPS receiver device receives information from the GPS satellite and calculates the geographical location. It can analyze the location and time information in all temperature conditions on the earth. Figure 10 refers to a GPS-G65 Module and its specification, it might seem that three sphere surfaces would be enough to solve for a position since space has three dimensions. However, a fourth condition is needed for two reasons. One has to do with position and the other is to correct the GPS receiver clock. Figure 11 shows the working flow of GPS. Check whether the GPS is turn On, if not turn on the GPS. Once the GPS is on it starts tracking the position of the soldiers according to the latitude and longitude of the earth field. The latitude and the longitude of the soldier are calculated accordingly and send these degrees to the Google server. The controller collects all the data (location address of the corresponding soldier) and transmits it to the receiver in the military unit.

Heartbeat Sensor NSK 22

Monitoring the heart rate of a person is more essential in the case of the war end soldiers. The principle behind the working of the heartbeat sensor is Photoplethysmograph. This principle states that the variations in the volume of blood flowing in the body could be measured by measuring the intensity variation of the light passing through it. By measuring the variations in the blood flow, one can calculate the heartbeat rate and the pulse rate of the person.The outlook of the heartbeat sensor is shown in Figure 12. The components of a heartbeat sensor are a light-emitting diode and detectors like a photodiode or light detecting resistor.Here the light is being illuminated inside the tissue and when the light hits the blood it is either absorbed or reflected. This reflected backlight is absorbed by the Light detecting

Figure 10.

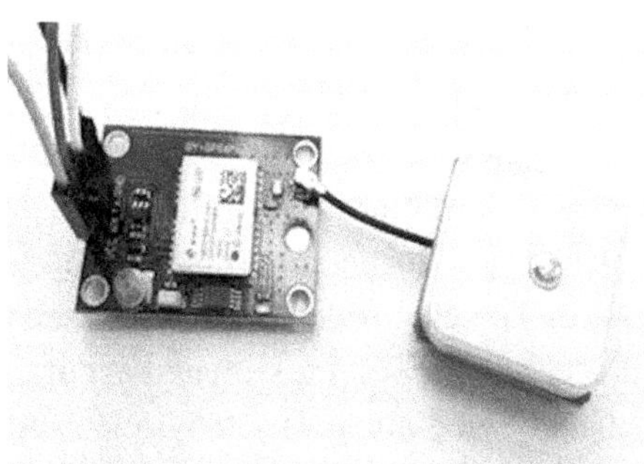

Voltage	3.7 VDC
Work current	<30 mA
GPS Accuracy	5-15m
GPS Accuracy	About 100m
Dimension	87(L)x41.6(W)x12H
GPS Frequency	1575 MHZ

Figure 11.

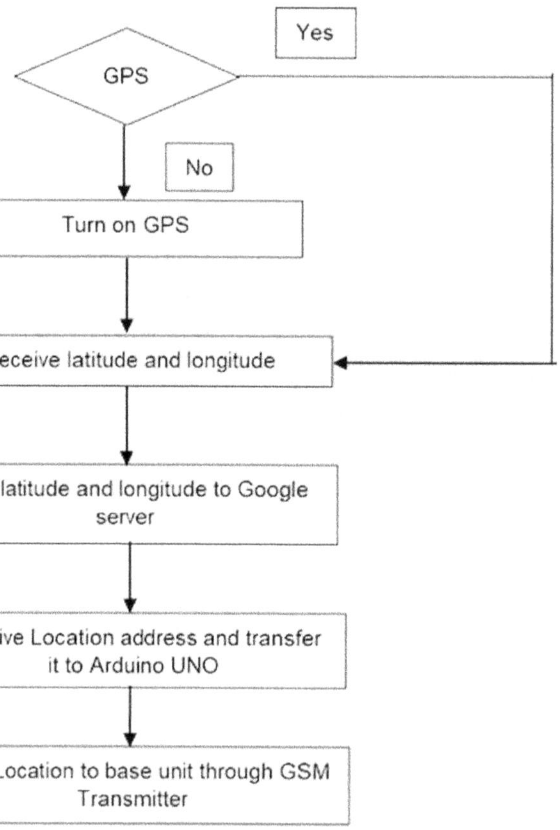

resistor and measured. This measured value is subjected to some calculations to find the exact heart rate and the pulse rate.Depending on the density of the tissue it absorbs the light inside and reflects the remaining.Figure 13 shows how the finger should be inserted inside the sensor for proper measurement of heartbeat and pulse rate.

ECG – AD8232 Monitor Sensor Module

The ECG Module transmits ASCII based control commands i.e. the UART module to the ECG Instrument. The ECG is implemented as a finite state machine. The ECG module is used to receive, check, extract and store the ECG lead data from incoming ECG datagram packet. Each packet contains one sample of each selected ECG leads. The ECG lead data memory is used to store the ECG values from a module. The data memory is split into 2 main sections with every section containing eight memory modules. Each memory module stores 250 ECG samples. The memory section areas used especially by the ECG lead data memory. ECG records the electrical activity is generated by the heart muscle depolarization; it propagates in electrical waves in the skin.The electrodes of the ECG sensor will conversion heart-beat to an electric signal. ECG Sensors are very lightweight, slim and accurately measure continuous heartbeat and give rate data of heartbeat. This device always uses by a trained doctor and

Figure 12.

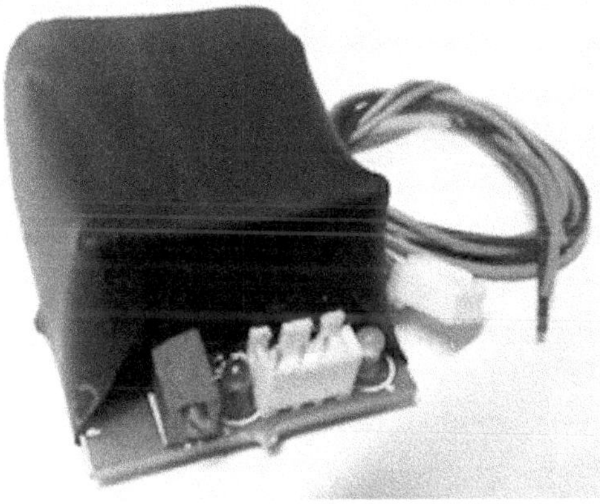

Figure 13.

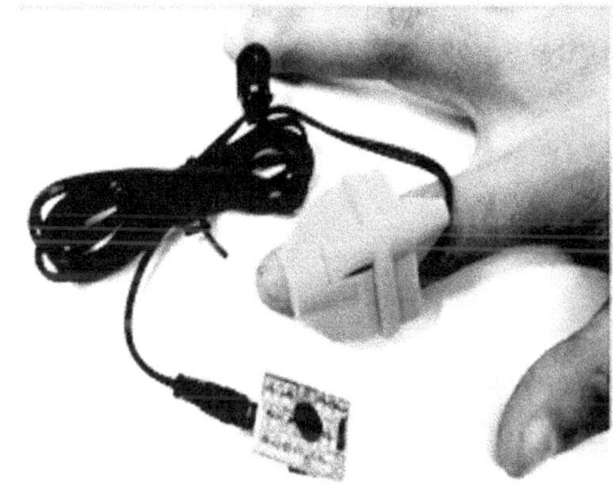

medical assistance. In Figure 14 Electrodes of ECG Sensor have 3 pins and connected by cable with 30 inches in length. It is making the ECG sensor easy to connect with the controller and placed at the wrist or pocket. The AD8232 module breaks out nine connections from the IC that you can solder pins, wires, or other connectors to SDN, LO+, LO-, Output, 3.3V, GND provide essential pins for interfacing this sensor with an Arduino. This ECG Sensor kit provides a 3 set pin which could be fixed in 3 different positions such as RA (Right Arm), LA (Left Arm), and RL (Right Leg) and measure accurate variations in the heart functioning. ECG sensor kit provides,an LED indicator light that will pulsate to the rhythm of a heartbeat. Figure 15 above the display of standard one cycle ECG signal from a heart-beat. From Figure15,one cycle of heartbeat consists of 3 different peaks namely P wave, QRS wave,and T wave. P wave portraits the propagation time of the impulse to both atria, which is then followed with a flat trend calledthe PR segment that is in consequence of the propagation of the electric impulse from atria to ventricles. The QRS complex wave follows the PR segmentwith three small wavesi.e. small Q wave, the high R wave, and the small S wave. This gives the information about the ventricular systole in consequence of the impulse propagation to the ventricles (Q wave), whereas the transmission to the whole tissue is caused by the R and S wave. The QRS complex wave provides information about fibrillation and arrhythmias, it can be helpful to analyze heart attacks. And then ST interval, it is following by the S wave and including with the T wave, it can point out the ischemia occurrences. It represents the period during which ventricles are contracting, which is the last stage of the heart cycle. The T wave permits one to have information about the cardiac hypertrophy, heart attacks, and ischemia. The inputs are taken from the sensor and electrodes for this sensor. ECG Sensor checks the heart-beat(rhythm) of the soldiers and sends data to Arduino. These data will be transferred to the receiver through Transmitter.

Communication Using GSM

A GSM Module isa GSM Modem (SIM 900) with different types of output taken from the board band RS232 Output to interface directly with a personal computer. For this project,we are connecting a GSM modem or module to Arduino to send and receive SMS at emergencies. This GSM Module with a Sim Card supports communication in a 900MHz band. In all the countries the minimum bandwidth required for communication over GSM network is 900MHz, Hence the use of this communication is more effec-

Figure 14.

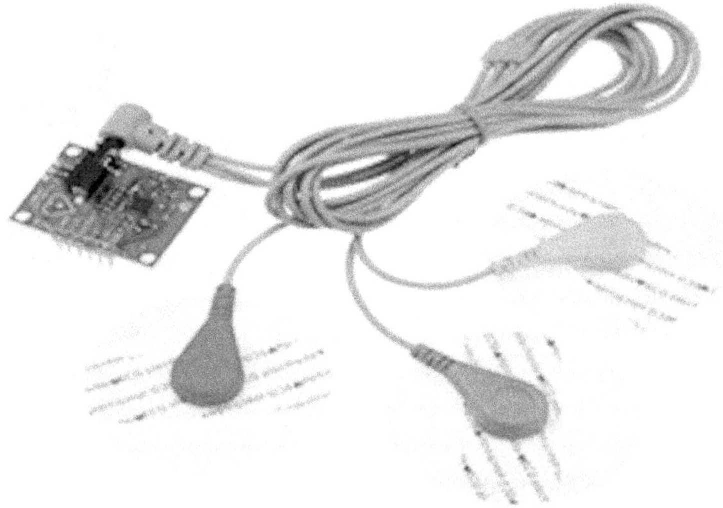

Figure 15.

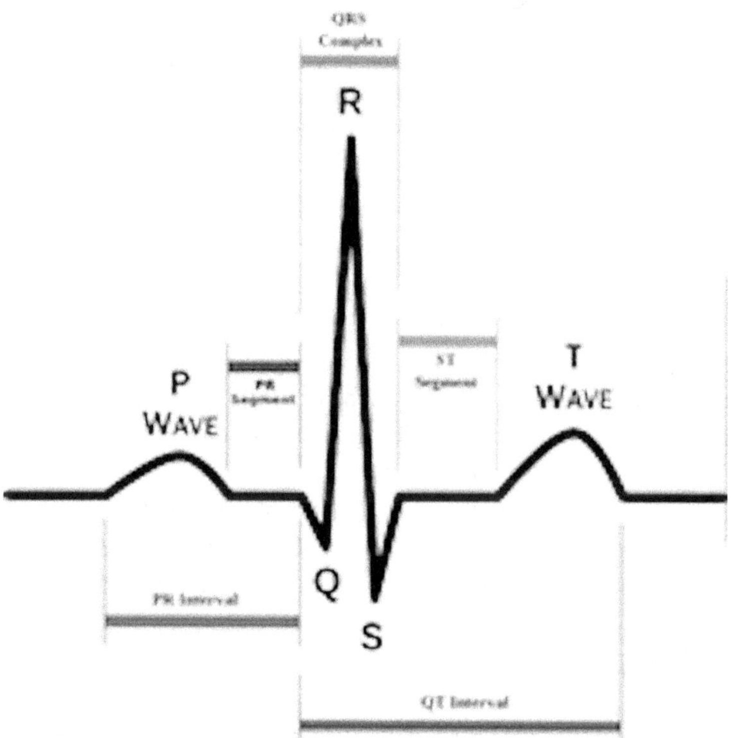

tive inemergencies. Figure 16depicts the GSM – SIM800C module that is to be connected to Arduino. In any case, the communication between Arduino and GSM module is serial then the serial pins of Arduino (Rx and Tx) are connected.

MILITARY BASE UNIT

In the Military base unit, the data's sent by the transmitter is received by the GSM receiver and the data are analyzed using CNN which is a pre-trained network. The working flow of the military base unit is shown below in Figure 17.

GSM Receiver

The GSM receiver receives the data that is being sent by the GSM transmitter and the data is fed into cloud IoT where the Convolutional Neural Networks is performed to analyze the data transferred by the GSM receiver. CNN is a pre-trained set of data where the features are first extracted from the signal. These features are then passed through the different layers of CNN as shown in Figure 18.

The pooling layer performs down-sampling operations which reduces the in-plane dimensionality and decreases the number of subsequent learnable parameters. And they are mapped by a subset of fully connected layers to the final outputs of the network.

Figure 16.

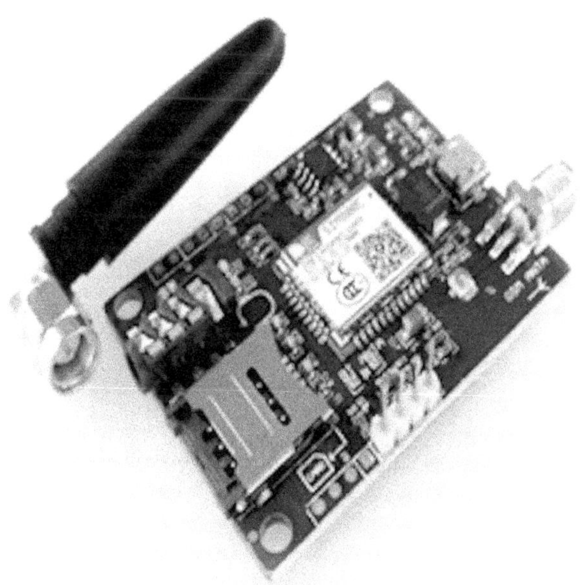

Figure 17.

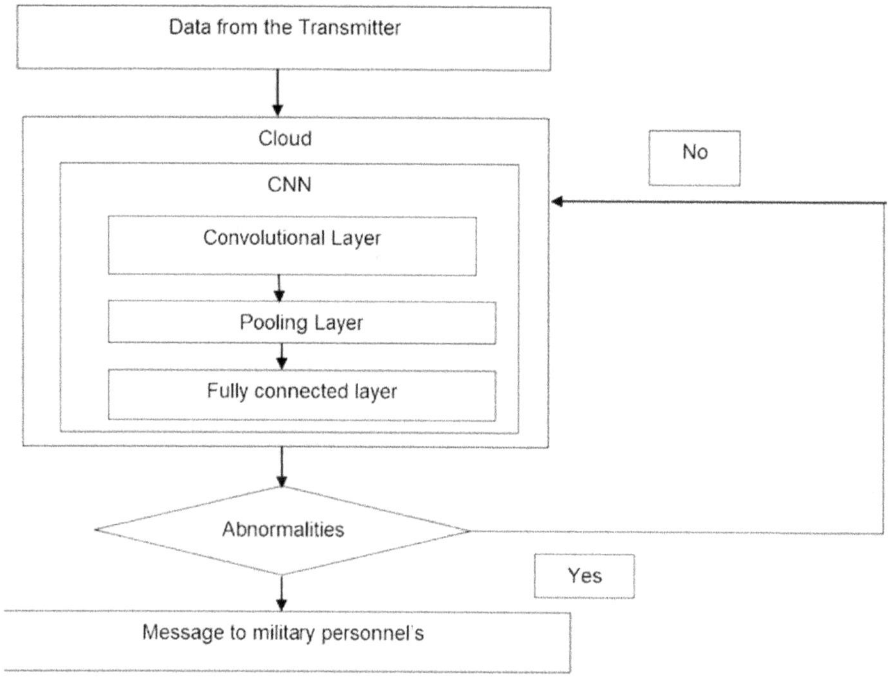

Figure 18.

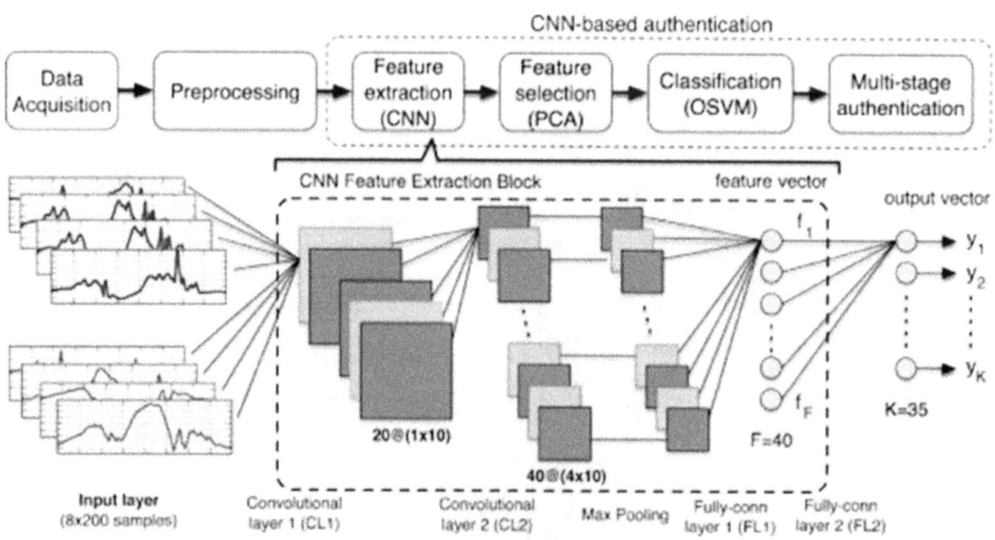

The Fusion of Sensor Data

In healthcare monitoring fusion of sensor data plays a vital role and it provides the physicians accurate and adequate diagnosis on the health condition based on the factors like effective estimation, classification and inferential data from medical sensors. Multi-sensor data fusion techniques can be well utilized for patient vital sign monitoring (VSM) systems because they can incorporate cognitive abilities through the classifiers. Moreover, using one specific type of sensor is not that beneficial to the system. Hence, we use multiple sensors with different characteristics which increases the potential of the system and gives an accurate response on the target. Some factors like inherent noise and Nyquist frequency may prevent the sensor from measuring the signal outside its bandwidth. Forinstance, some sensors like GPS sensors used for locating the position the target perform well in low frequencies whereas the accelerometer sensors will perform better in high frequencies.By measuring the displacement using both the GPS and accelerometer sensors and exploiting the both inputs will give an accurate value for the displacement. Data registration is the first step in multi-sensor data fusion process to collect the data from the various sensors and coordinate into a common system. Registration procedure could be carried out in 3-dimension, 2-dimension, and also in single dimension inputs.This data registration is achieved by searching the best resembling recordings of the sensor data's and are mapped onto a common frame based on their similarity. The factors influence the similarity criteria are template matching, control points, feature invariants, and regression. Mappingfunctions like bilinear, warping, or least square optimization could be used depending on the data type. The priority method used in this system for data fusion is Bayesian theory.The basic concept of the Bayesian theory is conditionalprobability that expresses the notion probability ofoccurrence of event x given event y, which is denotedas P(x|y). For data fusion, an expression for probability of hypothesis is given by Bayes' rule.The fundamental equation of Bayes' rule isgiven in equation below:

$$P(H_i|D) = [P(D|H_i)\, P(H_i)] \,/\, P(D) \quad (1)$$

Convolutional Neural Networks

Convolution Neural Network is a deep learning algorithm that takes in a set of input data, assign importance to various aspects/objects in the data and be able to differentiate one from the other. The pre-processing required in a convent is much lower as compared to other classification algorithms. More recently, the Convolutional neural network (CNN) has exploded in popularity and real-world applications. More recently, the Convolutional neural network (CNN) has exploded in popularity and real-world applications. The CNN merely provides a replacement category of NN that uses the conception of deep learning.CNN is one of the most recent breakthroughs in the area of computer vision, speech recognition, biomedical systems, and natural language processing. Unlike a normal NN, the layers of CNN can arrange neurons in three dimensions: width, height, and depth.Similarly, a 1D-CNN vibration-based technique was applied to wreck detection and localization in the period from the raw acceleration signals.The method was applied to large-scale test structures. It is proposed to incorporate sensor fusion by taking the advantage of CNN structure to achieve higher and more robust diagnosis accuracy.They analyzed each temporal and abstraction info of the information from multiple sensors for the coaching method of CNN. They pointed out that their method, compared with traditionalapproaches that use manual feature extraction, results in superior diagnosis performance. The advancements in computer vision with deep learning have been constructed and perfected with time, primarily over one particular algorithm- a Convolutional Neural Network. A Convolutional Neural Network consists of associate input associated with an output layer, as well as multiple hidden layers. From Figure 18 hidden layers of a CNN typically consist of Convolutional layers, RELU layer i.e. activation function, pooling layer, fully connected layers, and normalization layers. Convolutional layers apply a different stage of specific operation to the input, passes the result to the next layer. The convolution operation brings an answer to the current downside because it reduces the number of free parameters, permitting the network to be deeper with fewer parameters.

Training a Network

Training a network is a process of finding kernels in convolution layers and weights fully connected layers that minimize differences between output predictions and given ground-truth labels on a training dataset. Backpropagation algorithmic program is that the methodology normally used for coaching neural networks wherever loss performs and gradient descent improvement algorithmic program play essential roles.A model performance consists of explicit kernels and weights, which is calculated by a loss perform through forward propagation on a coaching dataset, and learnable parameters.Specifically, kernels and weights areupdated as per the loss worth through associate improvement algorithmic program known as backpropagation and gradient descent, among others.

Feature Extraction

Convolutional Neural Network (CNN) is a state-of-the-art learning network in deep learning technology. It is widelyused in image recognition, video classification, object localization and natural language processing (NLP), thanks to the rapid development of machine learning hardware and software. Compared with traditional neural networks, CNN has two advantageous characteristics, namely, local connectivity and weight sharing. Thus, it reduces the complexity of the network model and the number of weight parameters. Available informationis split into three sets: training, validation, and test set. A training set of data is employed to train a network, where loss values are calculated via forward propagation and learnable parameters are updated via backpropagation. A validation set is employed to monitor the model performance throughout the training process, fine-tune hyperparameters, and perform model selection. A test set is ideally used only once at the very end of the project to evaluate the performance of the final model that is fine-tuned and selected on the training process with training and validation sets. A CNN structure is made up of several convolutional layers, pooling layers and fully-connected layers. In Figure 19the work, we base the network design on LeNet-5. It has 7 layers excluding the output layer. We consider only a single BCG-sensor waveform, i.e. a 1-D signal, the size of the convolution kernel and some other parameters are adapted accordingly. Besides the input and output layers, the CNN has two convolutional layers (C1-C2) with ReLU nonlinear unit, two pooling layers (P1-P2) connected after C1-C2 and two fully-connected layers (F1-F2). The 732×1 dimension data is regarded as he extracted feature vector to be used in the subsequent classification processing by the ELM.All the above steps are described in Figure 19.

Figure 19.

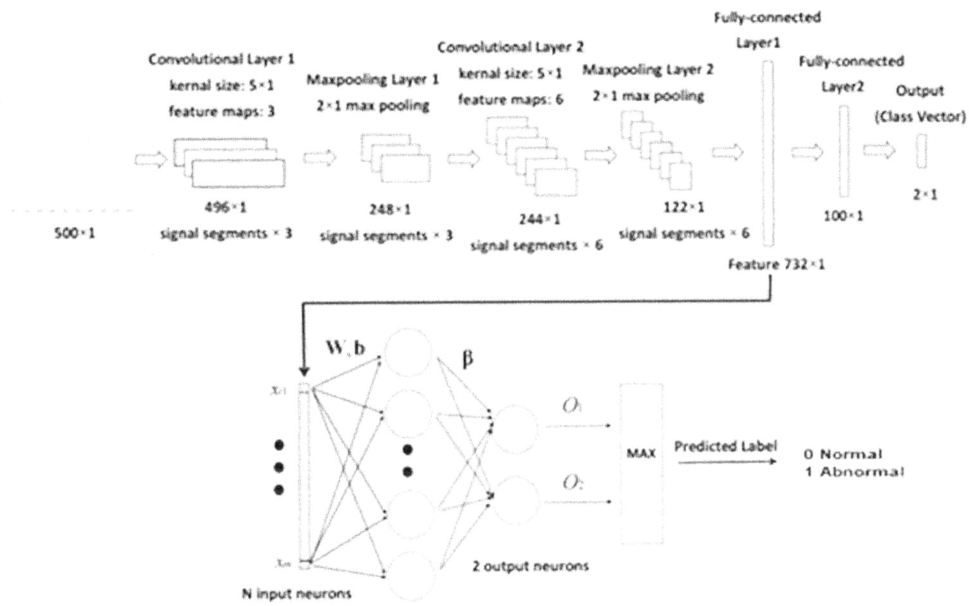

Analysis of the Collected Data

Figure 20 shows the working flow of health monitoring using CNN and the below steps illustrate the detailed procedure followed.

Step 1: The Sensor collects the health parameters, the ECG sensor collects the data based on the function of the heart, the temperature sensor collects the temperature of the human body.

Step 2: The parameters obtained are transmitted to Arduino, which transfers the data through the GSM transmitter.

Step 3: The transferred data are received through GSM receiver; these data are then fed into cloud IoT to perform CNN operation

Step 4: The CNN is pretrained with a dataset collected from the nearby private hospital with a data count of 6985 patients with different health parameters. The parameters mainly collected for this analysis are body temperature, blood pressure, heartbeat rate, and electrocardiogram output. Nearly 20 different features were extracted from the above -mentioned parameters. CNN is a pre-trained data, where already certain data are trained, tested and validated. The features are extracted first then the data are passed through different layers of CNN where the data is being analyzed, tested and validated.

Step 5: The output is classified into 3 different classes namely, Class A: Soldiers who are suffering from breathing suffocation and initial increase in values of the sensor data, Class B: Soldiers who are running out of breathe and facing high suffocation of inhalation along with increase or decrease of their body temperature and heart rate, Class C: Soldiers suffering from severe trauma and needed immediate assistance and first aid.

Step 6: After analyzing the correlational responses from the features extracted from the sensor values the 3 different threshold values for the 3 classes. If the analyzed value exceeds the threshold value the data collected is categorized into the 3 different classes and the alert messages are sent to the colonel, captain and the doctor in the military base camp.

Step 7: The messages sent to the military personnel are stated. Class A: initial trauma level, assistance required in few hours of time for the survival of the soldier, Class B: Trauma detected in the soldier end and he needs the first aid in few minutes so that he will be rescued, and Class C: High Trauma detected where, the soldier is under emergency situation and needed assistance immediately.

By using this the health parameters of the soldier are continuously monitored if any issues occur, they can be rescued easily. This helps to maintain the soldier's army safe with the reduction in death count and if the army persons are safe then our nation will be safe.

Figure 20.

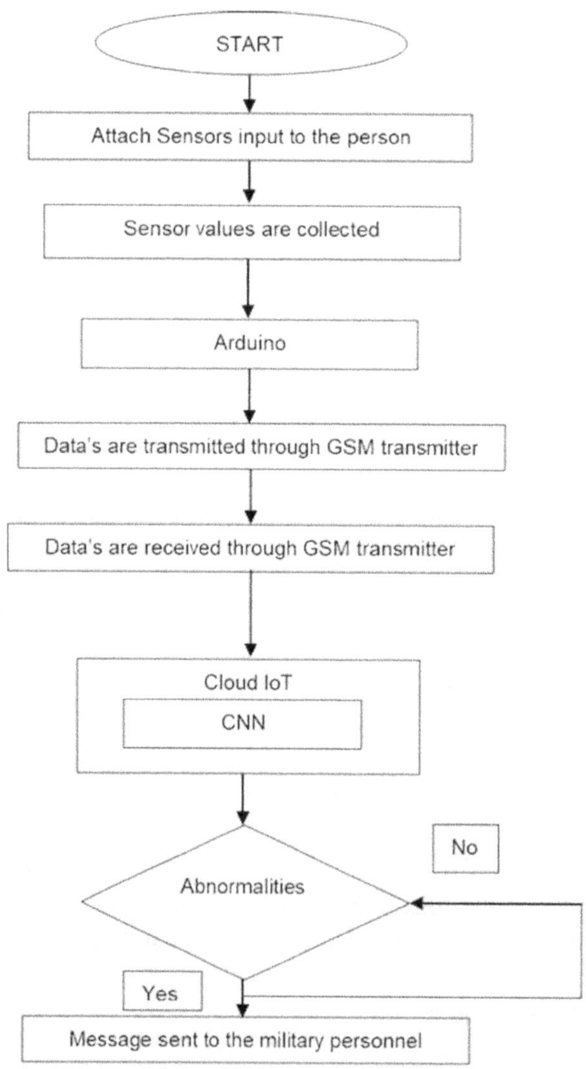

SOLUTIONS AND RECOMMENDATIONS

IoT Based Smart Jacket for Soldiers

Figure 21 shows the prototype constructed to implement a real-time smart jacket for soldiers which has various sensors placed on the board. The temperature sensor will sense the body temperature, pulse sensor will sense the blood flow of the heart, the ECG sensor will sense the heartbeat (rhythm) of the soldiers and the GPS sensor will track the location of the soldiers. This information is transferred to the Arduino board. The Arduino will get all the data and transfer the data through GSM to the base unit.

The various components in the experimental set up are connected to the Arduino controller and this is shown in Table 3. With the help of the sensors, the sensed readings will be notified in the user's device then the whole circuit is controlled based on the need of the field. This project has various sensor to monitor the solders. When the soldiers have any issue, it will get a notification the data will send through GSM to the military doctor and military colonel.

Military Unit Result

GSM is used to created viewing output in the mobile. To see the output Arduino board is connected with the GSM to send the data and it is shown in Figure 22. The sensor sends the reading to the Arduino board. The Arduino will get all the data for analysisand the analyzed data will be sent through the GSM to the captain of the camp whether the soldiers are in normal or anabnormal condition. The decision can be taken according to the sensor readings.

Figure 21.

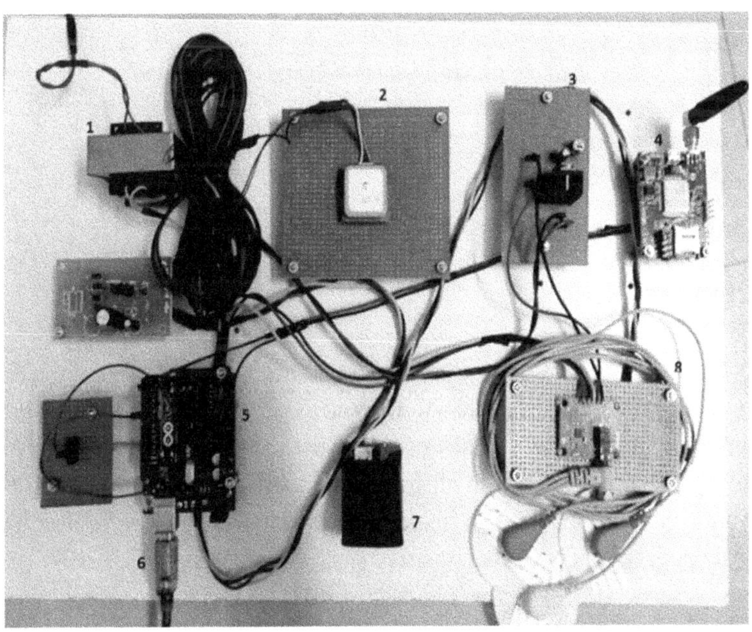

Table 3. Components Displayed on the Board

S.No	Name of the component
1.	Step Down Transformer Connected to 12V Power Supply.
2.	GPS Module – Connected to the 4th pin of Arduino Board.
3.	Relay – used to vary the input power for each sensor.
4.	GSM Module – Connected to the TX_1 pin of Arduino Board.
5.	Arduino UNO - Microcontroller board based on the ATmega328P.
6.	USB-Boot Loader – Used to load the program to controller.
7.	Heartbeat Sensor - Connected to the 8th pin of Arduino Board.
8.	ECG Module - Connected to the A_0 pin of Arduino Board.
9.	Temperature Sensor - Connected to the A_1 pin of Arduino Board.

Figure 22.

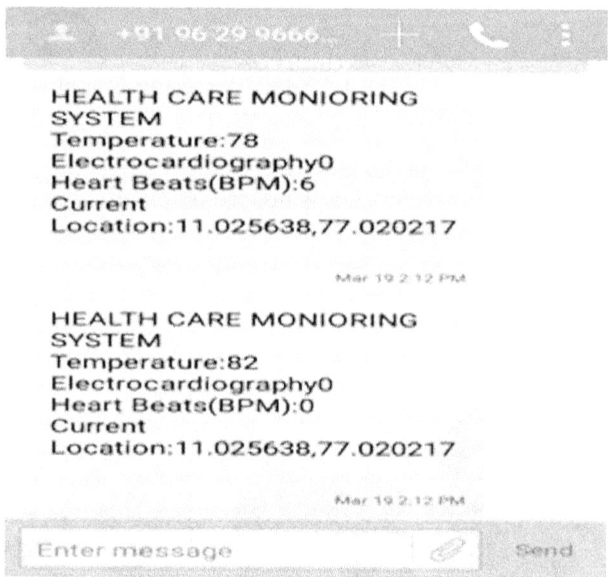
+91 96 29 9666...
HEALTH CARE MONIORING SYSTEM
Temperature:78
ElectrocardiographyO
Heart Beats(BPM):6
Current Location:11.025638,77.020217
HEALTH CARE MONIORING SYSTEM
Temperature:82
ElectrocardiographyO
Heart Beats(BPM):0
Current Location:11.025638,77.020217
Enter message
Send

Evaluation Parameter

Classification performance is measured using the four standard metrics found in the literature (Abraham, 2015): classification accuracy, sensitivity, specificity, and positive predictivity. While accuracy measures the overall system performance overall classes of beats, the other metrics are specific to each class and they measure the ability of the classification algorithm to distinguish certain events (Normal condition) from non-events (Abnormal condition). The respective definitions of these four common metrics using true positive (TP), true negative (TN), false positive (FP), and falsenegative (FN) are as follows:

- Accuracy is the ratio of the number of correctly classified patterns to the total number of patterns classified,

Accuracy = (TP+TN)/ (TP+TN+FP+FN) (2)

- Sensitivity is the rate of correctly classified events among all events,

Sensitivity = TP/ (TP+FN) (3)

- Specificity is the rate of correctly classified non-events among all non-events,

Specificity = TN/(TN+FP) (4)

- Positive Predictivity is the rate of correctly classified events in all detected events,

Positive Predictivity = TP/(TP+FP) (5)

Since there is a large variation in the different sensors data from different classes in the training/testing, sensitivity, specificity, and positive predictivity are more relevant performance criteria for medical diagnosis applications. The comparison of the proposed methods with the existing methods is given in Table 4.

Confusion Matrix

To analyze the performance of the classifier the confusion matrix is plotted and is shown in Figure 23. The confusion matrix also called the error matrix is a specific table layout designed for analyzing the performance of the CNN classifier algorithm which is used for the classification of the health condition of the soldier and takes a decision for the severity of the health issues. The Confusion matrix gives an overall accuracy of 97%.

F Score

F score or F Measure is a measure of accuracy in the statistical analysis of classification. The two identities that are used for calculating F Score are the Recall and the Precision where Recall is the ratio between number of positive results divided by number of all the relevant samples, and Precision is the

Table 4. Comparison with an existing system

Methods	Accuracy	Sensitivity	Specificity	Positive predictivity
AndoniElola et al.	93.5	94.1	92.9	82
Syed Umar Amin et al.	86.59	77.78	94	95.8
Fahmi Ben Rejabet al.	96.9	90.3	95.8	92.2
Proposed	97.1	80	88	91.459

Figure 23.

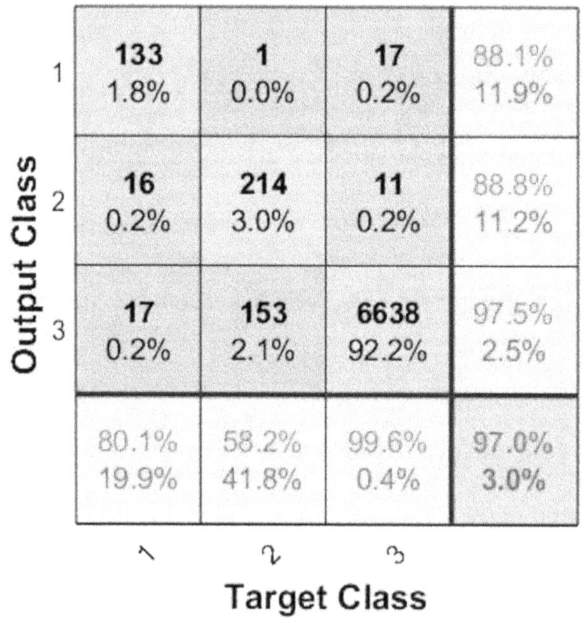

ratio of the correct positive results to the number of all positive results of the system. The formula for calculating the F Score is given below.

$$Fscore = 2x\frac{precision \times recall}{precision + recall}$$

where the precision value for this system is 91.46 and recall takes a value of 79.284. Applying the above values in F score formula we get a value of 84.937.

PRACTICAL CHALLENGES FACED DURING THE EXECUTION IN REAL-TIME

Physiological monitoring with smart jacketmeasures some of the vitalsigns like ECG, heart rate, respiratory rate, and skin temperature.The few challenges that are faced during the real-time implementation of this system are mentioned below:

- When the signal is received by a wireless node,it is degraded due to environmental factors like temporal physical obstructions due to deep fading.
- The long-term exposure of the electromagnetic signals from the bio sensors causes health hazards. Moreover, the biosensors are of large size and it requires specific on-body placement and specific posture to provide reliable measurements.

- Additional side-effects such as skin irritation or allergies should not arise when theECG system is used continuously. Commercial gel-adhesive sensors for ECG have been known tocause discomfort and irritation when used over long periods of time.

FUTURE RESEARCH DIRECTIONS

- It is expected that the health care system will be further aimed to implement more experiments and give more accurate results.
- The future scope of the system is to optimize classification algorithms for accurate results and classify different diseases.
- Accurate disease identification could be done using a greater number of sensors integrated into Nano level in the jacket.
- To reduce the circuit size and weight of the sensors integrated into the jacket.
- To reduce the hazards of the sensors on long time usage by reducing the power of the electromagnetic waves that are emitted from the biosensors.

CONCLUSION

IoT based smart health care monitoring system for war end soldiers using convolutional neural networking is used to reduce the death notification of the soldiers. It is achieved by the fusion of data from various sensors and at the soldier's jacket. The variations in sensor values will help us in classifying the data into various health conditions such as healthy, ill, abnormal and dead. Once the data has been collected and clustered, these clusters can be visualized for more instinctive summaries at the control unit. When soldier's health is in a dangerous situation the monitored parameters are sent from the wearable jacket to the base station. At the base station, the parameters are analyzed using the Convolutional Neural Networks. The hidden networks analyze the received parameters and give a prediction that the soldier is in a dangerous situation. Immediately the alert message along with the position of the soldier will be sent to the colonel, captain of the crew and the doctor at the military base station. This allows the rescue team to track the solider and recovery the solider with the medical first aid kit. The data received at the base station is highly secured with a high signal to noise ratio of 91% and theclassification algorithm gives an accuracy of 97% with reference to the confusion matrix. This makes the system more reliable and efficient with an F score of 84.937%.

REFERENCES

Ahanathapillai, V., Amor, J. D., Goodwin, Z., & James, C. J. (2015). Preliminary study on activity monitoring using an android smart-watch. *Healthcare Technology Letters*, *7*, 4456–4462. PMID:26609402

Amor, J. D. (2011). *Detecting and monitoring behavioral change through personalized ambient monitoring* (Ph.D. Doctoral Thesis). Institute of Sound and Vibration Research, University of Southampton.

Amor, J. D., Ahanathapillai, V., & James, C. J. (2014). Detecting and analyzing activity levels for the wrist a wearable unit in the USEFIL project. *Proc. XIII Mediterranean Conf. Medical and Biological Engineering and Computing*, 1201–1204. 10.1007/978-3-319-00846-2_297

Amor, J. D., Hattersley, J. G., Barber, T. M., & James, C. J. (2015). Characterization of wrist-a wearable activity measurement using whole-body calorimetry in semi-free-living conditions. *37th Annual International Conference in IEEE Engineering in Medicine and Biology Society, 5*, 2735–2738. 10.1109/EMBC.2015.7319205

Amor, J. D., & James, C. J. (2009). *Personalised ambient monitoring: accelerometry for activity level classification*. 4th European Conf. Int. Federation for Medical and Biological Engineering, Antwerp, Belgium.

Amor, J. D., & James, C. J. (2015). Setting the scene: Mobile and a wearable technology for managing healthcare and wellbeing. *37th Annual International Conference in IEEE Engineering in Medicine and Biology Society, 5*, 3752–3755. 10.1109/EMBC.2015.7320189

Awad, A., Mohamed, A., & El-Sheriff, A. A. (2013). Energy-efficient cross-layer design for a wireless body area monitoring networks in healthcareapplications. *IEEE 24th International Symposium on Personal, Indoor and Mobile Radio Communication, 6*, 1484-1489.

Ben Rejab, Nouira, & Trabelsi. (2014). Health Monitoring Systems Using Machine Learning Techniques. *Springer International Journal of Machine Learning, 10*, 234–251.

Ben Said, A., Mohamed, A., Elfouly, T., & Dennis, M. (2018). A Deep learning approach for Vital signs compressions and Energy Efficient delivery in m-health systems. *IEEE Journal of Translational Engineering in Health and Medicine, 6*.

Berlin, J. E., Storti, K. L., & Brach, J. S. (2006). Using activity monitors to measure physical activity in free-living conditions. *Journal of American Physical Therapy., 86*, 1137–1145. PMID:16879047

Bravata, D. M., Sundaram, V., & Gienger, A. L. (2007). Using pedometers to increase physical activity and improve health: A systematic review. *Journal of the American Medical Association, 298*(19), 2296–2304. doi:10.1001/jama.298.19.2296 PMID:18029834

Bernal, Yang, Li, Kumar, Madhvanath, Ramesh, & Bala. (2017). Deep TemporalMultimodal Fusion for Medical Procedure Monitoring using A wearable Sensors. *IEEE Transactions on Multimedia, 10*, 965–982.

Dennis, C. (2018). A systematic review of chronic disease management interventions in primary care. *BMC Family Practice, 19*(1). PMID:29316889

Easton, C., Philip, N., & Aleksandravicius, A. (2013). Validity of smartphone accelerometers for assessing energy expenditure during fast running. *XIII Mediterranean Conference on Medical and Biological Engineering and Computing*, 1911–1914.

Elola, Aramendi, Irusta, Picon, Alonso, Owens, & Idris. (2019). *Deep Neural Networks for ECG- Based Pulse Detection during Out-of-Hospital Cardiac Arrest*. Academic Press.

Gomez, J. (2016). Patient Monitoring System Based on Internet of Things: A survey. *Journal of Computer Networks, 11*, 532–550.

Grguric A. (2012). *ICT towards elderly independent living*. Research and Development Centre, Ericsson Nikola Tesla.

Hao, J. (2015). Image processing and transmission scheme based on generalized Gaussian mixture with opportunistic networking for a wireless sensor networks. *International Journal of Wireless Communication and Networking, 21*(1), 226–234. doi:10.118613638-015-0458-3

Hu, X., Wang, B., & Ji, H. (2013). A a wireless sensor network-based structural health monitoring system for highway bridges. *Computer-Aided Civil and Infrastructure Engineering, 10*, 1623–1637.

Humphereys, G. (2012). The health-care challenges posed by population aging. *Bulletin of the World Health Organization, 90*.

Hussein, M., Mohamed, A., & Alghoniemy, M. (2015). Scalable real-time energy-efficient EEG compression scheme for a wireless body areasensor network. *Journal of Biomedical Signal Processing Control, 19*, 122–129. doi:10.1016/j.bspc.2015.03.005

Jang, S. (2010). Structural health monitoring of a cable-stayed bridge using smart sensor technology: Deployment and evaluation. *Journal of Smart Structural System, 72*(8), 1156–1173.

Leidy, N. K., Kimel, M., Ajagbe, L., Kim, K., Hamilton, A., & Becker, K. (2014). Designing trials of behavioral interventions to increase physical activity in patients with COPD: Insights from the chronic disease literature. *Respiratory Medicine, 108*(3), 472–481. doi:10.1016/j.rmed.2013.11.011 PMID:24315467

Lynch, J. P., & Loh, K. J. (2006). A summary review of a wireless sensors and sensor networks for structural health monitoring. *Journal of Shock and Vibration, 4*, 2354–2362.

Majumdar, A., Gogna, A., & Ward, R. (2014). A low-rank matrix recovery approach for energy-efficient EEG acquisition for a wireless body area network. *Journal of Sensors, 14*(9), 15729–15748. doi:10.3390140915729 PMID:25157551

Marschollek, M., Goevercin, M., & Wolf, K. H. (2008). A performance comparison of accelerometry-based step detection algorithms on a large, non-laboratory sample of healthy and mobility-impaired persons. *Conference Proceedings; ... Annual International Conference of the IEEE Engineering in Medicine and Biology Society. IEEE Engineering in Medicine and Biology Society. Conference, 2008*, 1319–1322. PMID:19162910

Murphy, S. L. (2009). Review of physical activity measurement using accelerometers in older adults: Considerations for research design and conduct. *Preventive Medicine, 48*(2), 108–114. doi:10.1016/j.ypmed.2008.12.001 PMID:19111780

Najafi, B., Aminian, K., Loew, F., Blanc, Y., & Robert, P. A. (2002). Measurement of stand-sit and sit-stand transitions using a miniature gyroscope and its application in fall risk evaluation in the elderly. *IEEE Transactions on Biomedical Engineering, 49*(8), 843–851. doi:10.1109/TBME.2002.800763 PMID:12148823

Nangalia, V., Prytherch, D., & Smith, G. (2010). Health technology assessment review: Remote monitoring of vital signs current status and future challenges. *Journal of Critical Care, 14*(5), 552–565. PMID:20875149

Olivero, M., Tosi, D., & Perrone, G. (2018). *Low-cost fiber Bragg Grating vibroacoustic sensor for voice and heartbeat detection.* Academic Press.

Ou, J., & Li, H. (2010). Structural health monitoring in mainland China: Review and future trends. *Journal of Structural Health Monitoring, 3*(1), 874–890.

Pan, J., & Tompkins, W. (1985). A real-time QRS detection algorithm. *IEEE Transactions on Biomedical Engineering, 32*(3), 230–236. doi:10.1109/TBME.1985.325532 PMID:3997178

Prince, S. A., Adamo, K. B., Hamel, M. E., Hardt, J., Gorber, S. C., & Tremblay, M. (2008). A comparison of direct versus self-report measures for assessing physical activity in adults: A systematic review. *The International Journal of Behavioral Nutrition and Physical Activity*, 5. PMID:18990237

Ren, Jin, Chen, Ghayvat, & Chen. (2018). A Novel cardiac Auscultation monitoring system based a wireless sensing for healthcare. *IEEE Journal of Translational Engineering in Health and Medicine, 6*, 1324-1331.

Riazul Islam, S. M., Kwak, D., Humaun Kabir, M., Hossain, M., & Kwak, K. S. (2015). The Internet of Things for health care: A comprehensive survey. *IEEE Journal of Translational Engineering in Health and Medicine, 3*, 678–708.

Salih & Abraham. (2015). *Intelligent Decision Support for Real-time Health CareMonitoring System.* Afro-European Conference for Industrial Advancement.

Saxena, A., & Saad, A. (2017). Evolving an artificial neural network classifier for condition monitoring of rotating mechanical systems. *Journal of Applied Soft Computing, 7*(1), 135–154.

Shaladi, R., Alatshan, F., & Yang, C. (2015). An overview on the applications of structural health monitoring using a wireless sensor networks in bridge engineering. *International Conference in Advanced Science and Engineering Technology National Resources*, 19(3), 1542-1553.

Shelhamer, E., Long, J., & Darrell, T. (2017). Fully convolutional networks for semantic segmentation. *IEEE Transactions on Pattern Analysis and Machine Intelligence, 39*(4), 1753–1768. doi:10.1109/TPAMI.2016.2572683 PMID:27244717

Skulic, J., & Leung, K. K. (2015). Application of network coding in a wireless sensor networks for bridge monitoring. *Proceedings of IEEE 23rd International Symposium on Personal, Indoor and Mobile Radio Communication, 10*(1), 789–795.

Noel & Abdaoui. (2017). Structural Health monitoring using A Wireless Sensor Networks. *IEEE Journal of Communication, 19*(3), 1924–1936.

USEFIL. (2013). *USEFIL project.* Available at: http://www.usefil.eu/

World Health Organization. (2012). *Health Topics Ageing*. Available at: http://www.who.int/topics/ageing/en/

World Health Organization. (2013). *Physical Activity and Older Adults*. Available at: http://www.who.int/ dietphysicalactivity/factsheet_olderadults

Xna, S., & Lee, H.K. (2013). Neural network approach for damaged area location prediction of a composite plate using Electromechanical impedance technique. *Journal of Composite Science and Technology*, *56*, 794–804.

Ying, H., Schnitzer, A., Leonhardt, S., & Schiek, M. (2007). *Automatic step detection in the accelerometer signal.* Body Sensor Networks BSN2007, Aachen, Germany.

Zhu, Bojian, Li, Gu, & Yang. (2018). On the development of security monitoring system via a wireless sensing network. *Journal of a Wireless Communication Networking, 16*(6), 1685-1697.

Chapter 6
Wireless Body Sensor Networks for Patient Health Monitoring:
Security, Challenges, Applications
Security, Challenges, Applications
– IoT Healthcare Management

Bhanu Chander
https://orcid.org/0000-0003-0057-7662
Pondicherry University, India

ABSTRACT

Remote medical health management is the most attractive research field in the domain of WSN. Wireless body area network (WBAN) produces constant, unbroken observation of the patient. Basically, WBAN acts as the appliance of internet of things (IoT) which offers an opportunity to a medical examiner to supervise chronic disease. Dissimilar protocols, guidelines, policies have been developed and developing in the last decade. In WBAN, minute power sensor nodes deployed toward capturing unusual essential signs of patients at home, hospitals in support of analysis purpose and furthermore advise suitable procedures. The main goal of this chapter is to introduce a complete and advanced understanding of WBANs, energy savings methods, human activity monitoring procedures, challenges and research issues, applications, and a comprehensive literature survey.

DOI: 10.4018/978-1-7998-0261-7.ch006

INTRODUCTION

Wireless Body Area Networks (WBANs) is a combination of Wireless sensor nodes (WSNs) which capable of placed outside or inside the body of the patient/individual person and that in results shows observed or monitored functionalities along with adjoining conditions of the human body. The expansion and management of Wireless body area networks (WBAN) come into reality when the enlargement of wireless sensor networks (WSN) reach some level, hence WBAN recognized as sub-field in WSNs. Advanced development in wireless technology, Micro Electro Mechanical Systems (MEMS), Information Connection Technology (ICT) makes powerful healthcare category to compose effectively and efficiently furthermore endow with a variety of solutions and well-being services. WSNs come into view as a powerful as well as low cast platform for linking the physical world en route to the digital world. As a result of set-up at huge amount of tinny expensive sensor nodes in the observation area, we can check the adjacent atmosphere through systematically assembled sensed data which broadcast back to sink (Base station) in a wireless or wired configuration (Chris Otto et al., 2006; Chinmay et al., 2016; Kamta et al., 2019; Chinmay et al., 2013; Bhanu et al., 2018).

Day-by-day increase in population demanding speedy advances in healthcare costs. Healthcare system is progressive in the course of a revolution, in which unbroken regulation of inhabitant is achievable devoid-of hospitalization. Continuous innovations in sense mechanisms, nano-technologies, embedded systems, miniaturization, and wireless conversation technologies formulates that it is feasible to build a well-dressed system to examine actions of human being endlessly. E-health administration can go with Wireless Body Area Networks (WBAN) which shows empowering innovation, scientific knowledge, machinery performance, technology and attractiveness gaining day-by-day for the reason of its benefits. Sensors utilized to assemble sensitive, essential medical associated information/statistics of a patient moreover it can also applicable in sports to examine players' potentiality and strength. Wireless body area networks offer a guarantee to remodel health monitoring. In opposition, researchers/designers of such healthcare systems face a number of difficult tasks as they need to deal with incompatible requirements size, operating systems, exactness, and trustworthiness (Chris Otto et al., 2006; Chinmay et al., 2016; Kamta et al., 2019; Chinmay et al., 2013; Bhanu et al., 2018; Chinmay et al., 2013).

Internet of Things (IoT) is a combination of devices, actuators, and sensor nodes supervised in a distributed, comprehensive and omnipresent way. IoT exists in multiple applications, services in addition to the healthcare sector is not at all away from IoT rebellion (Jose-Luis et al., 2018). Along these lines, telemedicine plays the main role for expansion and improvement of IoT technologies in healthcare. Sensors which can easy way of use and remote monitoring are state-of-the-art of applications for IoT technologies. Remote monitoring distributed systems presented in universal level described in two types of architecture. One type is distributed system architecture provides storing behavior, biometric and context variable from profit-making sensors into appliances like a computer, Smartphone, and computers from there on producing complete exhaustive reports to support health-related decision making (Lin et al., 2004; Meneu T et al., 2011). The second type is automatically distributed system architectures broadcast captured data with the help of wireless technology, Wi-Fi, Bluetooth and ZigBee transmissions (Meneu T et al., 2011; Chris Otto et al., 2006). As the result of recent advancement in wireless communication technology, low power micro electro mechanical systems, miniaturization, and network technology now we have new enable and production called wireless sensor networks which proficient of autonomously monitoring and scheming surroundings (Chris Otto et al., 2006; Chinmay et al., 2016; Kamta et al., 2019).

Differentiation of WSN and WBAN

The problems and challenges faced by the Wireless Body Area Network (WBANs) are completely different from traditional wireless sensor networks (WSNs). In traditional wireless networks, a huge amount of sensor nodes monitor the large scale of the environment/surroundings. Coming to WBANs where patient/individual body offers a small atmosphere, surroundings, in addition, it reacts according to internal as well as external environment/surroundings behavior. While monitoring human body WBANs system requires more trustworthiness and accurateness because fake readings may cause wrong medical diagnosis especially on serious issues associated with heart working, blood pressure, etc., according to human behavior, movements and gestures sensor nodes have to move appropriately which is not available in most of traditional wireless sensor network applications (Later´ B et al., 2011; Rahat Ali Khan et al., 2018).

Some of challenging differentiations among WSN and WBAN (Chen M et al., 2011; Latre´ B et al., 2011; Negra R et al., 2016; Rahat Ali Khan et al., 2018):

1. *Number of Nodes:* WSNs consists of the huge amount of sensors then only we can cover large wide area whereas, WBANs consists of fewer sensors enough to monitor limited space (Human being).
2. *Size of Node:* WSN offers small size nodes but it mandatory depending on workload we can improve sensor size while WBAN mostly offers the small size of the sensor for human conformability.
3. *Monitoring:* WSN can monitor uncertain environments such as underwater monitoring, deep-forest monitoring, underground mines (Oil, Salt, and Gold), etc., WBAN can only make to monitor human body physiological parameters like heart-beat monitoring, body parts monitoring.
4. *Replacement of Node:* In WSN, some nodes may not work properly because of un-natural things happen in those surroundings which can easily replace. In WBAN replacement of node is very difficult which may lead to false readings.
5. *Task of Node:* In WSN we assign a committed task to one group of nodes, coming to WBAN each node can assign multiple tasks.
6. *Scale:* In WSN transmission scale is in-between meters to kilometers, whereas in WBAN transmissions scale up to centimeters to meters to reduce the energy usage which is very important in WBAN.
7. *Energy Scavenging Source:* Traditional WSN energy sources are wind and solar whereas WBAN it has energy sources from motion, vibration movement, thermal heat, thermoelectric generators.
8. *Channel:* Most of WSN applies Industrial scientific and medical bands which provide a free radio band with comprehensive accessibility. Optical, infrared communications are some other usable transmission technologies. Coming to WBAN it uses the medical channel, ISM, body surface, etc.
9. *Node Life Tome:* Node lifetime in WSN is depending on the application which environment we monitoring, mostly the life of node is in months/ years. WBAN it reduces to days/months only.
10. *Accuracy of the Result:* WSN accuracy depends on node redundancy and scalability, WBAN node accuracy depends on fall detection and robustness.
11. *Network Topology:* In WSN applications network topology we likely to be fixed and static, moreover WSN has three very special topologies namely pre-deployment, re-deployment, and post-deployment. WBAN network topology is more variable due to gestures and body movements.
12. *Power Demand:* WSN demands large power supply whereas WBANs demands very low power supply.

13. *Security:* WSN security plays an important role because to make a good decision making the quality of data is important; coming to WBAN security levels takes very high to protect patient information.
14. *Wireless Technology:* In WSN various technology are available some are Bluetooth, Zigbee, Wireless local area network; general packet radio services many more. In WBAN Low power technology required.
15. *Impact of Loss Data:* With the help of redundant node data loss will be compensated in WSN but in WBAN data loss will significantly effect on decision making.
16. *Data Rates:* WSN data rate is in Homogenous form coming to WBAN data rate is in Non-Homogenous form.

Node Taxonomy in WSNs, WBANs

In WBAN sensor node notably classified based on their performance role in the network functionality and performance. See Fig. 3. WBAN and Wearable sensing devices and services (Rahat Ali Khane et al., 2018; Latre´ B et al., 2011; Negra R et al., 2016).

1. *Sensor:* In the view of WBANs, sensor monitors certain kind of parameters from patients' body either outside or inside. When there is any physical charge occurred on human body sensor automatically collect reacted information and this reacted information transformed through wireless media for proper decision making. Ambient, bio-kinetics are some examples for sensors utilized as a part of a patient's body parts or part of person wrist watch, headphones or portable and permits checking wirelessly anyplace, whenever needed. An accessible sensor as part of WBANs listed as follows temperature sensor, DNA sensor, humidity, blood pressure, Spiro-meter, ECG and EMG, DNA and CO2 gas sensor, EEG and so on.
2. *Actuator:* Actuator receives information/data from the sensor after that collaborates with the user. Generally, actuator awards feedback by acting on sensor information/data like the exact dosage of medicine into the individual/patient body in ubiquitous medical apps.
3. *Personal Device:* Personal device is responsible for connecting with other clients by accumulating the data provided by the sensor and actuator. Screen/LED is located on a personal device or actuator to advise the client. Gateway, sink, body control unit is some personal devices applicable in WBAN.
4. *Implant Node:* Nodes which are implanted within the patient/individual, underneath the skin, inside the body tissue are named as implanted nodes.
5. *Body Surface Node:* As the name suggests these body surface node mostly placed on the surface or outside of the human body and node may keep away from the human body like 2-4 cm away from the patient.
6. *External Node:* Implanted nodes are not connected with patient/individuals body somewhat placed couple of centimeters (5cm or more) away from the body.
7. *Relay node:* Relay node same as intermediate nodes, it has two nodes namely parent node, child node, and they displacement messages. Basically whenever any of nodes reaches its final limit, at that point data/information forward handled by an alternate node before it reaches personal device (PD).

8. *Coordinator:* Coordinator works as gateways or it simply resembles with another WBAN. One that wants to communicate with other remaining nodes makes usage of PDA well-known as WBAN Coordinator.
9. *End Node:* End node do not have the ability to transform messages between nodes, they are restricted to perform their inserted applications.

BODY AREA SENSOR NETWORK

Body sensor networks communicate with existing systems such as portable devices, medical database storage, and medical representatives and also with loved ones. The main function of wireless body sensors is making available data/information to body aggregators that play a vital role in managing body function. As shown in figure 1 a wireless body area sensor networks (WBASN) communication architecture consists or equipped with the wireless sensor placed on the human body. These sensor nodes can be electromyography, blood pressure measuring and heart rhythm measuring sensor nodes. The aggregated valuable data of sensor nodes transformed to the nearest base station or personal servers. Likewise, all the data recorded from deployed sensors are collected by the base station is transformed into medical data storage for further analysis's and to medical representatives for immediate precautions. While designing a WBAN we must be careful that when a person is in moving scenario, figure/body is also in movement hence for the period of that time the arrangements of sensors involved may possibly modify so WBASNs are not regarded to be an as static node. The communication performed in WBASNs is divided into three categories (See Fig. 1. WBASN communication structural design) in category 1 we talk about sensor nodes communications, in category 2 we talk about multiple access points, personal

Figure 1.

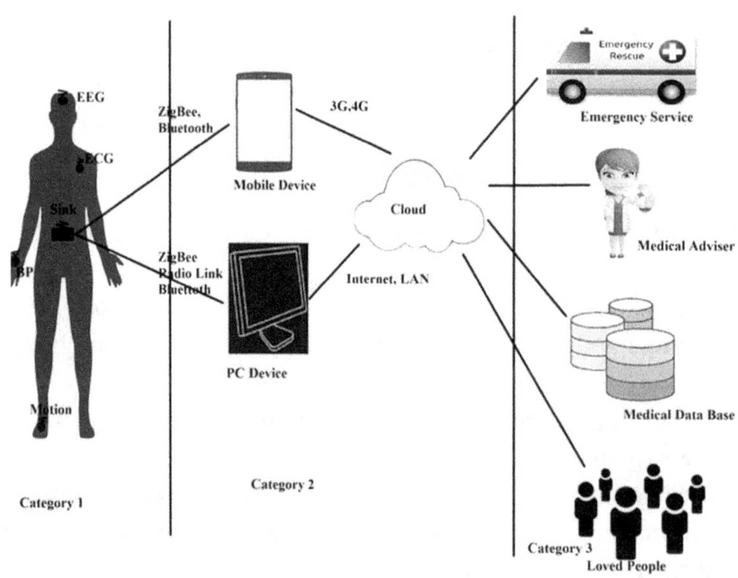

devices, etc. Finally in category 3 we talk about communication with medical representatives and medical data storage for analysis purpose (Meneu T et al., 2011; Jose-Luis et al., 2018; Chris Otto et al., 2006; Rahat ali Khan et al., 2018; Mark A Hanson et al., 2009; Chinamy et al., 2019; Sravanth et al., 2019).

Category 1 Communication

In Category 1 communication, the main role played by sensor nodes. It happens only between the sensors and sinks nodes. Sensing is the fundamental task of sensor nodes and quality of sensor node heavily depends upon industrial advances in signal conditions; signal nano-technology, controls, micro electro mechanical systems (Rahat ali Khan et al., 2018). There are three main categories of sensor used in WBAN namely physiological sensors- measure body temperature, blood pressure, signals related to electromyography and electrocardiography. Bio-kinetic sensors - measure angular rotation and acceleration derived from human body movement. Ambient sensors-measure adjacent situations like pressure, temperature levels. Communication range in category 1 is something like 2 meters around the human body. WSNs and WBASNs node communication is necessary for node synchronization with other nodes, devices. WBANS is more unique that they confine communication radius, limiting transmission range reduce nodes power consumption and interference among BASNs. WSNs sensor node communicates over radio frequency channel between 175 MHz to 2.4GHz, unlike traditional WSNs, WBASNs challenged by dramatic attenuation result by body shadows, line of sight disturbances, continuous movements, and high path loss. Maintain quality of services over traditional WSNs, WBASNs requires many approaches such as multi input-multi output, adaptive channel coding, novel transceiver architecture, transmission scaling etc (Meneu T et al., 2011; Jose-Luis et al., 2018; Chris Otto et al., 2006; Rahat Ali Khan et al., 2018; Mark A Hanson et al., 2009).

Because of short-range communication, we prefer Zigbee and Bluetooth are the most preferred communication technologies used in this category. Compare to traditional WSNs, in WBASNs we use little number sensors so it requires specific placement, quality of data will be degraded if we place sensors in ineffective places and human/sensor movements also significantly degrade the performance of the sensor. The sensed observations, physical conditions of patients are forward to sink nodes which are located near to sensor nodes. The main assignments facing sink nodes are buildup the composed data and broadcast it on the road to category 2 devices.

Category 2 Communication

Category 2 communication modeled among sink node and one or more personal devices/access points. There will be specific infrastructure for deploy personal devices, access points and they may place directly into a dynamic environment so that may help in handling critical or disaster situations. The main objective of category 2 is inter-linkage between dissimilar types of networks that can straightforwardly available like the mobile network to BASNs, computer system to BASNs. Wireless expertise's like Bluetooth, radio frequency, 3G, 4G, Zigbee, cellular, wireless LAN are preferable communication technologies used in category 2 (Rahat Ali Khan et al., 2018).

Category 3 Communication

In Category 3 communication, medical sensors deliver the collected data to the recipients with the help of the internet or any other network. The recipients could be doctor/nurse, loved ones, ambulance moreover data could be saved in a recipients database or in medical data storage with profile name of the patient. Based on that message doctor can notify patient condition going to be worst and necessary precautions will be formulated prior-to patients arrive at the hospital. The medical database is the most important component this include profile and medical history of the patient. So doctors can easily notify emergency status with a message or internet service. However, depending on the application or emergency situations sink node directly transform data to a medical data store instead of communicating with the access point.

Hierarchical Aggregation

Sensor nodes data processing reveals important information on specific sensor locality. However, information may also come from the relationship between multiple sensor nodes over time. For example, sensor node verifies new coming data with own stored old data may possibly give some kind of idea about the particular locality and sensor node verify its own combined data with neighboring data give some kind of idea about that same locality (Mark A Hanson et al., 2009). So in WBASNs body area data collector has the significant responsibility of combining data/information from multiple sensors deployed on the human body. Basically data collector has high range resource facilities and superior energy competence than sensor nodes; in addition, it creates Connectivity Bridge between body sensors and higher level infrastructures. Data aggregator also allows user interfaces and can pass its own sensing capabilities. Communication technologies like Bluetooth, wireless technology, IEEE 802.11 and interactive user interfaces similar to touch screen, embedded microprocessors make personal computers, mobile phones, and personal digital assistants are attractive hosts for body area data collection. Data processing at each data aggregator will reveal progressive relation between body sensors with the help of sophisticated and dedicated data mining techniques. If available data is as large as possible data aggregator will provide much accurate relationship for WBANs but data aggregator need higher data rates, hardware and software interoperate throughout numerous levels of interactions to share information (Jose-Luis et al., 2018; Chris Otto et al., 2006; Rahat Ali Khan et al., 2018; Mark A Hanson et al., 2009).

Topology

As we know Computer network technology contains some notable topologies like bus, star, tree, mesh, and hybrid but among this star, mesh and combination of star-mesh topology show promises for meeting needs of the body sensor network. In a star network, all body sensors connect with one body collection agent, which allocate for huge data rate throughput by simplified routing. Moreover having one central body collection agent, it leads one single network failure; to overcome failure star-mesh topology extends the typical star topology furthermore to construct mesh network surrounded by central coordinators. The failure of one central coordinator does not affect the overall performance of network moreover star-mesh topologies link aggregators and bridge networks starting one body area network to another body area network or with wider area networks (Chris Otto et al., 2006; Mark A Hanson et al., 2009).

Storage

Compare to Traditional sensor nodes, WBASNs are very smaller and they have very limited memory capacity. MRAM, RARAM are some nonvolatile memories powered by micro-electro industries. Most importantly on-node storage preferable solution for achieving greater aggregation, flexibility and thereby increase battery life moreover on-node data storage will increase the BASNs functionality. Some healthcare appliances prefer cache data until body channel conditions more positive for transmission. So, the provisional cache could extend battery life through lessen bit errors or form factor.

From all of the above discussion, we can conclude that the environment beyond the WBANs is also considered. The same measurements should be extended toward a surrounded atmosphere that would unite thousands of devices to increases facilities of healthcare system furthermore make possible long distance, remote wellness program in favor of hard-to-reach patients. Therefore well-organized methods/ techniques could be employed beyond WBASN environment moreover suitable mechanisms should be preferred for various issues like security, energy efficiency and coverage, and data rate.

SECURITY SERVICES IN WIRELESS BODY AREA SENSOR NETWORK

A recent development in the fields of wireless communication technology and body area sensor network various kind of medical area networks built to supervise, observe wellbeing position of patients/ individuals in real time. Here IoT healthcare environment wearable, medical wireless sensor nodes deployed in different approaches such as installed in offices, being attached at persons clothes or body parts, home, public facilities to monitor the motion, changes in position of patient furthermore health data accumulated by sensors are transformed into a medical database store accessed by health-protection providers, shared by government agencies, patients, researchers, insurance agencies. Meanwhile transmitting as well as analysis processing of medical data at healthcare systems three main security problems will occur first, diversity of intrusion methods- where healthcare system is collection of data transmission modes, topologies, and simple interaction requirements among devices but most of those be various category of sensor nodes, therefore, the corresponding system can molest by a variety of network communication attacks. Second, diversification of attackers- healthcare is very important monitoring system which collects huge needful information attracts all domain people includes intruder who wants to strike back. The third one, specialized attacks- from the beginning healthcare system attacked in many ways especially targets on certain system function or feature. This kind of attacks is very important than traditional attacks (Abdullah et al., 2016). There are dissimilar types of attacks and threats for collected, stored data associated with patient/individual expressed by WBAN can be stolen or compromised. Attacks are simply categorized into two categories passive attack and negative attacks. The expressed ideas of data/information in WBANs create employing security as well as privacy difficult. Encryption, decryption techniques of cryptography related algorithms are picking up for maintenance of access control to sheltered privacy of patient data/information. Security and secure exchange of data is undoubtedly the key importance of WBAN. The appropriate level of privacy, integrity, authenticity must be provided to patient data. Moreover, only an authenticated person should be permissible to access composed information/data. Therefore permission is also a necessary principle in security perspective. More importantly, when we talk about WBAN setting, security protocols must be in lightweight nature so that we easily run on the wireless body, wearable or implanted sensors.

Replaying

In reply attack, the main attention of the attacker is to stop sensor node working. An attacker may possibly resent digital data signal, at the beneficiary side, mentioned repeated data shows as valid. As we know transfer and receiving a part in a conversation that exhausts power supply of sensor node. Hence assuming that attacker introducing continuous recap messages, the intention is exhaust energy of sensor node so that it will stop working.

Eavesdropping

Eavesdropping is secretly capturing communication with no knowledge of two actual entities whose take part in that transmission set-up. WBANs sensor exchange confidential data in radio signals where attacker easily interrupts those radio signals and capture information between the nodes.

Impersonation Attack

Impersonation attack is someway different from other attacks; in this invader effectively understand uniqueness/identity regarding one of the valid entities of a network or transmission protocol. In case any invader impersonates or eavesdrop information/data of valid entity and stoles information/data, the invader can easily formulate to misuse or criminal use.

Message Corruption

In Message corruption attack, the attacker not only eavesdrops but also changes or modifies partial/full data which cause for message corruption. Such data is not more useful for processing. In WBAN message corruption significantly affect patient/individual diagnosis process.

Forged Base Station Attack

As we know WBAN has relatively miniature-sized set-up, so there is a possibility of things similar to forged base attack will occur. Compare to WSN where base station has a large capacity of resources and processor which is mostly not easily available for any kind of attack, coming to WBANs which consists of the small network which creates lots of chance to forge base station. The attacker can accumulate sensitive information by dumping legitimate sensor nodes that are in the actual monitoring sector.

Data Integrity

Whenever data/information transformed or exchanged through insecure channel data may modify or changed moreover sometimes data simply deleted. It is the truth that in WSNs it is very tough to find error-free transmission. To protect data/information while in transmission mode where data can be remodeled, error control will be guaranteed via data integrity. Simply data integrity is a process of confirmation that data packets which are part of communication are not altered by opponents.

Data Confidentiality

About confidential data/information could accomplish via defending against illegible entities. Here an authoritative person can also entail protecting data from further external networks. In the view of the health care system, it is a very significant problem and proper principle must be taken so we are able to defend patient/individual information among bordering or external networks. With the help of secure algorithms and shared secret keys, we can easily obtain data confidentiality.

Data Availability

Data availability provides conformation moreover makes the work/function comfortable the same as it constructed in advance for patient/individual security. Healthcare system must provide data availability when it requires moreover required services can be carried out anytime, anyplace throughout an emergency. Switching network is also important when some network does not work properly because of external or internal behavior that direct to loss of existence of individual/patient.

Scalability

Healthcare system contains various patients' related information; shared access control systems have to be flexible with a number of patients. More importantly, low consumption and storage data are required which easily set-up and reformed for the superior end result.

Cryptographic Techniques

Encryption decryption techniques of cryptography play the main role in data confidentiality by employing algorithms like advanced encryption standard (AES), Data encryption standard (DES), Diffie-hellman key exchange protocols, secure hash algorithms, etc.

Data Privacy

In data privacy only approved and legitimated persons can utilize accumulated patient data or information. When patient data or information reveal to illegitimate inhabitants/people it will guide to numerous uncertainty situations because patient information is a dreadfully sensitive issue. A phantom routing protocol is essential in WBAN in order to achieve privacy of source location.

ENERGY EFFICIENT WIRELESS BODY AREA NETWORK

Compare to sensor nodes of traditional WSNs, WBANs sensors are supposed to be relatively small and that instructs a noticeable problem. In particular, the sensors used in medical and healthcare systems energy resources are very small. A network technology which contains sensors energy efficient is one of the main issues in its core operation. Especially in healthcare IoT systems, we need increased data rates for emerging problems thus it increases overall energy consumption. However with the help of some advanced energy efficient routing protocols, energy scavenging technologies and some advanced architecture techniques we can reduce energy consumption (Süleyman Mahircan Demir 2018). Nowadays, emerging healthcare systems employed with new innovative technologies or architectures like cyber-physical systems, cloud, Internet of Things may increase required communication technologies, processing tasks which eventually increase power consumption. However, in these type methods, we only consider perimeters of WBANs only; associated networks and technologies are not taken into consideration. There must be a particular method which read body constraints similar to blood pressure, heart rate and pulse rate, etc. hence, WBAN much not affected by the external affairs. A wide variety of technologies utilized in healthcare systems need better data rate, as a result, they consume more energy, and in fact, it placed us to think about new better battery technologies, devices with greater resources while the sizes of devices kept as small as possible and energy harvesting technologies. In traditional WSNs, sensor node consumes more energy for communication or data transmission than computational processing and it has been proved by many researchers. Coming to WBANs, where we require more number of transmission and receptions take place because human activity correlated data should be collected consistently and continuously (E. Ibarra et al., 2016; F. U. Qureshi et al., 2017; Suleiman et al., 2018).

Nowadays energy flow-studies have become important research area and it is not only strict to the fulfillment of ambient energy resources, progress performances but also on probable to restore the batteries that principally useful to wireless body area networks (WBANs). However, the capacity of power affords by batteries has some restrictions such as the range of communication and onboard features of WBANs. Here unadventurously, the battery is used to make available energy toward WBAN's. For the most part, battery changing and recharging are unworkable in WBAN's applications moreover facing momentous tribulations in particular for biomedical applications. So, there are numerous works are proposed, done and going on to overcome limitations on energy scavenging interface circuits with dissimilar productivities (Süleyman et al., 2018). Ever-increasing size and capacity of batteries is not an optimal solution because simultaneously it increases the cost and weight. So current researches mostly focus on removing the batteries from WBAN's (E. Ibarra et al., 2016; F. U. Qureshi et al., 2017).

Recently the demand for advanced technology has tremendously amplified; mentioned demand is accompanied by the development of industrial groups. Energy seriously important for modern society started with this point energy saving, harvesting notions attract ample concentration to overcome energy-related dilemma as well as save resources for the next upcoming generations. IoT is somewhat a combination of physical devices from microelectronic circuits to wide range devices in consequence of internet (A. Muhtaroglu et al., 2017). Recently Cisco a multinational american company which produces hardware networking products stated that the amount of overall allied devices in 2010 was 12.5 billion and it is probable to see mention number to move 50 billion in coming 2020. It also stated that a number of connected devices for one human being will change from 1.84 to 6.58 for the above mentioned period (D. Evans et al., 2011). These allied devices have the capability to collect, store, process, send and receive data with help of internet can change of daily lifestyle and guide us in our routine life. As discussed WSNs are a subpart of the Internet of Things (IoT) technology. WSN is collections of hundreds to thousands of tiny sensors which can easily deploy in uncertain environment moreover nodes have different sensing capabilities, energy resources, and data handling capacity and communication limits. WSNs are mostly used in monitoring uncertain physical environments, security, and surveillance, industrial applications, transport, and entertainment. As a result of these advantages, researches start utilizing WSNs in healthcare systems which called as wireless body area networks. Many investigation/researches illustrate that diseases can effortlessly be stopped if they detect in premature stages. So deployment of WBANs is to inspect uncharacteristic situations happening in the human body and provide appropriate decision makings can improve the quality of human life (Suleyman et al., 2018; A. Muhtaroglu et al., 2017; U. Qureshi et al., 2017; D. Evans et al., 2011; Akash et al., 2019).

Energy Saving Methods

The goal of energy scavenging is expand battery life or restores battery from ultra-low-power electronic systems. It is necessary to discover available resources in favor of energy scavenging circuits, in addition, evaluate whether the subsequent technology is helpful for a definite application. Universally, solar, mechanical movements/vibrations, thermal, and mostly radio frequency resources are exploited to produce electrical power/energy. Mechanical movements/vibration based energy generation divided into three main classes, those are piezoelectric, electromagnetic and electrostatic (A. Harb et al., 2011; H. Rashidzadeh et al., 2016). But it is the most serious criteria to ensure whether the specific definite energy scavenging system satisfactory for particular WBANs appliance. Moreover, output power, physical size, characteristics of the harvesting circuits, power resource extraction capacity play an important position for the potential application which should be carefully monitored.

In generally convoluted systems that have more interface circuits will constantly diminish the effectiveness of circuit, the output of micro scavenging circuit transform among micro-watts to milli-watts that is all most extremely lesser to run a system. So the integration of these circuits may reduce cost, size and increase the efficiency of the circuit. Classification of micro scavenging depending upon the source types some of them mentioned here

Photovoltaic Energy Scavenging (PV)

Basically PV energy scavenging generates energy from outside source either sunlight or artificial light to fabricate electricity. PV cells composed with semiconductor materials which absorb light source from the outside world (Suleyman et al., 2018; C. Gould et al., 2016). In this method, we use the effect of the p-n junction where semiconductor releases electrons from the absorbed light source, those released electron collected at electrodes to create voltage difference. Because of the result of varying temperature and irradiance the output characteristic of the PV cell non-linearly changes, it is very hard to get optimal current levels and voltage at harvester to obtain maximum power (D. Brunelli et al., 2008). So here we apply maximum power point tracking (MPPT), it has two structures with a digital signal processor or microprocessor, another without digital signal processor or microprocessor. (A. Liberale et al., 2014) authors propose a method for energy scavenging, especially for WBAN applications. In this harvester system, there is no battery, energy is stored in a super capacitor, once it founds enough power, it will send and receive data from collated by sensor nodes. The main goal of the proposed system is to work in indoor conditions. But because of its small size of super capacitor, it produces low leakage current. (W. Y. Toh et al., 2014) authors propose a system Flexible energy harvesting (FEH) mechanism as energy storage, which uses the ultra-low-power management system specially designed on flexible printed circuit board (PCB). Results of experiments indicate that wearable WBANs able to monitor temperature read data and transmit back to the base node using wireless communication even though in typical indoor condition.

Thermoelectric Energy Scavenging

Thermoelectric energy generators extract power from temperature differences; clearly, the generator produces electrical energy by using the temperature gradient between hot and cold surfaces. These generators contain both p and n-type semiconductors connected in two ways electrically in series way thermally in a parallel way. However, thermoelectric energy scavenging is less intermittent because they work as long as temperature difference across their surfaces, stationary structure, and easily scalable and moreover long lifetime makes them very attractive principally for Body area networks applications (Süleyman et al., 2018). However thermoelectric need an interface circuit to boost the output voltage in order to make the voltage level high enough to drive a sensor node? This type of harvesting methods is more convenient in wireless body area networks applications since the human body can help to constantly produce differences between hot and cold surfaces on generators. (D. C. Hoang et al., 2009) describes a Thermoelectric based system for WBANs. They use the accelerometer to detect any fall event. Power is stored in a capacitor to have a higher energy level which is necessary to power loads. Power storage and release events are controlled by two MOSFET. (R. Kanan et al., 2016) presented a new energy harvesting method using a bracelet type device to boost sensor using a thermal generator, sensor accumulated data sent to smart-phone for continuous monitoring.

Piezoelectric Energy Scavenging for WBAN

Mechanical movements or vibration are one of the sources for energy harvesting. Piezoelectric is a renowned technique which typically used in WBANs applications in the recent era. Generator stimulates current in the coil when there is relative motion among coil and magnetic field that motion is created by movement or vibration mechanism. Separation of charge is the principle in piezoelectric energy scavenging and it's calculated as coupling factor, which shows how much amount of mechanical energy transformed into electric energy (C. Lu et al., 2011). (I. Mahbub et al 2016) designed piezoelectric transducer based model for low breathing problem. This model is employed as a wearable device around the chest same as a belt, transducer gets charge in reaction to trembling created in inhalation/breathing. Transducer utilized as a sensor, no need for static power moreover inhalation data is composed in actual fact without any disturbance created to patient. This kind of piezoelectric energy scavenging is very much optimistic for WBAN applications.

Radio Frequency Energy Scavenging

Radio signals always reachable in air exceptionally in big cities. Capturing radio signals with help of antenna the procedure of RF energy scavenging is begin. Confined RF signals reformed into DC with the help of different techniques depending on the application. This type of energy harvesting does not affect the environmental conditions so easily applicable to WBAN applications. TV band 41MHz to 950 MHz, ISM band 2.4 GHz, GSM 0.85-0.90 GHz, and 1.8GHz to 1.9 GHz, 3G band, Wi-Fi band 2.45GHz to 5.8GHz, 4G band, CDMA band are some resources for Radiofrequency energy scavenging. (A. Shirane et al., 2015) authors presented power management unit based on RF energy harvesting for battery limited WBANs. The designed PMU has a suitable duty cycle process; it has two operations energy charging and discharging times. The availability of RF signals amplifies the significance, potential of

RF schemes in favor of both WSN and WBAN. But one drawback low output voltages and power is still an intensive research area, there is some more area like multi-band RF energy harvesting, RF circuits, wearable antennas are made the possibility of attracting WBANs applications.

Hybrid Energy Scavenging

Recent researches/studies on energy scavenging found that combinational models similarly hybrid energy harvesting systems to soak energy from sources in order to satisfy the demand of WBANs and which can produce great results compare with other technologies. RF-PZT, TEG-F, and PZT-TEG are some notable hybrid systems which can reduce communication range as well as on-board features of WBAN. Furthermore, its new research area and mainly focused on combinations of two energy harvesting models in future we can see these types of models with high voltage output and power concentration compared to single resource harvesting. Additionally, the use of multiple sources could be an advantage if one source not working properly another source use for continuous operation to power WBAN. (S.-W. Wang et al., 2011) proposed completely new hybrid energy harvesting by employing both TEG along with a solar cell to pull-out needed energy. Gained energy of TEG transform toward sensor but its limited, here solar cell provides power for both sensor and electric ADC, RF circuits. However, for better efficiency and power productivity hybridization is one of the futures trading technologies to energy harvesting. It absolutely guarantees technology which will boost communication range of WBAN.

NECESSARY REQUIREMENTS FOR ADOPTION OF WIRELESS BODY AREA NETWORK

Adoption and diffusion of BAN depend upon factors that involve both consumers and manufacturers. Value, security, privacy, compatibility, safety and ease of use are some user consumer requirements which are explained below (Negra R et al., 2016; Ullah S et al., 2012).

1. Specific goal value may depend on many factors such as internal, external factors, assessment ability but overall the concept of BASN must improve its user's quality life.
2. Quality of data is very important in healthcare for appropriate decision making. Unauthorized access, exploitation of system function could make brutal cost. Security measures such as authentication, accessibility will prevent such brutal cost.
3. BASN entrust with potentially sensitive information regarding people. Encryption technique is necessary for protecting sensitive data and encryption techniques must be resource-aware. Both technical and non-technical solutions are required to achieve user privacy, BASN package needs to attention against not noticeable medical conditions.
4. Arranged BASN nodes must cooperate with other BASN nodes, existed inter-BASN networks and electronic record systems. For this high standard communication protocols and data, formats are needed.
5. Wireless body sensors, wearable sensors, and implanted sensors need to be biocompatible in order to prevent harm to users/individuals.
6. Wearable and body sensors need to be small in size, easy to employ, stylish in looks, few in numbers.

Beyond these consumer requirements, BASN manufactures in order to get products in the market they will face expensive regulatory processes. After development, WBASN system will involve in complex web of stockholders such as physicians, users, researchers, emergency services and so on, each stockholder create and derive value for BASN systems Those derived values create complex relationships such as ownership and liability issues (Negra R et al., 2016; Ullah S et al., 2012).

APPLICATIONS

As a result of current research advancement and market demands, Body area network (BAN) research concentrated on healthcare applications, recognizing weakness about classical patient/individual data composed works, conditional observation and irregular samplings. WBAN continuously capture a variety of qualitative information from different sensor nodes for longer periods. Combinations of both medicinal and non-medicinal appliances regarding WBANs boost the quality of human life. Researches continuously working for heart regulation, drug delivery, and deep brain stimulation moreover BASN technology help to protect humans from life-threatening environments like soldiers taken away battleground, space, and deep sea explodes. Continuous monitoring, early assistance, and detection of disease, feedback of post-surgery are some of the healthcare application areas of WBAN. Nonmedical applications include movement and gesture detection for assisting player behavior in gaming, assistance in driving, cognitive recognition and many more. WBAN has a wide variety of applications such as military, sports, healthcare, entertainment and many others some of them listed below for your understanding (Rahat Ali Khan et al., 2018; Jose-Luis et al., 2018; Sourav et al., 2018).

Medicinal Applications

WBAN has the ability to transfer healthcare since it recommends sophisticate and monitoring data in real life. As per the reports from world health organization (WHO) more than 2.5 billion people will be beyond the age of 60 years and there were about to 17.7 million cardiovascular diseases, higher than 422 million inhabitants agony from diabetes. Dieses like asthma, cancer and parkinson's are fatal, which can prevent if we detect them at the right time. With the help of WBAN application, we can reinforce the healthcare system so it can valuable in premature detection of any kind of diseases. Moreover, according to the reports, compulsory medical procedures might be taken to avoid diseases before it attacks (Rahat Ali Khan et al., 2018; Jose-Luis et al., 2018).

Asthma Monitoring

Air pollution, weather changes are the two most crucial reasons linked to the asthma disease, nowadays asthma become as common diseases because of increasing environmental pollution and it turns to fatal if not treated in the right time. Asthma infected patient need to take timely precautions before it turns to an allergy (Chen M 2011). WBAN based asthma monitoring systems backing the asthma patients in early recognition of dangerous situations. WBAN sensor can also detect factors or agents which influence the cause of allergy which is helpful for people who suffer from asthma.

Sports Training

Besides wellbeing monitoring of individual and critical patients from life-threatening issues, WBANs be able to bring into play for uninterrupted and isolated monitoring where the health is essential. Fields consist of players in dissimilar sports, aircraft pilots; astronauts, etc need WBANs to handle critical issues of individuals. Heart rate, body temperature, blood glucose, respiratory rates are important in health monitoring of athletes, sports players/members. More clearly at some stage in training time as well as during game time, athlete or player observed for their performance so based on those training test achievements they could be preferred or drop from a game. Observed standards saved as acknowledgment for future prospect in-order to make the player to skilled and to give the first-rate comeback.

Fall Detection

Fall detection system is real-time wearable and alarm notification system. It has wearable indolence sensor node outfitted by tri-axial accelerometer detecting and recognizing a different kind of fall detections with the help of personal mobile device employed at the wrist. This kind of device very helpful for old-age people who can move but fall down anyplace due to their illness or dotage.

Sleep Monitoring

Healthful sleep is important on the way to sustain mental and physical strength; it's a basic and fundamental need to human. If human lack of sleep several diseases and fatalities will occur. Narcolepsy is a neurological disease which influences the management of sleep as well as sleeplessness (Latre´ B 2011). In fact, large numbers of people affected by sleep disorders because of work stress, increasing the usage of modern technology devices (mobile phone). Polysomnography (PSG) analytical technique employed to monitor sleep disorders furthermore saves observed sleep information as feedback for doctors in future response. Researchers keep working on WBAN architectures for observing sleep disorders and applying sensors nodes to reduce the complexity of wired PSG.

Cardiovascular Diseases (CVD)

Cardiovascular is one of the leading causes of death all over the world. As we know one of the foremost purposes of WBAN is premature recognition of regular working and medical abnormalities. Heart attack (Myocardial infarction) is the most deadly one for people deaths. In case uncharacteristic conditions are examined on a standard basis, the outcome of heart attack can be condensed via WBAN technology.

Cancer Detection

Cancer is also one of the leading deaths of people globally. WBAN sensors have the capability to monitor cancer cells efficiently moreover proficient to make a diagnosis tumors devoid-of biopsy.

Diabetes Control

Diabetes is nothing but the process of the patient/individual body loses the capacity to control/operate insulin. Present surveys show that diabetes caused deaths constantly increasing moreover the number of inhabitants having diabetes is predicted to reach 458 million by the year 2010. With the assist of employed body sensor nodes, we can evaluate the diabetic level.

Patient Monitoring

Physical monitoring /activities turn to more important since they are related to health position. Activity monitoring easily achieved by WBAN systems which have the potential to allow internetworking with other networks or devise such as the Internet of Things (IoT).

Telemedicine System

The ambient assisted living (AAL) aim toward a focus on utilizes promising information and transmission technology. BASN connects electronic components to make available continence to consumers.

Non-Medicinal Applications

A little-noted non-medicinal application of WBANs are described below

Biometrics

WBAN for nonmedical applications mostly used for security purpose such as banking sector, locking and unlocking bank locker, smart phones, and other security devices. For secure transactions, bio-related signs work out to create a digital signature.

Entertainment Applications

WBAN also attractive for various fields like sports and entertainment. Several types of music can be twisted on home base applications by monitoring face gestures and some kind of video may probably start playing on a TV monitor during work-out.

CHALLENGES AND OPPORTUNITIES

1. IoT devices in health-protection systems remain an interesting objective for cybercriminals because IoT devices have weak security measurements. Securities with privacy are two central concerns in Healthcare IoT. Because healthcare systems in IoT use context, personal information, locations of patients in order to provide services. By using some simple hardware or software we cannot defend attacks on them. For example, an attacker can effortlessly examine the physical activity of the patient. Fake IoT services, for instance, whenever one mechanism wants to connect with another

mechanism or access point there are some possible choices to choose fake service that offers best signals. So adversaries can easily access sensitive information of patients and also stored data in medical data storages. So research community should focal point on increasing efficient privacy and security protocol mechanism for healthcare IoT systems (Sur S et al., 1993; Abdullah wan et al., 2016; Rahat Ali Khan et al., 2018).

2. Expansion of protracted linkage of lifespan enlarge the network presentation, there is need for continual study on energy responsive routing procedures for WBAN.
3. Data privacy is greatly compromised since patient data are top secret, so it is essential to improve safety measures mutually in the system and in the repositories.
4. Human body posture is one the critical challenge in IoT healthcare systems. The nodes which are deployed for this purpose are communicated via line of sight, line of sight is one type of propagation where both transmitters, as well as the receiver, must be in outlook to each other without any disturbances then only they can able to transmit and receive data. But due to various positions of patients during sleeping, sitting positions and more challenging one is patients body movements (while moving human middle body makes different angles so sensor cannot communicate with other sensors appropriately) signal transmission could be inconvenience, due to inconvenient in line of sight they cannot able to communicate properly (Rahat Ali Khan et al., 2018).
5. Execution of Machine learning techniques for data preprocessing, compression and predictive analysis for health management information in WBAN need to progress more.
6. Impeding cognitive radio technology into healthcare sensor nodes, it would be helpful to provide great application development. For example with the help of cognitive radio technology sensor node can turn on and off based on some definite perspective of users, as a result, some energy can be saved (Sur S et al., 1993; Abdullah wan et al., 2016; Rahat Ali Khan et al., 2018).
7. Network transformation interruptions mostly done because of huge frame structures which require higher bandwidth which was not available in WBAN. Sometimes medical information needed immediate retrospective actions to threatening health conditions of patients. With the help of data compression and preprocessing techniques bandwidth usage can be reduced.
8. Energy consumption is also important challenging in WBAN, where sensor nodes need energy for its every sensitivity actions and communications. More work has to done on energy efficient and sensor protocols should be made more limelight. With the help of energy scavenging technologies we can to improve the battery lifetime (Sur S et al., 1993; Abdullah wan et al., 2016; Rahat Ali Khan et al., 2018).
9. In some recent works accuracy of healthcare system improved with the help of amalgamation of multi-sensor BSN. But the amalgamation of multi-data from multiple-sensor nodes, sensor nodes sources will become a challenging task. So research can focus on developing efficient techniques for improving amalgamation of BSN data (Abdullah wan et al., 2016; Rahat Ali Khan et al., 2018).
10. Sensors improve the technical feasibility of healthcare systems however designers face a number of problems while design such as size, ease of use, reliability so the research community must focus on these design issues. Moreover, low latency of 5G has the potentials to be transmitted over mobile networks. Combination of such advanced technologies can help in real time lower risk operations.
11. Much more important challenge task in WBAN which makes every research group busy is how sensors in BSN use gain study temperature of the body to convert into an energy source (Rahat Ali Khan et al., 2018; Sur S et al., 1993).

CONCLUSION

The chapter has provided comprehensive reports on WBAN devices for supervise human activity monitoring. Description of Architectures, Applications, energy saving methods along with security issues, applications, and challenges provided. Above mentioned sections contain energetic area of research. Numerous research works to be done in the areas of light weight, energy saving and high performance wireless devices to monitor dissimilar human activities. As a result of various innovations in IoT, communication facilities, cloud computing, machine learning, artificial intelligence expectations regarding extension of WBAN will be likely to explode. But still there are issues in security and energy efficiency of nodes.

REFERENCES

Abdullah, W. A. N., Yaakob, N., & Elobaid, M. E. (2016). Energy efficient remote healthcare monitoring using IoT: a review of trends and challenges. In *Proceedings of the international conference on the Internet of Things and cloud computing*. New York: ACM. 10.1145/2896387.2896414

Akash,, G., Chakraborty, C., & Bharat, G. (2019). Medical Information Processing Using Smartphone Under IoT Framework. *Springer: Energy Conservation for IoT Devices, Studies in Systems. Decision and Control, 206*, 1–26.

Amin, N. U., & Asad, M. C. (2013). An authenticated key management with rekeying for secured body sensor networks based on Hybrid cryptography. *ICNC, 9th IEEE international conference.*

Bandodkar, A. J., Jia, W., Yardimci, C., Wang, X., Ramirez, J., & Wang, J. (2015). Tattoo-based noninvasive glucose monitoring: A proof-of-concept study. *Analytical Chemistry, 87*(1), 394–398. doi:10.1021/ac504300n PMID:25496376

Bluetooth. (2017). *Bluetooth technology*. Retrieved from https://www.bluetooth.com/

Brunelli, Benini, Moser, & Thiele. (2008, March). An efficient solar energy harvester for wireless sensor nodes. *Design, Automation and Test in Europe*, 104-109.

Chakraborty, Gupta, & Ghosh. (2016). Mobile Telemedicine Systems for Remote Patient's Chronic Wound Monitoring. In *M-Health Innovations for Patient-Centered Care*, (pp. 217-243). IGI Global.

Chakraborty, C. (2019). Mobile Health (m-Health) for Tele-wound Monitoring. *IGI: Mobile Health Applications for Quality Healthcare Delivery, Ch., 5*, 98–116.

Chakraborty, C., Gupta, B., & Ghosh, S. K. (2014). Mobile metadata assisted community database of chronic wound images. *Wound Medicine, 6*, 34–42. doi:10.1016/j.wndm.2014.09.002

Chander & Kumaravelan. (2018). One class outlier detection Using SVM formulations in WSN harsh environments. *International Journal of Recent Technology and Engineering, 7*(4).

Chander. (2018). A Analysis of machine learning in WSN. *International Journal of Engineering & Technology, 7*(4).

Chen, M., Gonzalez, S., Vasilakos, A., Cao, H., & Leung, V. C. M. (2011). Body area networks: A survey. *Mobile Networks and Applications*, *16*(2), 171–193. doi:10.100711036-010-0260-8

Chinmay, C. B. G., & Ghosh, S. K. (2013). A Review on Telemedicine-Based WBAN Framework for Patient Monitoring. *Telemedicine Journal and e-Health*, *19*(18). PMID:23841489

Choong, C. L., Shim, M. B., Lee, B. S., Jeon, S., Ko, D. S., Kang, T. H., ... Im, J. (2014). Highly stretchable resistive pressure sensors using a conductive elastomeric composite on a micropyramid array. *Advanced Materials*, *26*(21), 3451–3458. doi:10.1002/adma.201305182 PMID:24536023

Chortos, A., & Bao, Z. (2014). Skin-inspired electronic devices. *Materials Today*, *17*(7), 321–331. doi:10.1016/j.mattod.2014.05.006

Demir. (2018). Energy Scavenging Methods for WBAN Applications: A Review. *IEEE Communications*, 1558-1748.

DeVaul, R., Sung, M., Gips, J., & Pentland, A. (2003). MIThril applications and architecture. *SeventhIEEE International Symposium on Wearable Computers*, 4-11. 10.1109/ISWC.2003.1241386

Dohler, D., Michael, P., & Binder, W. H. (2017). CuAAC-based click chemistry in self-healing polymers. *Accounts of Chemical Research*, *50*(10), 2610–2620. doi:10.1021/acs.accounts.7b00371 PMID:28891636

Edwards. (2012). Wireless sensors relay medical insight to patients and caregivers. *IEEE Signal Process. Magzine.*, *29*(3), 8–12.

Eom, J., Jaisutti, R., Lee, H., Lee, W., Heo, J. S., Lee, J. Y., ... Kim, Y. H. (2017). Highly sensitive textile strain sensors and wireless user-interface devices using all-polymeric conducting fibers. *ACS Applied Materials & Interfaces*, *9*(11), 10190–10197. doi:10.1021/acsami.7b01771 PMID:28251848

Evans, D. (2011). *The Internet of Things - How the Next Evolution of the Internet is Changing Everything.* White Paper. Cisco Internet Business Solutions Group (IBSG).

Fernández, L., Blasco, J.M., & Hernández, J.F. (2009). *Wireless sensor networks in ambient intelligence. Book Wireless Sensor Networks in Ambient Intelligence City*. Univ. Politécnica de Valencia: Technologies for Health and Well-being Institute ITACA.

Gould, C., & Edwards, R. (2016). Review on Micro-Energy Harvesting Technologies. *51st International Universities Power Engineering Conference (UPEC)*, 1-5.

Hanson, Powell Jr., Barth, & Ringgenberg. (2009). *Body Area Sensor networks: Challenges and opportunities.* IEEE Computer Society.

Harb. (2011). Energy harvesting: State-of-the-art. *Renewable Energy*, *36*, 2641-2654.

He, D., Ye, R., Chan, S., Guizani, M., & Xu, Y. (2018). Privacy in the Internet of Things for Smart Healthcare. *IEEE Communications Magazine*, *56*(4), 38–44. doi:10.1109/MCOM.2018.1700809

Hoang, D. C., Tan, Y. K., Chng, H. B., & Panda, S. K. (2009). Thermal energy harvesting from human warmth for wireless body area network in medical healthcare system. In *International Conference on Power Electronics and Drive Systems (PEDS)* (pp.1277-1282). Academic Press. 10.1109/PEDS.2009.5385814

Ibarra, E., Antonopoulos, A., Kartsakli, E., Rodrigues, J., & Verikoukis, C. (2016). QoS-aware energy management in body sensor nodes powered by human energy harvesting. *IEEE Sensors Journal, 16*(2), 542–549. doi:10.1109/JSEN.2015.2483064

Jingwei Liu, K. S. K. (2010). Hybrid security mechanisms for wireless body area networks. *Second Int. Conf. Ubiquitous Future Networks*, 98–103. 10.1109/ICUFN.2010.5547221

Jose-Luis, B.-M. (2015). *Wearable Sensors Integrated with Internet of Things for Advancing eHealth Care Sensors*. MDPI.

Kamta & Chakraborty. (2019). A Novel Approach Toward Enhancing the Quality of Life in Smart Cities using Clouds and IoT-Based Technologies. Springer: Digital Twin Technologies and Smart Cities, 1-17.

Kanan & Bensalem. (2016). Energy harvesting for wearable wireless healthcare systems. *IEEE Wireless Communications and Networking Conference.*

Kanaparthi, S., & Badhulika, S. (2017). Low cost, flexible and biodegradable touch sensor fabricated by solvent-free processing of graphite on cellulose paper. *Sensors and Actuators. B, Chemical, 242*, 857–864. doi:10.1016/j.snb.2016.09.172

Kanaparthi, S., Sekhar, V. R., & Badhulika, S. (2016). Flexible, eco-friendly and highly sensitive paper antenna based electromechanical sensor for wireless human motion detection and structural health monitoring. *Extreme Mech. Lett, 9*, 324–330. doi:10.1016/j.eml.2016.09.007

Khan & Pathan. (2018). The state-of-the-art wireless body area sensor networks: A survey. *International Journal of Distributed Networks, 14*(4).

Latre´, B., Braem, B., Moerman, I., Blondia, C., & Demeester, P. (2011). A survey on wireless body area networks. *Wireless Networks, 17*(1), 1–18. doi:10.100711276-010-0252-4

Le, X. H., Khalid, M., Sankar, R., & Lee, S. (2011). An Efficient Mutual Authentication and Access Control Scheme for Wireless Sensor Network in Healthcare. *Journal of Networks, 27*, 355–364.

Li, R. Z., Hu, A., Zhang, T., & Oakes, K. D. (2014). Direct writing on paper of foldable capacitive touch pads with silver nano wire inks. *ACS Applied Materials & Interfaces, 6*(23), 21721–21729. doi:10.1021/am506987w PMID:25365734

Liberale, Dallago, & Barnabei. (2014). Energy harvesting system for wireless body sensor nodes. *IEEE Biomedical Circuits and Systems Conference (BioCAS) Proceedings*, 416-419. 10.1109/BioCAS.2014.6981751

Liu, Y., Wang, H., Zhao, W., Zhang, M., Qin, H., & Xie, Y. (2018). Flexible, Stretchable Sensors for Wearable Health Monitoring: Sensing Mechanisms, Materials, Fabrication Strategies and Features. *Sensors (Basel), 18*(2), 645. doi:10.339018020645 PMID:29470408

Lu, C., Raghunathan, V., & Roy, K. (2011). Efficient design of micro-scale energy harvesting systems. *IEEE J. Emerging Sel. Topics Circuits Syst, 1*(3), 254–266. doi:10.1109/JETCAS.2011.2162161

Mahbub, Wang, Islam, Pullano, & Fiorillo. (2016). A low power wireless breathing monitoring system using piezo electric transducer, *IEEE International Symposium on Medical Measurements and Applications. (MeMeA)*, 1-5.

Malhi, S. C., Mukhopadhyay, S. C., Schnepper, J., Haefke, M., & Ewald, H. (2012). A Zigbee-based wearable physiological parameters monitoring system. *IEEE Sensors Journal*, *12*(3), 423–430. doi:10.1109/JSEN.2010.2091719

Mazzeo, A. D., Kalb, W. B., Chan, L., Killian, M. G., Bloch, J. F., Mazzeo, B. A., & Whitesides, G. M. (2012). Paper-based, capacitive touch pads. *Advanced Materials*, *24*(21), 2850–2856. doi:10.1002/adma.201200137 PMID:22539155

Muhtaroglu. (2017). Micro-scale energy harvesting for battery less information technologies in Energy Harvesting and Energy Efficiency: Technology. *Methods and Applications, 37*, 63-85.

Negra, R., Jemili, I., & Belghith, A. (2016). Wireless body area networks: Applications and technologies. *Procedia Computer Science*, *83*, 1274–1281. doi:10.1016/j.procs.2016.04.266

Otto, C., & Milenković, A. (2006). System Architecture of a Wireless Body Area Sensor network for Ubiquitous Health Monitoring. *Journal OF Mobile Multimedia*, *1*(4), 307–326.

Patel, S., Park, H., Bonato, P., Chan, L., & Rodgers, M. (2012). A review of wearable sensors and systems with application in rehabilitation. *Journal of Neuroengineering and Rehabilitation*, *9*(1), 21. doi:10.1186/1743-0003-9-21 PMID:22520559

Qureshi, F. U., Muhtaroğlu, A., & Tuncay, K. (2017). Near-optimal design of scalable energy harvester for underwater pipeline monitoring applications with consideration of impact to pipeline performance. *IEEE Sensors Journal*, *17*(7), 1981–1991. doi:10.1109/JSEN.2017.2661199

Rajagopal, M. K., & Rodriguez-Villegas, E. (2013). Towards wearable sleep diagnostic systems for point-of-care applications. *Proceedings of the 2013 IEEE point-of-care healthcare technologies (PHT)*. 10.1109/PHT.2013.6461276

Rashidzadeh, H., Kasargod, P. S., Supon, T. M., Rashidzadeh, R., & Ahmadi, M. (2016). Energy harvesting for IoT sensors utilizing MEMS technology. *2016 IEEE Canadian Conference on Electrical and Computer Engineering (CCECE 2016)*. 10.1109/CCECE.2016.7726622

Shirane, Ito, Ishihara, & Masu. (2015). An RF energy harvesting power management circuit for appropriate duty-cycled operation. *Japanese Journal of Applied Physics*, *54*(4S), 04DE11.1-04DE11.6. March.

Sourav, Chakraborty, & Sumit. (2018). A Survey on IoT based Traffic Control and Prediction Mechanism. In *Internet of Things and Big data Analytics for Smart Generation, Intelligent Systems Reference Library*. Springer.

Sourav, Chakraborty, & Paul. (2019). Programming Paradigm and Internet of Things. In A Handbook of Internet of Things & Big Data. CRC.

Sravanth, C. C., & Anudeep, B. G. (2019). Classification Algorithms for EEG-based Brain-Computer Interface: A Review. IGI Global.

Sur, S., Crotty, T. B., Kephart, G. M., Hyma, B. A., Colby, T. V., Reed, C. E., ... Gleich, G. J. (1993). Sudden-onset fatal asthma: A distinct entity with few eosinophils and relatively more neutrophils in the airway submucosa? *The American Review of Respiratory Disease*, *148*(3), 713–719. doi:10.1164/ajrccm/148.3.713 PMID:8368644

Toh, W. Y., Tan, Y. K., Koh, W. S., & Siek, L. (2014). Autonomous wearable sensor nodes with flexible energy harvesting. *IEEE Sensors Journal*, *14*(7), 2299–2306. doi:10.1109/JSEN.2014.2309900

Tzanis, G. (2018). Healthcare data analysis in the Internet of things era. In D. B. A. Khosrow-Pour (Ed.), *Encyclopedia of information science and technology* (4th ed.; pp. 1984–1994). Hershey, PA: IGI Global. doi:10.4018/978-1-5225-2255-3.ch172

Ullah, S., Higgins, H., & Braem, B. (2012). A comprehensive survey of wireless body area networks. *Journal of Med Systems, 36*(3), 1065–1094.

Wang, S.-W., Im, J.-P., & Cho, G.-H. (2011). Dual-input dual-output energy harvesting DC-DC boost converter for wireless body area network. In *IEEE Biomedical Circuits and Systems Conference (BioCAS)* (pp.217-220). IEEE. 10.1109/BioCAS.2011.6107766

Chapter 7
Methodical IoT-Based Information System in Healthcare

Ambika Nagaraj
Department of Computer Applications, SSMRV College, Bangalore, India

ABSTRACT

Elderly monitoring has become essential to provide comfort and flexible life for the aged. Internet of things is a field that aids in providing accurate information through communication. Using these devices, emergency alerts can be raised. The chapter provides an assistance model that aids the caretakers and doctors to provide appropriate action during emergencies. Different conditions of the patient are considered to analyze the working of the system. The work shows considerable amount of flexibility from the previous system.

INTRODUCTION

Elderly monitoring is essential in today's world. Smart equipment can be used to supervise the object of interest and alert the necessities in time. According to the world health organization report, the elderly in South-East Asian region is rising at the rate of 6% in comparison to the world population (McEvedy, Colin, & Jones, 1978). The report claims to double from 12% in 2015 to 22% in 2020. The life expectancy of the elderly will outnumber the infants below the age of 5 years. According to the recent survey 125 million people are aged 80+ onwards. Due to various reasons some of the elderly are subjected to stay alone and look after themselves. The elderly are liable to frail and hence require help (Chakraborty, B., & S.K., 2016) (C, B, & S.K., 2014) (G, Chakraborty, & G, 2019) from others. Some of the common disorders in this category of humans are hearing loss (Boi, et al., 2012) (Weinstein, E., Spitzer, & Ventry, 1986), back/neck pain (Bressler, B., Keyes, Rochon, & Badley, 1999) (Lavsky-Shulan, Wallace, Kohout, Lemke, Morris, & Smith, 1985), diabetes (Meneilly, S., & Tessier, 2001) and so on. These elderly are

DOI: 10.4018/978-1-7998-0261-7.ch007

reluctant to many kinds of fatal conditions like Alzheimer disease (Devanand, Taylor, Gurland, Wilder, Stern, & Mayeux, 1996), stroke (Draper, Poulos, Cole, Poulos, & Ehrlich, 1992), heart attacks (Piller, et al., 2006), etc which requires immediate attention.

Internet-of-things (Pang, et al., 2015) aids in providing an appropriate measure for these kinds of situations. IoT devises aids in better communication through web applications and mobile devices to the respective personnel. Using these communicating devices, the elderly whether indoor/outdoor will be under continuous surveillance. These devices provide alert to the receptor in case of emergencies. They also provide time-to-time information of the observed object. Many suggestions are provided by various authors (Abbate, Stefano, Avvenuti, Corsini, Light, & Vecchio., 2010). The authors in (Nasution, Hans, & Emmanuel, 2007) have considered only the indoor environment and provided their suggestions limited to that environment. Both indoor and outdoor environment (Bourouis, Abderrahim, Feham, & Bouchachia, 2011) (Mainetti, Patrono, Secco, & Sergi, 2016) are considered in some works. Considering outdoor environment the personnel has to be in constant vigilance. Each work provided by various authors addresses different issues or provides a better improvement over the other. The authors in (Mishra, Lin, & Chang, 2014) have addressed cardiac patients. In (Ani, Krishna, Anju, Aslam, & Deepa, 2017) the authors have considered the stroke patients and their monitoring.

Many kinds of wearables (Basanta, Huang, & Lee, 2016) are used by the authors. We-watch wristband is used to provide the solution to elderly monitoring in (Pinto, Sandro, Cabral, & Gomes, 2017). In (Shehab, Ismail, Osman, Elhoseny, & El-Henawy, 2017) a wearable ring device is used to monitor the health of the elderly. The devices are not required in some of the suggested work(Wang, Yuxi, Wu, & Ni, 2017). Each work consists of its own way of measuring and concluding the situation of the personnel. In (Chandel, Sinharay, Ahmed, & Ghose, 2016) the authors have used fall, immobility, step count and stride length are the basic events that are observed. In (Foroughi, Homa, Aski, & Pourreza, 2008) different poster-based events are used to detect the fall of the target.

The monitoring of the personnel using different methodology is suggested. The work is the outline of different components or the functionalities to be used to bring in a betterment to the personnel. The proposed study has incorporated additional functionalities to improve the performance of the previous system (Dziak, Jachimczyk, & Kulesza, 2017). The advantage of the system is it can incorporate new findings in the device and avail updated options to the personnel. The available case studies are considered to gain a better understanding of the system. The previous methodologies used by various personnel are compared against the existing scenario to accommodate the methodologies. New advance methodologies certified are considered to give the best assistance to the personnel. The work provides better flexibility compared to the previous system. The proposed work obtains 8% effectiveness and 12% better usage of new methodologies compared to (Dziak, Jachimczyk, & Kulesza, 2017). It obtains 3% more effectiveness and 1.67% better usage of new methodologies compared to (Bourouis, Abderrahim, Feham, & Bouchachia, 2011). The paper is divided into six sections. Literature survey is detailed in section 2. The drawbacks in (Dziak, Jachimczyk, & Kulesza, 2017) are discussed in section 3. Modified system design is suggested in section 4. Analysis w.r.t flexibility and updating new methodologies is provided in section 5. Future scope and research challenges are discussed in section 6. The work is concluded in section 7.

BACKGROUND

The proposed work suggests the outline to be considered to bring in effectiveness and flexibility in the system. The work incorporates analyzing different case studies, the use of previously adopted methodologies in different scenarios. The work also suggests using the new methodologies which can be availed by using IoT. The present section provides using the different methodologies to bring the suggestions into play. The methodologies suggested can be implemented by many kinds of devices and the authors suggest using different kinds of methodologies with various types of equipment to avail betterment for the personnel. The suggestion aids in monitoring process (Nguyen, Hong, Mirza, Naeem, & Nguyen, 2017) (Odunmbaku, Rahmani, Liljeberg, & Tenhunen, 2015) and alerting the respective in times of emergencies (Kleinberger, Becker, Ras, Holzinger, & Müller, 2007). The brief explanation of them is provided in this section.

Indoor Surveillance

In (Foroughi, Homa, Aski, & Pourreza, 2008) home surveillance scenario is considered. The work focuses on different poster-based events to detect the fall of the target. Three types of fall are detected using the suggested work. Many postures normal and abnormal were considered. The knowledge database consisted of ten different kinds of postures. The background estimation procedure was conducted by analyzing the motion in the given time frame window. The obtained silhouette was analyzed with the video sequences. The procedure aims to analyze the detected motion from abnormal. Temporal changes in head position are considered. The extracted image is fed into multilayer perceptrons (MLP) neural network (Karlik & Olgac, 2011) to determine fall.

The authors in (Nasution, Hans, & Emmanuel, 2007) considered the indoor environment. A single fixed camera was used to monitor the target of interest. The authors used the background subtraction method (Stauffer & Grimson, 1999) developed by Stauffer and Grimson to segment the moving object. The methodology is based on the assumption that the elderly will remain in a static position for a long time. Horizontal and vertical projection histograms are used to extract the foreground object. The angle between the last position and the new position is measured and analyzed. The histogram obtained is used as an input to the classifier. K-NN algorithm (Keller, M., Gray, & Givens, 1985) along with evidence accumulation methodology (Wagenmakers, et al., 2004) is used by the classifier. The implementation of the work was done using the OpenCV library. 12-16 frames/second was made to run on Intel Centrino Duo 1.83 GHz laptop. 30 video clips of 2 minutes of duration were used in the implementation. The distance between the camera and the person considered was 3 – 6 meters. The system was able to recognize five poster-based events. An average of eight frames as necessary to be accumulated to analyze an event. The work was able to recognise 93.21% of cameral events.

A smart home system is suggested by authors in (Arcelus, Amaya, Jones, Goubran, & Knoefel, 2007). Artificial Intelligence (AI) expert system (Fox, 1990) is recommended in this work. The dynamic architecture aims in applying the regular behavior and the ones observed over time. The system aids in making decisions on elderly status and physiological condition. Two systems were used – the lited pathway is used to guide the elderly in the dark and Austco DCS-2000 Dementia care system (Arcelus, Jones, Goubran, & Knoefel, 2007) is used to monitor the adult behavior. The Austco system consists of bed exit sensor, door reed switch, and passive infrared sensor. The knowledge database has sixteen different behaviours stored in it. The system makes a comparison of the behavior to the pre-defined behavior to detect the variation. The abnormalities are detected using the four-tier system – mild abnormality, caution, high alert, and emergency. In case of emergency, the direct line emergency services are availed by the system. In rest of the cases, the family member and the caretaker are alerted.

The authors in (Wang, Jin, Zhang, Li, Lee, & Sherratt, 2014) have proposed an enhanced system to monitor the elderly. The work is focussed on the changes that happen when the fall happens. Impact magnitude, trunk angle, and after-event heart rate are considered to derive conclusions. Signal magnitude vector is calculated considering the 3D axis. Different postures are gauged using three-axis and common changes. Based on the gauged outcomes emergency cases are listed.

The authors in (Ray & P, 2014) Home health hub Internet-of-things (IoT) is suggested. The layered based model consists of dependency and interconnectivity of biosensors, microcontroller, communication channels, applications, internet, and gateway. The architecture is designed to bring in mobility, flexibility and economical. The physiological sensing layer is used to sense physiological activities. The sensed data is later transmitted to the upper layers. Local communication layer mediates the data sent by the physiological layer to the upper layers. Information processing layer consists of a microcontroller that aids in processing the data. Internet application layer aids in conveying the information to any device using the internet facility. User application layer aids in providing visualization of the received message.

The smart home system was suggested by the authors in (Ghayvat, Mukhopadhyay, Gui, & Suryadevara, 2015). The system developed is reliable, efficient, flexible and economical. The nodes deployed are heterogeneous in nature. The readings are collected based on object usage and movement. The system is designed with two stages. The nodes are deployed to perform multiple activities in multiple events. Zigbee Technology (Farahani, 2011) is used to bring the thought into play. The central coordinator node collects the readings from the sensors. The coordinator node transmits the aggregated data to the home gateway. Data logging, data extraction, and data storage are some of the activities performed by the nodes.

Outdoor/Indoor Surveillance

A real-time mobile health system to monitor the elder patients is suggested in (Bourouis, Abderrahim, Feham, & Bouchachia, 2011). Both indoor and outdoor environments are considered. A bio-signal sensor is used to keep a tab on the patient's activities. Three major components make up the architecture. The wireless body area network worn by the patients monitor the activities of the same and transmit appropriate signals to the intelligent center node (ICN) through Bluetooth (Bray & Sturman, 2001) communication protocol. The star topology aids in communicating the signal to ICN. The second component after receiving the signal communicates with the intelligent center server (ICS). General packet radio service/ universal mobile telecommunication system (GPRS/UMTS) (Halonen, Romero, & Melero, 2004) is used to communicate. After receiving the readings the ICS makes a comparison to the pre-existing conditions and recommendations. The authenticated family member can check the status of the elderly through the web application. If an abnormal situation is detected the alert message is sent to the medical practitioner for assistance. Nokia Smartphone N95 is used as ICN in the work. The system works on Symbian v 9.2 based on S60 interface. Python programming is used to bring the work into play. Nonin sensors and Smartphone integrated sensors are managed using BT connections. MySQL database is used in the work. Apache server is used to connect the web application to the readings.

In (Ani, Krishna, Anju, Aslam, & Deepa, 2017) the suggestion is provided to minimize the future recurrence of stroke in patients. The system is a monitoring and diagnostic prediction tool. The system continuously monitors the patient's condition and transmitted to the cloud. The parameters received are analyzed and cross-verified against normal values. Any change observed is notified using SMS or email service. The classification algorithm is used to develop the prediction model. The hardware layer consists of Arduino mega microcontroller, pressure sensor, heartbeat sensor, and sugar sensor. The application layer consists of a web application, cloud server, and algorithm design. The web application is used to view and manipulate patient's records using a web application. The cloud is used for storing and analyzing data. This analyzed data is cross-verified against the testbed data to alert the respective during any variation. Different classification methodologies are used. The naive Bayesian classifier (Domingos & Pazzani, 1997) uses class conditional independence methodology. The values of predictors of the class are independent of each other. Random forest method (Albert, et al., 2008) utilizes multiple machine learning algorithms to end up in good prediction. The methodology is basically used for classification and regression. The subsets of data lead to a decision tree. Another approach used is K nearest neighbor method (Cunningham & Delany, 2007). The neighbors cast votes based on which classes are classified. The distance function is used to complete the procedure. The fourth classification is decision tree classification (Friedl & Brodley, 1997). Based on the relevant set of features a solution is proposed. Multiple classifiers are generated using different samples to reduce the variance of the prediction is bagging classification.

The authors in (Jimenez, Freddy, & Torres, 2015) have suggested building an Adhoc health care monitoring system. The technology build uses the current technology used in patients home. An addition or editing is done to create runtime alerts. The psychological parameters and environmental conditions are considered to create alerts. The system provides alerts to the relatives or the doctors connected with the patient. The essential medical attention required is alerted to the personnel's respective so that they can further with their set of actions. A sensor-tag is used for implementation purpose. CC2451 (Baoding & Liu, 2010) is a power-optimized true system-on-chip. It is a solution for Bluetooth with low energy working and proprietary 2.4 GHz applications. It gathers ambient data using Bluetooth sensor embedded inside them. The technology is based on a wireless sensor network where the sensors are equipped with the job to sense the environment, process the data and transmit them to the respective pre-defined destination. An application developed on the smartphone is used to access the necessary data by the concerned person. The tag is enabled to collect data like temperature, humidity, pressure, gyroscope, magnetometer and accelerometer (Bagala, et al., 2012). The tag is an energy-effective device. The battery of the device is capable of lasting for a long time. In the implementation, the authors have used smart sensor type chest belt to monitor the heart rate. The device monitors the heart rate and reports the readings. The smartphones are used as a gateway in the implementation to gather data from the patient's residence. The gateway is capable of converting data sensors to Extensible Messaging and Presence protocol messages (Nie, 2006). The software uses a special extension to do so. The software of the gateway uses Extensible Messaging and Presence protocol account to connect to the server. The server has XEP-0326 extensions. The system hence assures security between the two while transmitting the messages. The clyster technology (Waher, 2014) is used by the server. This technology enables the registration of new sensors. The system facilities the availability of the readings sensed by the sensors immediately. The technology aids in creating and modifying the model using new attached sensors. The server supports using sharing the sensors among the patients.

In (Park.S.J., et al., 2017) the authors have suggested a proactive measure to care stroke victims. The system captures the brain images, body movement signals. It does signal analysis, communication and detection and warning procedure. The authors have surveyed the occurrence of the medical emergency in case of stroke victims. The system consists of smart wearable devices that collect the parameters, notify the respective and alert the medical personnel in case of abnormalities. Some of the applications include Electro Cardiogram (ECG) for drivers that aid in preventing accidents. The system detects the heart signals, alerts the same when they lose track in case of sleep.

In (Baldiseera, Andrea, & M.Camarinhamatos, 2016) the authors have proposed a personalized and evolutionary care service model. The system collaborates with the network, context awareness (Abowd, Dey, Brown, Davies, Smith, & Steggles, 1999) and Internet-of-things. The Collaborative model is based on A Reference model for collaborative networks (ARCON reference model) (Camarinha-Matos, Afsarmanesh, Ermilova, Ferrada, Klen, & Jarimo, 2008) and ambient assisted living ecosystem context. The collaborative business ecosystem model supports integrated services to acquire agility. The system consists of a service composition model which can be single or collaboration of many entities. The work considers the variation of scenario and hence context awareness model is considered. The sub-system aids in adapting the service to the needs of the elderly, environment and the elderly life context. The assistance service provider shall analyze the situation and evolve with the model that suit the requirements. The system provides its suggestion to the elderly with the experimentation period. During this tenure, multisource information activity collects sensed data from multiple devices and helps the service provider support activity to store a new description in the service catalog. The received data is analyzed and suggestions are provided to the Elderly living environment customers.

A human monitoring system was proposed in (Shehab, Ismail, Osman, Elhoseny, & El-Henawy, 2017). The system aids in minimizing the overall cost for the users. Group of sensors is used to accomplish the job. A wearable ring device is used to monitor the health of the elderly. The system consists of three types of communications- device to device, the device to mobile and the hybrid sub-system.

In (Mainetti, Patrono, Secco, & Sergi, 2016) the authors have suggested Ambient assisted living for the elderly. The system provisions the elderly to take care of themselves without much intervention or monitoring. The system into the monitoring process continuously, checking the health status of the elderly by obtaining data from multiple sources. Environmental sensors and medical devices provide their aid in accomplishing the task. The system guarantees to localize the elderly in both indoor and outdoor environment. The remote reasoning system aids in analyzing and generating alerts of the elderly. The alerts are used to trigger a signal to the family member of the accident.

A daily monitoring system is suggested by the authors to care for the elderly (Kim, Seo, & Seo, 2016). The system consists of two sub-systems. IoT assisted living space is provided that encompasses contactless sensors gathering its readings from the environment. The system provides triggers in case of emergencies. The emergency gateway collects the data and generates alerts. It communicates with the daily monitoring server. The daily activity monitoring server aids in collecting data, events and user management. It also performs activity analysis and reporting. The work is also into the estimation of unexpected situation and hence aids in betterment.

Elderly monitoring service is suggested in (Miori & Russo, 2017). The environmental and physical user data is collected. The system called a smart-smile is a set of sub-modules. These modules act as a gateway to the interface. The gateways are designed to manage its defined set of functionalities. Interactions happen in three ways. The user can use his tablet, Smartphone (Abbate, Stefano, Avvenuti, Corsini, Light, & Vecchio., Monitoring of human movements for fall detection and activities recognition in elderly care using wireless sensor network: a survey., 2010) or a web interface to interact with the system. This kind of interaction is classified as indirect interaction. the second kind of interaction is when the devices get activated by the user's behavior. This kind of interaction is called the involuntary device interaction. Direct device interaction is where the occupant acts directly by touching some device.

The authors in (Almeida, Fiore, Mainetti, Mulero, Patrono, & Rametta, 2017) have aimed to create innovative frameworks. ICT tools are services are utilized to detect earlier detection of risk related population. Personalized intervention aids in improving the quality of life by bringing out positive behavioral changes. A set of geriatric factors and sub-factors are used as quantitative indicators. The aggregated values influence the factors with low-level abstractions and a large basin of sources. Low-level elementary actions (LEA) detect the behavior of the elderly. Person LEA tracks the mobility of the object, collects data w.r.t Smartphones and the number of visits it has paid. Home LEA is used to track the object in the home environment. It watches the usage of home appliances. City LEA is used to track the object indoor and outdoor environment.

The authors have suggested (Mishra, Lin, & Chang, 2014) to investigate the feasibility of implementing cognitive interference device. The interference algorithm is used in the work. An artificial neural model with different configurations is used to map the cognitive interference device functions. This procedure aids in minimizing the device prediction error. The intelligence and self-learning capabilities aid the monitoring process. The activity interference framework is used to analyze the brainwave patterns.

A novel signal quality-aware IoT enabled ECG telemetry system is suggested by authors in (Satija, Barathrum. Ramkumar, & Manikandan, 2016). The system is used for continuous cardiac monitoring. The suggested paradigm improve resource/network/bandwidth utilization, improves accuracy and reliability. The system reduces cloud server bandwidth, treatment cost, and traffic load. Three sub-modules are defined in the work. ECG signal sensing module, automated signal quality assessment module and signal quality-aware ECG analysis and transmission modules are the three sub-modules designed. The system is into detecting flat-line detection, abrupt baseline wanders extraction and high-frequency noise detection/extraction. The same is used to calculate signal quality index to assess the clinical acceptability of ECG signals.

Various technologies of devices are integrated with (Basanta, Huang, & Lee, 2016) to build an effective system. Wearable devices, biosensors and sensor network aid in the process. Real-time activity is monitored effectively in the system. The system connects the respective in times of emergency. The system consists of a central decision unit that detects an emergency and alerts the respective. The system analyzes the situation and makes a record of the same. The system also aids in managing the daily routine. The system provides remainder providing the details to the respective. The system increases efficiency and accessibility. It improves comfort and safety managing the routine activities.

The authors in (Chandel, Sinharay, Ahmed, & Ghose, 2016) have suggested the three-layered framework. Fitness monitoring and elderly care are the mottoes of the work. Fall, immobility, step count and stride length are the basic events observed. Inertial measurement units (embedded or wearable) form is used to collect readings. The sensors pre-process and transmit the data to the gateway and later to the cloud-based repository.

A set of heterogeneous system is used in (Ghose, Sinha, Bhaumik, Sinha, Agrawal, & Choudhury, 2013). In UbiHeld system, the occupant is expected to carry the Smartphone all the times with a few exceptions. Kinect is used to detect the sleeping patterns, watching TV, sitting idle of the occupant. Inertial sensors are used to cover other indoor activities.

A well-defined Ambient An assisted living system is suggested in (Mainetti, Luca, Patrono, Secco, & Sergi, 2017). The system is capable of capturing the data of the adults in the city premises and the home environments. The funded project City4Age is suggested to provide flexibility in monitoring the object of interest. Innovative framework on ICT tools is created. The service is enabled to serve European cities. The system is designed to detect early detection of risk related to frailty and Mild cognitive impairment (MCI) (Petersen, Smith, Waring, Ivnik, Tangalos, & Kokmen, 1999). The proposal aims to intervene to help the elderly population to improve their life. It also promotes positive behavioral changes. The proposal aims to activate urban communities. The social and health services are facilitated using the suggestions. The cognitive impairments services are also included in this project.

The motto of the project (Mainetti, Luca, Patrono, Secco, & Sergi, 2017) is to make the city enabled to take care of the elderly population by playing its major role in early detection of the ailment. The system is designed to initiate the cities to collect the data of the elderly randomly. The collected data is utilized in two ways. The data is used to identify the segments of the population under risk. Using the first set of data, the individuals are monitored coming under the risk category. The second category aims at detecting negative traits in behavior in the monitored individuals. The collected data falls into four categories. First category filters data related to user body activates. Regulars like sleep, walk, and motion is monitored to classify them as user motility category. The set of data is obtained by measuring the location of the individual which is categorized into indoor/outdoor localization category. This category includes locations like individual home, shopping mall, streets, parks, etc. The third category filters the data w.r.t indoor and outdoor environments. Temperature, humidity, and luminosity fall into this category. The fourth category is user-environment interaction category. The data related to the user environment is filtered and put into this category of data set. Using home application service and public services fall into this category. The system consists of two major components. The local environment building block is responsible to collect data from the sensors deployed in the network. This collected data is furnished to the upper layers. The task is accomplished without considering sensor technology and communication protocols used in the procedure. The cloud building block is the second component of the system. Low-level elementary actions contain the basic user actions, information related to time and position of action. The Low-level elementary actions transmit the collected details to cloud building block using REST API's. The other computations are completed by cloud building block. The segment is into measuring the changes in behavior using daily indicators. Some of the instances include the average speed of walking, number of walks, the number of visited shops, etc. The risk to the elderly is calculated based on the readings provided by the daily indicators. This data is availed to city4Aged platform.

The authors in (Khoi, Manh, Saguna, Mitra, & Åhlund, 2015) have suggested a remote health monitoring system. The designed system consists of many protocols placed in the lower layers. This methodology aids in effectively transmitting data to the remote servers. The system architecture consists of five layers namely sensing layer, home gateway, network infrastructure, cloud computing (Hayes, 2008) and application layer. Home automation devices such as actuators and sensors make up the sensing layer. The authors suggest using Radio Frequency Identification (RFID) (Finkenzeller, 2010), accelerometers in this layer. Data collection, filtering, encryption, and pre-processing and performed in-home gateway layer. OpenHAB (Bruce, 2015), middleware is used to integrate the system with home applications. The collected data from the home gateway is transmitted to the monitoring side. Technologies like WiFi (Balasubramanian, Mahajan, & Venkataramani, 2010) and Ethernet (Metcalfe & Boggs, 1976) can be utilized to do so. This data transmitted is received by the cloud. The sub-system uses different algorithms, dedicated software to extract what is required. The system is into storage and analytics after the filtration process. The application layer is the topmost layer of the system. This layer uses a web interface to interact with users. Using this layer the users will be able to read the sensor readings. The readings can aid in attending emergency situations, generating a summary report and monitoring the health condition of the adult.

A precise reconcilement is made between evidence theory with the frequentist approach of probability calculus by authors in (Sebbak, Faouzi, & Benhammadi, 2017). Combining beliefs are used to form the solution to the disadvantages created by evidence theory and its derivatives. Non-normalized conjunctive (Martin, Osswald, Dezert, & Smarandache, 2008) and majority rules are merged to bring in better work. The approach redistributes global conflict. The rule is based on normalization of the sum of masses mixed with the masses of majority rule. The masses of conjunctive consensus operation are also fused to the set. The authors have considered a simple implementation of shifting health monitoring to more personalized care. The authors have suggested two methodologies to do so. The first method suggests using external wearable sensors. The system uses embedded inertial sensors that aid in connecting it to the Smartphone. The activities the system focussed on include sleeping, exercising, watching television and fall detection. The data from the sensors are collected and transmitted to the Smartphone. The aggregated data is later used to recognize the activity, aggregation and generating inferences. Based on the deduction made the doctors can monitor the readings from anywhere. Using the accelerator sensor, Smartphone and heart rate monitor can provide an accurate scenario of the situation. Analyzing the situation the system sends an alert in case of emergency to the registered hospital and the caregiver.

In (Pinto, Sandro, Cabral, & Gomes, 2017) the authors have utilized we-watch wristband to provide the solution to elderly monitoring. The waistband is capable of collecting the data from the sensors w.r.t humidity, temperature, and many other environmental changes. The received signal strength indicator is collected. The system connects to We-care board using User Datagram Protocol (UDP) socket with the UDP server running on We-watch gateway. The sensors are provided their own roles to collect the necessities. The system consists of the push button which is used by the personnel to alert the caregiver. The received signal strength indicator value is used to trace the elderly. The on-board buzzer aids in dealing with a situation like out-of-range and disconnections. The accelerometer is used to detect the fall detection of the personnel. The device also keeps a tab on the activities of the personnel. The sensors are also provided the responsibility to monitor the body temperature of the elderly. The system provides an alert if the wristband is tried to be detached from the personnel.

The authors in (Hsieh, Yi-Zeng, & Jeng, 2018) suggested feedback optional flow convolution neural network system. The object recognition model has two learning stages. the Interest of point histogram is used in the detector model. The sub-system derives efficient features and transmits them as input to the convolution layer. The system uses back-propagation computation (Suresh, Omkar, & Mani, 2005). The motion object boundary is detected using this computation. The statistical Euclidean distance (Johnson & Wichcrn, 2002) of the histogram is calculated using feedback mechanism scheme of the optical flow vector. The required data is extracted using the back-propagation algorithm. The optimal flow feedback scheme is used to identify moving objects. A human is detected using temporal and facial information.

The authors in (Kelly, Tebje, Suryadevara, & Mukhopadhyay, 2013) have used the low-cost ubiquitous network to monitor the regulars. In the suggested work wireless sensor network and Zigbee technology are combined. The end devices are responsible to collect the data and transmit it to the coordinator. The Zigbee protocol translates the Zigbee data format to internet protocol format. The system is designed to measure electrical parameters and gain control over domestic objects. The system avoids complications by eliminating the monitoring process by multiple systems. The Zigbee sensors are used to gather information from the environment. The topology varies with the distance between the sensors and the coordinator. A star topology is formed if the sensor and coordinator distance is reachable. The system uses mesh topology in other cases. The sensor uses hop technology to transmit its data to the coordinator. A wired serial connection is provided between the router and the coordinator. The routers behave as IoT gateways. They aid in connecting internet protocol V6 and Zigbee network. A virtual private network is used to handle a private network. The server aggregates the data provided by the gateway and makes it possible for the user to view the readings. This setup is used to design intelligent smart homes. Sensing unit one does the monitoring process. The IoT interface is used to monitor water temperature in the hot water cylinder, the temperature of water in the solar water heater, the amount of current supplied and light intensity. Sensing unit two takes care of home appliances. The current and voltage parameters are measured by this unit. The power consumption of a particular device is recorded. Environment condition generated readings are measured by sensing unit three. Light intensity, humidity, and temperature are some of the parameters on which the third sensing unit works. Using these reading a control over remote monitoring (Fattah, Sheik, Sung, Ahn, Ryu, & Yun, 2017) and controlling of applications is made possible. Table 1 provides the characteristics of the work suggested by different authors, time and space complexity.

The authors in (Bourke, O'brien, & Lyons, 2007) recorded eight different kinds of fall. They include forward fall, backward fall, left fall, right fall, performed with legs straight and flexed. The work consisted of false triggering of the threshold fall detection procedure. The activities of daily life can aid in creating false triggering events. These eight instances were understood and fall detection procedure was suggested. Trial-axial accelerometer sensor at the trunk and thigh provided the resultant signal. The root of the sum of squares of the three signals from tri-axial accelerometer was calculated to arrive at the resultant signal.

In (Chen, Kwong, Chang, Luk, & Bajcsy, 2005) the authors have suggested using the computer to computer the fall detection. The accelerated data can be computed at the mobile motto or can take base station assistance. Pattern matching is used to conclude the fall detection. After affirmation, the mobile motto can alert the respective base station. This base station can forward the alert to the emergency center. The norm of the three axes is considered. The mobile mottos compute the three accelerometers.

Table 1. Characteristics of the contribution with time and space complexity made by various authors

Contribution	Characteristics of the work	Time complexity	Space complexity
(Foroughi, Homa, Aski, & Pourreza, 2008)	Time frame window is considered to detect fall; temporal head changes are considered; video sequences are analyzed; MLP neural network is used to analyze the position by providing the collected data as input	$O(n^2 logn)$	O(nlogn)
(Nasution, Hans, & Emmanuel, 2007)	Indoor environment is considered Background subtraction method is utilized Horizontal and vertical histograms are used to extract the foreground image. KNN algorithm is used as the classifier	$O(n^2)$	O(n)
(Arcelus, Amaya, Jones, Goubran, & Knoefel, 2007)	The system assists the elderly in the dark environment 16 behaviors are considered in the proposed work. The system works in four stages are namely caution, mild abnormality, high alert, and emergency.	$O(n^2 log\ n)$	$O(n^4)$
(Bourouis, Abderrahim, Feham, & Bouchachia, 2011)	Both indoor and outdoor environments are considered in the study TheWeb application is available for the caregiver to check the readings.	O(log n)	$O(2^n)$
(Wang, et al., 2014)	Impact magnitude, trunk angle, and the after-event heart rate are considered to derive conclusions. Different postures are gauged using the three axis and common changes	$O(n^3)$	$O(2^n*n^2)$

continued on the following page

Table 1. Continued

Contribution	Characteristics of the work	Time complexity	Space complexity
(Ray & P, 2014)	Home health hub IoT is suggested The layered based model consists of the dependency and interconnectivity of biosensors, microcontroller, communication channels, applications, internet, and gateway.	$O(n^2)$	$O(n^3)$
(Ani, Krishna, Anju, Aslam, & Deepa, 2017)	The Suggestion is provided to minimize the future recurrence of stroke in patients. The system continuously monitors patients condition and transmitted to the cloud. The parameters received are analyzed and cross-verified against normal values.	$O(n \log n)$	$O(n^2)$
(Jimenez, Freddy, & Torres, 2015)	The technology build uses the present technology used in patients home. An addition or editing is done to create runtime alerts.	$O(2^n)$	$O(n)$
(Park.S.J., et al., 2017)	Suggested a proactive measure to care, stroke victims. It does signal analysis, communication and detection and warning procedure.	$O(n^2)$	$O(n \log n)$
(Baldiseera, Andrea, & M.Camarinhamatos, 2016)	The system collaborates with network, context awareness and Internet-of-things. The assistance service provider shall analyze the situation and evolve with the model that suit the requirements. Multisource information activity collects sensed data from multiple devices and helps the service provider support activity to store a new description in the service catalog.	$O(n^3)$	$O(n^4 \log n)$
(Shehab, Ismail, Osman, Elhoseny, & El-Henawy, 2017)	A wearable ring device is used to monitor the health of the elderly. The system aids in minimizing the overall cost for the users	$O(n \log n)$	$O(n^2)$
(Mainetti, Patrono, Secco, & Sergi, 2016)	The system aids in minimizing the overall cost for the users The system provisions the elderly to take care of themselves without much intervention or monitoring.	$O(n)$	$O(n^2)$
(Kim, Seo, & Seo, 2016)	encompasses contactless sensors gathering its readings from the environment	$O(n^2)$	$O(n)$
(Ghayvat, Mukhopadhyay, Gui, & Suryadevara, 2015)	The system developed is reliable, efficient, flexible and economical The nodes are deployed to perform multiple activities in multiple events. Data logging, data extraction, and data storage are some of the activities performed by the nodes.	$O(n^2 \log n)$	$O(n^4)$
(Miori & Russo, 2017)	Both direct and indirect interaction is available in this system.	$O(n \log n)$	$O(n^2)$
(Almeida, et al., 2017)	The system is into earlier detection of risk related population. A set of geriatric factors and sub-factors are used as quantitative indicators. Track the object in an indoor and outdoor environment.	$O(2^n)$	$O(\log n)$
(Mishra, Lin, & Chang, 2014)	The system is used for continuous cardiac monitoring. The system reduces cloud server bandwidth, treatment cost, and traffic load. The system is into detecting flat-line detection, abrupt baseline wanders extraction and high-frequency noise detection/extraction.	$O(n^2 \log n)$	$\Omega(\log n)$
(Basanta, Huang, & Lee, 2016)	Wearable devices, biosensors and sensor network aid in the process. Real-time activity is monitored effectively in the system.	$O(\log n)$	$O(n^2)$
(Chandel, Sinharay, Ahmed, & Ghose, 2016)	Fall, immobility, step count and stride length are the basic events observed. Inertial measurement units (embedded or wearable) form is used to collect readings.	$O(n^2)$	$O(n \log n)$
(Ghose, et al., 2013)	The occupant is expected to carry the Smartphone all the times with a few exceptions. Kinect is used to detect the sleeping patterns, watching TV, sitting idle of the occupant. Inertial sensors are used to cover other indoor activities.	$O(n \log n)$	$O(n^4)$
(Mainetti, Patrono, Secco, & Sergi, 2016)	The system is capable of capturing the data of the adults in the city premises and home environments. The proposal aims to intervene to help the elderly population to improve their life. It also promotes positive behavioral changes.	$O(n! * n^4)$	$\Omega(n^4 \log n)$
(Khoi, Manh, Saguna, Mitra, & Åhlund, 2015)	Suggested remote health monitoring system. The readings can aid in attending emergencies, generated a summary report and monitoring the health condition of the adult	$O(n \log n^2)$	$O(n^4)$
(Sebbak, Faouzi, & Benhammadi, 2017)	A precise reconcilement is made between evidence theory with the frequentist approach of probability calculus The activities the system focussed on include sleeping, exercising, watching television and fall detection.	$O(n^3)$	$O(n^2 \log n)$
(Pinto, Sandro, Cabral, & Gomes, 2017)	we-watch wristband to provide the solution to elderly monitoring The system provides an alert if the wristband is tried to be detached from the personnel. The system consists of the push button which is used by the personnel to alert the caregiver. The received signal strength indicator value is used to trace the elderly.	$O(2^n)$	O(2[illegible] n^2)
(Bourke, O'brien, & Lyons, 2007)	The work consisted of false triggering of the threshold fall detection procedure. This aided in arriving at the resultant signal that provided the actual fall.	$O(n \log n^2)$	$O(n^3 \log n)$
(Chen, Kwong, Chang, Luk, & Bajcsy, 2005)	Pattern matching is used to conclude fall detection. After affirmation, the mobile motto can alert the respective base station. This base station can forward the alert to emergencies center. The norm of the three-axes are considered. The mobile mottos compute the three accelerometers.	$O(\log n)$	$O(n^2)$

MAIN FOCUS OF THE CHAPTER

In (Dziak, Jachimczyk, & Kulesza, 2017) suggested the outline methodology be used in elderly monitoring. The system is beneficial in both indoor and outdoor surveillance. Two major subsystems- Problem formulation and product development are utilized. The first stage is the combination of need definition, requirement formulation, and feasibility assessment. Stakeholders, future users, and designers also are part of the system. The work lacks the following-

- It does not make any mapping with the scenarios with the previous records. Mapping with the previous case studies aids in choosing better methodologies adopted in similar scenarios.
- It does not try to incorporate the new methodologies. The new methodologies aids in the betterment of the personnel. Using IoT aids in regular updating of the system with the respective scenarios. This methodology aids in bringing better usage of the present technology.

MODIFIED SYSTEM DESIGN

Monitoring the elderly is leading to many challenges. The previous system proposed (Dziak, Jachimczyk, & Kulesza, 2017) the authors have proposed a design to aid indoor and outdoor activities. Two major subsystems- Problem formulation and product development are utilized. The first stage is the combination of need definition, requirement formulation, and feasibility assessment. Stakeholders, future users, and designers also are part of the system. The proposed system suggests a better approach where the system will have a store related data from prior-knowledge.

Figure 1. flow chart of modified design system

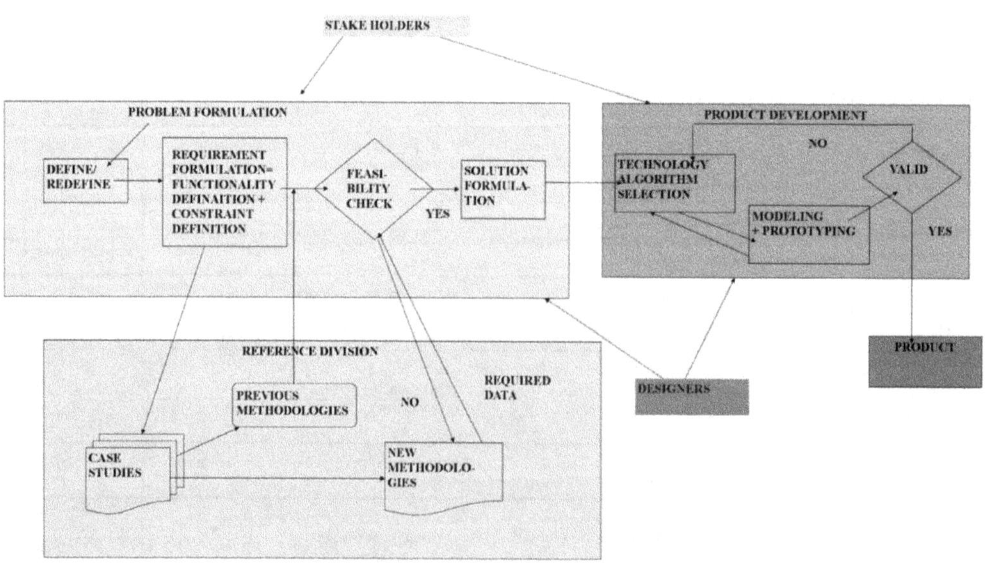

The system is utilized by the stakeholders. The stakeholders include the patient's doctor, family member, and the governess. The stakeholders are given access to study the previous history with a similar scenario. The family member can take appropriate action after understanding the scenario. The system consists of three major divisions-

Problem Formulation

The system is used by stakeholders, future users, and designers. Each has its priorities and necessities. The system has to be designed considering all the essentials listed by the user set. The personnel may be a cardiac patient (Mishra, Lin, & Chang, 2014) or stroke patient (Ani, Krishna, Anju, Aslam, & Deepa, 2017). The system has to consider these constraints before defining. This is the stage where any of the stakeholders queries the system for the answers. The patient's doctor can query the system for the appropriate measure at different stages of medication. The patient's family member or the governess can query in for assistance and take appropriate action. This subsystem has four stages-

- *Need definition / redefine* – The family member can place his query to the system w.r.t to the recovery duration, the procedure followed and so on. The respective doctor or consultant will provide with appropriate answers during the design process. This aids the family members in times of emergencies.
- *Requirement formulation* – The functionality procedure is provided to the system with its constraints (Lin, Chiu, Hsiao, Lee, & Tsai, 2006). Several constraints like fall detection, monitoring the elderly in multi-environment w.r.t cost and lifetime can be included. The patient may have some complications which can be provided as constraints as a query to the system. The family member can provide their queries like time duration for the procedure to be followed, medication procedure and duration.
- *Solution formulation* – The appropriate solution is provided considering the suggestion provided by the system. The solution can be the old methodologies (Abbate, et al., Monitoring of human movements for fall detection and activities recognition in elderly care using wireless sensor network: a survey., 2010) followed or the new methodologies (Jalal, Ahmad, Kamal, & Kim, 2014) suggested. The accuracy rate of the solution to be considered (Rashidi, Parisa, & Mihailidis., 2013) of the elderly is searched for to suggest the solution.

Reference Division

This division is composed of three sections namely case study, new methodologies, and previous methodologies. The reference section is used to provide accurate answers to the query. The section is created by previous analysis, the case studies are evaluated, and the methodologies for the same are stored for future purpose.

- *Case studies* –The stakeholder when queries the system, the system makes a query to the reference division. Similar case studies are extracted. The methodologies used are exacted and an appropriate one is recommended. If any advanced solution is devised the same is stored in new methodologies. The solution is suggested accordingly. In (Bourke, O'brien, & Lyons, 2007) false triggering of threshold fall detection procedure was considered and a new mechanism was suggested.

- *Previous methodologies* – After the system extracts a similar case study, the system searches for the methodologies (Blinman, King, Norman, Viney, & Stockler, May 2012) used. The results of the same are analyzed to obtain a solution. If the methodology is accurate for the situation, the same is suggested. For instance, if the required scenario is indoor and outdoor monitoring done is mass, (Mainetti, Luca, Patrono, Secco, & Sergi, 2017) can be considered. The system is capable of capturing the data of the adults in the city premises and the home environments.
- *New methodologies* –The new methodology is the set of inventions made accordingly to the present time and situation. If the methodology suggested by previous methodology sub-division is inappropriate to the present situation of the patient or if it is not existing, then the new methodology is looked into for the answers. The system is connected to the internet. As the new inventions are certified the same is updated in the system.

Product Development Stage

This is the stage where the product is evolved using different methodologies and algorithms. This stage consists of three sub-divisions namely technology and algorithm selection, modeling and prototyping and checking for validity.

- *Technology and algorithm selection* –The technology (Gaddam, Anuroop, Mukhopadhyay, & Gupta, 2011) (Costa, Castillo, Novais, Fernández-Caballero, & Simoes, 2012) and the appropriate algorithm has to be suggested based on the appropriate solutions chosen. Technology represents the different ways of handling the situation. Appropriate algorithms have to be suggested to bring the technology into play. Algorithm selection has to also address time duration, the amount of medication to be done and the tenure the medication has to be continued. The algorithm also suggests the different stages of medications to be considered.
- *Modelling and prototyping*-The solution provided is followed and the case study for the future users is fed into the system. The different stages outcome whether it is an indoor/outdoor environment (Bourouis, Abderrahim, Feham, & Bouchachia, 2011) is modeled with the recovering stages.
- *Validation* – The stakeholders consider the design provided by the designer and if found appropriate go ahead with approving the same.

ANALYSIS

Different scenarios are considered to analyze the system. The assisted methodologies with previous findings and new findings are listed out. Assuming different postures (Iazzi, Rziza, & Thami, 2018) (Fan, Kaibo, Wang, Hu, & Dou, 2017) (Noury, et al., 2007) (Mubashir, Muhammad, Shao, & Seed, 2013) are analyzed to build the model. Compared to the previous work (Dziak, Jachimczyk, & Kulesza, 2017), the proposed work has incorporated some add-ons. The same is represented in table 2.

Providing Flexibility and Effectiveness to the System

In (Bourouis, Abderrahim, Feham, & Bouchachia, 2011) the authors consider making a comparison to pre-existing conditions (previous methodologies) and recommendations (new methodologies). In (Bourouis, Abderrahim, Feham, & Bouchachia, 2011) three different components are used. The wireless body area network worn by the patients monitor the activities of the same and transmit appropriate signals to the intelligent center node (ICN) through Bluetooth communication protocol. The star topology aids in communicating the signal to ICN. The second component after receiving the signal communicates with the intelligent center server (ICS). General packet radio service/ universal mobile telecommunication system (GPRS/UMTS) is used to communicate. After receiving the readings the ICS makes a comparison to the pre-existing conditions and recommendations. The authenticated family member can check the status of the elderly through the web application. If an abnormal situation is detected the alert message is sent to the medical practitioner for assistance. Nokia Smartphone N95 is used as ICN in the work. But the system does not consider using the case studies and mapping it to a similar scenario. The same effect can be brought into play by using different types of equipment.

The suggestions provided in (Dziak, Jachimczyk, & Kulesza, 2017) is restricted to certain limitations. The situation does not remain the same for all the elderly. Hence some amount of flexibility has to be provided in their supervision. In case of emergencies, if the appropriate solution is not available, the system should provide some alternate measure to take the situation under control. The proposed system provides a variety of solutions – old methodologies and new inventions that provides 8% increase in flexibility. Comparing the proposed work with the methodology used in (Bourouis, Abderrahim, Feham, & Bouchachia, 2011) the proposed work provides 3% more effectiveness and flexibility.

Figure 2. Comparison of flexibility provided between two systems

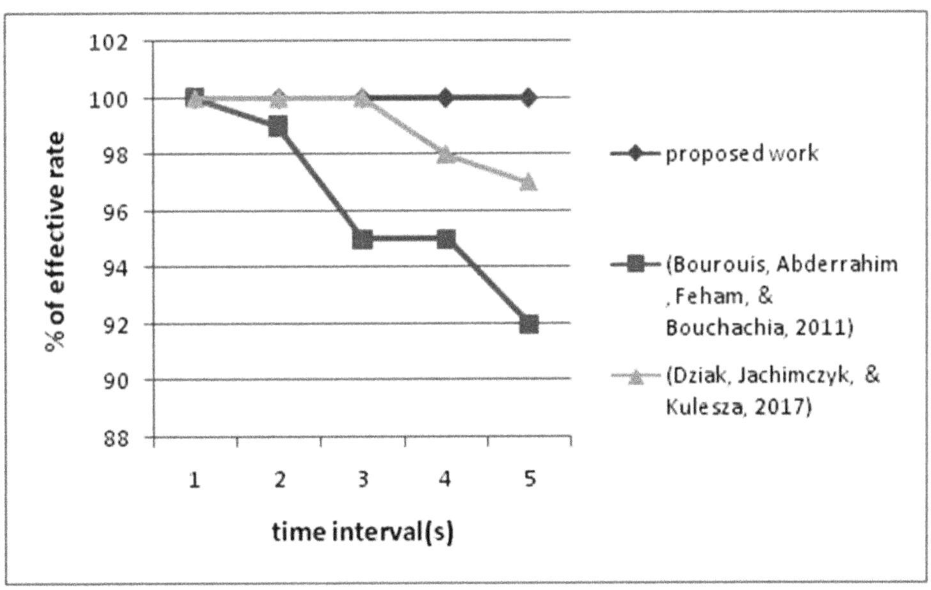

Availing New Inventions

The system accommodates new certified inventions into its system. As the server connected to the application installs the respective invention, the same is reflected in the IoT device. Hence updated methodology can be availed for betterment. The proposed work provided 12% of updated methodologies compared to (Dziak, Jachimczyk, & Kulesza, 2017). In (Bourouis, Abderrahim, Feham, & Bouchachia, 2011) the new methodologies are considered but the scenario mapping is not provided in the system. Hence the proposed work provides 1.67% more usage of present technologies aiding in the betterment of the personnel.

Future Scope And Research Challenges

The proposed system has made improvements to the suggested work (Dziak, Jachimczyk, & Kulesza, 2017). To the existing suggestions provided by the author, the proposed work fuses using previous case studies and new designed tested methodologies to provide better comfort and care to the elderly. The system can be further improved by some add-ons-

- The huge amount of case studies storage is always a challenge. Managing them and availing the methodologies on time can be considered in future work.
- Internet connectivity always is a problem. Designing the module which gets along and serves the purpose can be considered.

Figure 3. Comparison of the previous work with proposed work w.r.t. updated methodologies

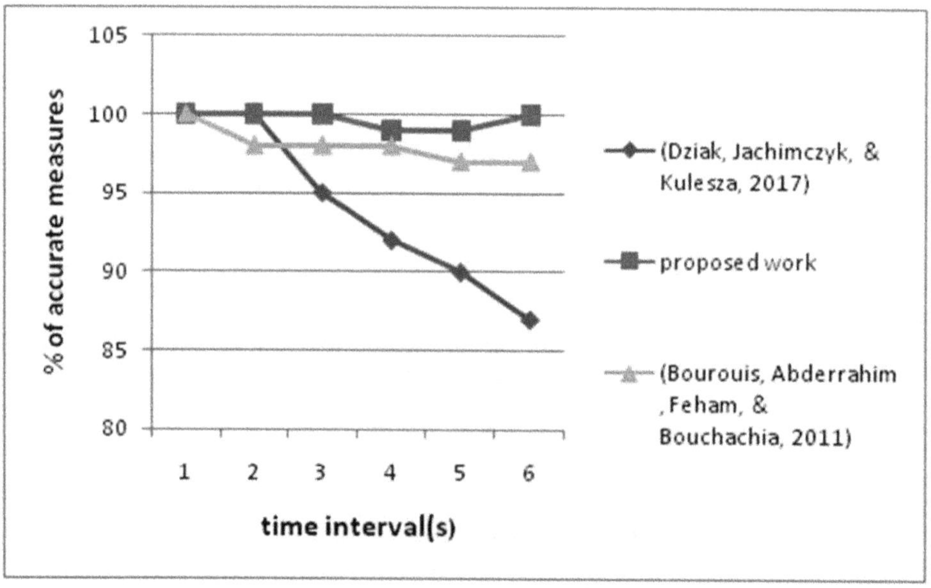

CONCLUSION

Elderly monitoring is one of the challenges in today's life. As for the lifespan of the elderly increase, the situation may lead them to stay alone or they may come up with several complications. The competition with time has made the families neutral and hence has also affected the elderly population. Internet-of-things is providing the answers to the problem by devising a solution to cater to the needs of the elderly. The caretakers or the family members can aid in time to the needs of the elderly. The proposed work has surveyed several works of the previous authors. To provide them accurate solution the proposal is suggested. The developed system aids in providing the elderly with a flexible measure so, that the medication in case of emergencies can be provided on time. The proposed work obtains 8% effectiveness and 12% better usage of new methodologies compared to (Dziak, Jachimczyk, & Kulesza, 2017). It obtains 3% more effectiveness and 1.67% better usage of new methodologies compared to (Bourouis, Abderrahim, Feham, & Bouchachia, 2011).

REFERENCES

Abbate, S., Avvenuti, M., Corsini, P., Light, J., & Vecchio, A. (2010). Monitoring of human movements for fall detection and activities recognition in elderly care using wireless sensor network: a survey. *Wireless Sensor Networks: Application-Centric Design.*

Abbate, S., Avvenuti, M., Bonatesta, F., Cola, G., Corsini, P., & Vecchio, A. (2012). A smartphone-based fall detection system. *Pervasive and Mobile Computing*, *8*(6), 883–899. doi:10.1016/j.pmcj.2012.08.003

Abowd, G. D., Dey, A. K., Brown, P. J., Davies, N., Smith, M., & Steggles, P. (1999). Towards a better understanding of context and context-awareness. In *International symposium on handheld and ubiquitous computing* (pp. 304-307). Springer. 10.1007/3-540-48157-5_29

Albert, J., Aliu, E., Anderhub, H., Antoranz, P., Armada, A., Asensio, M., ... Zapatero, J. (2008). Implementation of the random forest method for the imaging atmospheric Cherenkov telescope MAGIC. *Nuclear Instruments & Methods in Physics Research. Section A, Accelerators, Spectrometers, Detectors and Associated Equipment*, *588*(3), 424–432. doi:10.1016/j.nima.2007.11.068

Almeida, A., Fiore, A., Mainetti, L., Mulero, R., Patrono, L., & Rametta, P. (2017). An IoT-Aware Architecture for Collecting and Managing Data Related to Elderly Behavior. *Wireless Communications and Mobile Computing*, *2017*, 1–18. doi:10.1155/2017/5051915

Ani, R., Krishna, S., Anju, N., Aslam, M. S., & Deepa, O. S. (2017). Iot based patient monitoring and diagnostic prediction tool using ensemble classifier. In *International Conference on Advances in Computing, Communications and Informatics (ICACCI)* (pp. 1588-1593). Udupi, India: IEEE. 10.1109/ICACCI.2017.8126068

Arcelus, A., Jones, M. H., Goubran, R., & Knoefel, F. (2007). Integration of smart home technologies in a health monitoring system for the elderly. In *21st International Conference on Advanced Information Networking and Applications Workshops (AINAW'07)* (*vol. 2*, pp. 820-825). Niagara Falls, Canada: IEEE. 10.1109/AINAW.2007.209

Arcelus, A., Jones, M. H., Goubran, R., & Knoefel, F. (2007). Integration of smart home technologies in a health monitoring system for the elderly. In *21st International Conference on Advanced Information Networking and Applications Workshops (AINAW'07)* (pp. 820-825). Niagara Falls, Canada: IEEE. 10.1109/AINAW.2007.209

Bagala, F., Becker, C., Cappello, A., Chiari, L., Aminian, K., Hausdorff, J. M., ... Klenk, J. (2012). Evaluation of accelerometer-based fall detection algorithms on real-world falls. *PLoS One*, *7*(5), e37062. doi:10.1371/journal.pone.0037062 PMID:22615890

Balasubramanian, A., Mahajan, R., & Venkataramani, A. (2010). Augmenting mobile 3G using WiFi. In *Proceedings of the 8th international conference on Mobile systems, applications, and services* (pp. 209-222). ACM.

Baldiseera, A. T., & Camarinhamatos, L. (2016). towards a collaborative business ecosystem for elderly care. In Doctral conference on computing, electrical and industrial systems (pp. 24-34). Cham: Springer.

Baoding, Z., & Liu, J. (2010). A kind of design schema of wireless smart water meter reading system based on zigbee technology. *International Conference on E-Product E-Service and E-Entertainment* (pp. 1-4). Henan, China: IEEE.

Basanta, H., Huang, Y.-P., & Lee, T.-T. (2016). Intuitive IoT-based H2U Healthcare System for Elderly People. In *13th International Conference on Networking, Sensing, and Control* (pp. 1-6). Mexico: IEEE. 10.1109/ICNSC.2016.7479018

Blinman, P., King, M., Norman, R., Viney, R., & Stockler, M. R. (2012, May). Preferences for cancer treatments: An overview of methods and applications in oncology. *Annals of Oncology: Official Journal of the European Society for Medical Oncology*, *23*(5), 1104–1110. doi:10.1093/annonc/mdr559 PMID:22234737

Boi, R., Racca, L., Cavallero, A., Carpaneto, V., Racca, M., Dall' Acqua, F., ... Odetti, P. (2012). Hearing loss and depressive symptoms in elderly patients. *Geriatrics & Gerontology International*, *12*(3), 440–445. doi:10.1111/j.1447-0594.2011.00789.x PMID:22212622

Bourke, A. K., O'brien, J. V., & Lyons, G. M. (2007). Evaluation of a threshold-based tri-axial accelerometer fall detection algorithm. *Gait & Posture*, *26*(2), 194–199. doi:10.1016/j.gaitpost.2006.09.012 PMID:17101272

Bourouis, A., Feham, M., & Bouchachia, A. (2011). Ubiquitous mobile health monitoring system for elderly (UMHMSE). *International Journal of Computer Science & Information technology*, *3*(3), 74-82.

Bray, J., & Sturman, C. F. (2001). *Bluetooth 1.1: connect without cables.* Pearson Education.

Bressler, B. H., Keyes, W. J., Rochon, P. A., & Badley, E. (1999). The prevalence of low back pain in the elderly: A systematic review of the literature. *Spine*, *24*(17), 1813. doi:10.1097/00007632-199909010-00011 PMID:10488512

Bruce, J. (2015). *Getting Started with OpenHAB Home Automation on Raspberry Pi.* Academic Press.

C, C., B, G., & S.K., G. (2014). Mobile metadata assisted community database of chronic wound. *Int. Journal of Wound MEDICINE, 6*, 34-42.

Camarinha-Matos, L. M., Afsarmanesh, H., Ermilova, E., Ferrada, F., Klen, A., & Jarimo, T. (2008). ARCON reference models for collaborative networks. *Collaborative Networks: Reference Modeling*, 83-112.

Chakraborty, C. B., G., & S.K., G. (2016). Mobile Telemedicine Systems for Remote Patient's Chronic Wound Monitoring. In M-Health Innovations for Patient-Centered Care (pp. 217-243). IGI.

Chandel, V., Sinharay, A., Ahmed, N., & Ghose, A. (2016). Exploiting IMU Sensors for IOT Enabled Health Monitoring. In *First Workshop on IoT-enabled Healthcare and Wellness Technologies and Systems* (pp. 21-22). Singapore: ACM. 10.1145/2933566.2933569

Chen, J., Kwong, K., Chang, D., Luk, J., & Bajcsy, R. (2005). Wearable sensors for reliable fall detection. In *IEEE Engineering in Medicine and Biology 27th Annual Conference* (pp. 3551-3554). Shanghai, China: IEEE.

Costa, Â., Castillo, J., Novais, P., Fernández-Caballero, A., & Simoes, R. (2012). Sensor-driven agenda for intelligent home care of the elderly. *Expert Systems with Applications*, *39*(15), 12192–12204. doi:10.1016/j.eswa.2012.04.058

Cunningham, P., & Delany, S. J. (2007). k-Nearest neighbour classifiers. *Multiple Classifier Systems*, *34*(8), 1–17.

Devanand, D. P.-X., Taylor, S., Gurland, B. J., Wilder, D., Stern, Y., & Mayeux, R. (1996). Depressed mood and the incidence of Alzheimer's disease in the elderly living in the community. *Archives of General Psychiatry*, *53*(2), 175–182. doi:10.1001/archpsyc.1996.01830020093011 PMID:8629893

Domingos, P., & Pazzani, M. (1997). On the optimality of the simple Bayesian classifier under zero-one loss. *Machine Learning*, *29*(2-3), 103–130. doi:10.1023/A:1007413511361

Draper, B. M., Poulos, C. J., Cole, A. M., Poulos, R. G., & Ehrlich, F. (1992). A comparison of caregivers for elderly stroke and dementia victims. *Journal of the American Geriatrics Society*, *40*(9), 896–901. doi:10.1111/j.1532-5415.1992.tb01986.x PMID:1512385

Dziak, D., Jachimczyk, B., & Kulesza, W. J. (2017). IoT-Based Information System for Healthcare Application: Design Methodology Approach. *Applied Sciences*, *7*(6), 596. doi:10.3390/app7060596

Fan, K., Wang, P., Hu, Y., & Dou, B. (2017). Fall detection via human posture representation and support vector machine. *International Journal of Distributed Sensor Networks*, *13*(5). doi:10.1177/1550147717707418

Farahani, S. (2011). *ZigBee wireless networks and transceivers*. Newnes.

Fattah, S., Sung, N.-M., Ahn, I.-Y., Ryu, M., & Yun, J. (2017). Building IoT services for aging in place using standard-based IoT platforms and heterogeneous IoT products. *Sensors (Basel)*, *17*(10), 2311. doi:10.339017102311 PMID:29019964

Finkenzeller, K. (2010). *RFID handbook: fundamentals and applications in contactless smart cards, radio frequency identification and near-field communication*. John Wiley & Sons. doi:10.1002/9780470665121

Foroughi, H., Aski, B. S., & Pourreza, H. (2008). Intelligent video surveillance for monitoring fall detection of elderly in home environments. In *11th international conference on computer and information technology* (pp. 219-224.). Khulna, Bangladesh: IEEE.

Fox, M. S. (1990). AI and expert system myths, legends, and facts. *IEEE Intelligent Systems, 1*, 8–20.

Friedl, M. A., & Brodley, C. E. (1997). Decision tree classification of land cover from remotely sensed data. *Remote Sensing of Environment, 61*(3), 399–409. doi:10.1016/S0034-4257(97)00049-7

G, A., Chakraborty, C., & G, B. (2019). Medical Information Processing Using Smartphone Under IoT Framework. In *Energy Conservation for IoT Devices, Studies in Systems, Decision and Control* (Vol. 206, pp. 283-308). Springer.

Gaddam, A., Mukhopadhyay, S. C., & Gupta, G. S. (2011). Elder care based on cognitive sensor network. *IEEE Sensors Journal, 11*(3), 574–581. doi:10.1109/JSEN.2010.2051425

Ghayvat, H., Mukhopadhyay, S., Gui, X., & Suryadevara, N. (2015). WSN- and IOT-Based Smart Homes and Their Extension to Smart Buildings. *Sensors (Basel), 15*(5), 10350–10379. doi:10.3390150510350 PMID:25946630

Ghose, A., Sinha, P., Bhaumik, C., Sinha, A., Agrawal, A., & Choudhury, A. D. (2013). UbiHeld - Ubiquitous Healthcare Monitoring System for Elderly and Chronic Patients. In *1st Workshop on Human Factors and Activity Recognition in Healthcare, Wellness and Assisted Living* (pp. 1255-1264). Zurich, Switzerland: ACM.

Halonen, T., Romero, J., & Melero, J. (2004). *GSM, GPRS and EDGE performance: evolution towards 3G/UMTS*. John Wiley & Sons.

Hayes, B. (2008). Cloud computing. *Communications of the ACM, 51*(7), 9–11. doi:10.1145/1364782.1364786

Hsieh, Y.-Z., & Jeng, Y.-L. (2018). Development of home intelligent fall detection IoT system based on feedback optical flow convolutional neural network. *IEEE Access: Practical Innovations, Open Solutions, 6*, 6048–6057. doi:10.1109/ACCESS.2017.2771389

Iazzi, A., Rziza, M., & Thami, R. O. (2018). Fall detection based on posture analysis and support vector machine. In *4th International Conference on Advanced Technologies for Signal and Image Processing (ATSIP)*. Sousse, Tunisia: IEEE. 10.1109/ATSIP.2018.8364462

Jalal, A., Kamal, S., & Kim, D. (2014). A depth video sensor-based life-logging human activity recognition system for elderly care in smart indoor environments. *Sensors (Basel), 14*(7), 11735–11759. doi:10.3390140711735 PMID:24991942

Jimenez, F., & Torres, R. (2015). Building an IoT-aware healthcare monitoring system. In *34th International Conference of the Chilean Computer Science Society (SCCC)* (pp. 1-4). Santiago, Chile: IEEE.

Johnson, R. A., & Wichern, D. W. (2002). *Applied multivariate statistical analysis* (Vol. 5). Upper Saddle River, NJ: Prentice hall.

Karlik, B., & Olgac, A. V. (2011). Performance analysis of various activation functions in generalized MLP architectures of neural networks. *International Journal of Artificial Intelligence and Expert Systems, 1*(4), 111–122.

Keller, M. J., Gray, M. R., & Givens, J. A. (1985). A fuzzy k-nearest neighbor algorithm. *IEEE Transactions on Systems, Man, and Cybernetics, SMC-15*(4), 580–585. doi:10.1109/TSMC.1985.6313426

Kelly, T., Suryadevara, N. K., & Mukhopadhyay, S. C. (2013). Towards the implementation of IoT for environmental condition monitoring in homes. *IEEE Sensors Journal, 13*(10), 3846–3853. doi:10.1109/JSEN.2013.2263379

Khoi, M. N., Saguna, S., Mitra, K., & Åhlund, C. (2015). Irehmo: an efficient iot-based remote health monitoring system for smart regions. In *17th International Conference on E-health Networking, Application & Services (HealthCom)* (pp. 563-568). Boston, MA: IEEE. 10.1109/HealthCom.2015.7454565

Kim, H.-S., Seo, J.-S., & Seo, J. (2016). A Daily Activity Monitoring System for Internet of Things-Assisted Livingin Home Area Networks. *Iranian Journal of Electrical and Computer Engineering, 6*(1), 399–405.

Kleinberger, T., Becker, M., Ras, E., Holzinger, A., & Müller, P. (2007). Ambient intelligence in assisted living: enable elderly people to handle future interfaces. In *International conference on universal access in human-computer interaction* (pp. 103-112). Springer. 10.1007/978-3-540-73281-5_11

Lavsky-Shulan, M., Wallace, R. B., Kohout, F. J., Lemke, J. H., Morris, M. C., & Smith, I. M. (1985). Prevalence and functional correlates of low back pain in the elderly: The Iowa 65+ Rural Health Study. *Journal of the American Geriatrics Society, 33*(1), 23–28. doi:10.1111/j.1532-5415.1985.tb02855.x PMID:3155530

Lin, C., Chiu, M., Hsiao, C., Lee, R., & Tsai, Y. (2006). Wireless health care service system for elderly with dementia. *IEEE Transactions on Information Technology in Biomedicine, 10*(4), 696–704. doi:10.1109/TITB.2006.874196 PMID:17044403

Mainetti, L., Patrono, L., Secco, A., & Sergi, I. (2017). An IoT-aware AAL System to Capture Behavioral Changes of Elderly People. *Journal of Communications Software and Systems, 13*(2), 68-76.

Mainetti, L., Patrono, L., Secco, A., & Sergi, I. (2016). An IoT-aware AAL system for elderly people. In *2016 International Multidisciplinary Conference on Computer and Energy Science (SpliTech)* (pp. 1-6). Split, Croatia: IEEE. 10.1109/SpliTech.2016.7555929

Martin, A., Osswald, C., Dezert, J., & Smarandache, F. (2008). *General combination rules for qualitative and quantitative beliefs.* Infinite Study.

McEvedy, C., & Jones, R. (1978). Atlas of world population history. Harmondsworth, UK: Penguin Books Ltd.

Meneilly, S. G., & Tessier, D. (2001). Diabetes in elderly adults. *The Journals of Gerontology. Series A, Biological Sciences and Medical Sciences, 56*(1), M5–M13. doi:10.1093/gerona/56.1.M5 PMID:11193234

Metcalfe, R. M., & Boggs, D. R. (1976). Ethernet: Distributed packet switching for local computer networks. *Communications of the ACM, 19*(7), 395–404. doi:10.1145/360248.360253

Miori, V., & Russo, D. (2017). *Improving life quality for the elderly through the Social Internet of Things (SIoT). In 2017 Global Internet of Things Summit (GIoTS)* (pp. 1–6). Geneva, Switzerland: IEEE.

Mishra, N., Lin, C.-C., & Chang, H.-T. (2014). Cognitive Inference Device for Activity Supervision in the Elderly. *The Scientific World Journal*, 1–12. PMID:25405211

Mubashir, M., Shao, L., & Seed, L. (2013). A survey on fall detection: Principles and approaches. *Neurocomputing, 100*, 144–152. doi:10.1016/j.neucom.2011.09.037

Nasution, H. A., & Emmanuel, S. (2007). Intelligent video surveillance for monitoring elderly in home environments. In *9th Workshop on Multimedia Signal Processing* (pp. 203-206). IEEE. 10.1109/MMSP.2007.4412853

Nguyen, H. H., Mirza, F., Naeem, M. A., & Nguyen, M. (2017). A review on iot healthcare monitoring applications and a vision for transforming sensor data into real-time clinical feedback. In *21st International Conference on Computer Supported Cooperative Work in Design (CSCWD)* (pp. 257-262). Wellington, New Zealand: IEEE. 10.1109/CSCWD.2017.8066704

Nie, P. (2006). *An open standard for instant messaging: eXtensible Messaging and Presence Protocol (XMPP). In TKK T-110.5190 Seminar on Internetworking* (pp. 1–6). Helsinki University of Technology.

Noury, N., Fleury, A., Rumeau, P., Bourke, A., Laighin, G., & Rialle, V. (2007). Fall detection-principles and methods. In *29th Annual International Conference of the IEEE Engineering in Medicine and Biology Society* (pp. 1663-1666). Lyon, France: IEEE.

Odunmbaku, A., Rahmani, A. M., Liljeberg, P., & Tenhunen, H. (2015). *Elderly monitoring system with sleep and fall detector. In International Internet of Things Summit* (pp. 473–480). Cham: Springer.

Pang, Z., Zheng, L., Tian, J., Kao-Walter, S., Dubrova, E., & Chen, Q. (2015). Design of a terminal solution for integration of in-home health care devices and services towards the Internet-of-Things. *Enterprise Information Systems, 9*(1), 86–116. doi:10.1080/17517575.2013.776118

Park, S.J., Subramaniyam, M., Kim, S.E., Hong, S., Lee, J.H., & Jo, C.M. (2017). Development of the elderly healthcare monitoring system with IoT. *Advances in Human Factors and Ergonomics in Healthcare*, 309-315.

Petersen, R. C., Smith, G. E., Waring, S. C., Ivnik, R. J., Tangalos, E. G., & Kokmen, E. (1999). Mild cognitive impairment: Clinical characterization and outcome. *Archives of Neurology, 5*(3), 303–308. doi:10.1001/archneur.56.3.303 PMID:10190820

Piller, L. B., Ford, C. E., Davis, B. R., Nwachuku, C., Black, H. R., Oparil, S., ... Probstfield, J. L. (2006). Incidence and predictors of angioedema in elderly hypertensive patients at high risk for cardiovascular disease: A report from the Antihypertensive and Lipid-Lowering Treatment to Prevent Heart Attack Trial (ALLHAT). *Journal of Clinical Hypertension, 8*(9), 649–658. doi:10.1111/j.1524-6175.2006.05689.x PMID:16957427

Pinto, S., Cabral, J., & Gomes, T. (2017). We-care: An IoT-based health care system for elderly people. In *IEEE International Conference on Industrial Technology (ICIT)* (pp. 1378-1383). Toronto, Canada: IEEE. 10.1109/ICIT.2017.7915565

Rashidi, P., & Mihailidis., A. (2013). A survey on ambient-assisted living tools for older adults. *IEEE Journal of Biomedical and Health Informatics, 17*(3), 579-590.

Ray, & P, P. (2014). Home Health Hub Internet of Things (H 3 IoT): An architectural framework for monitoring health of elderly people. In *International Conference on Science Engineering and Management Research (ICSEMR)* (pp. 1-3). Chennai, India: IEEE.

Satija, U., Barathram, R., & Manikandan, M. S. (2016). Real-Time Signal Quality-Aware ECG Telemetry System for IoT-Based Health Care Monitoring. *IEEE Internet of Things*, 1-9.

Sebbak, F., & Benhammadi, F. (2017). Majority-consensus fusion approach for elderly IoT-based healthcare applications. *Annales des Télécommunications*, *72*(3-4), 157–171. doi:10.100712243-016-0550-7

Shehab, A., Ismail, A., Osman, L., Elhoseny, M., & El-Henawy, I. (2017). Quantified self using IoT wearable devices. In *International Conference on Advanced Intelligent Systems and Informatics* (pp. 820-831). Cham: Springer.

Stauffer, C., & Grimson, W. (1999). Adaptive Background Mixture Models for Real-time Tracking. In *IEEE Computer Society Conference on Computer Vision and Pattern Recognition* (Vol. 2, pp. 246-252). Fort Collins, CO: IEEE. 10.1109/CVPR.1999.784637

Suresh, S., Omkar, S. N., & Mani, V. (2005). Parallel implementation of back-propagation algorithm in networks of workstations. *IEEE Transactions on Parallel and Distributed Systems*, *16*(1), 24–34. doi:10.1109/TPDS.2005.11

Wagenmakers, E.-J., Steyvers, M., Raaijmakers, J. G. W., Shiffrin, R. M., van Rijn, H., & Zeelenberg, R. (2004). A model for evidence accumulation in the lexical decision task. *Cognitive Psychology*, *48*(3), 332–367. doi:10.1016/j.cogpsych.2003.08.001 PMID:15020215

Waher, P. (2014). Securing the Life Cycle of Things. *Internet of Things using Thing Registries.*

Wang, J. (2014). An enhanced fall detection system for elderly person monitoring using consumer home networks. *IEEE Transactions on Consumer Electronics*, *60*(1), 23–29. doi:10.1109/TCE.2014.6780921

Wang, Y., Wu, K., & Ni, L. M. (2017). Wifall: Device-free fall detection by wireless networks. *IEEE Transactions on Mobile Computing*, *16*(2), 581–594. doi:10.1109/TMC.2016.2557792

Weinstein, E. B., Spitzer, J. B., & Ventry, I. M. (1986). Test-retest reliability of the Hearing Handicap Inventory for the Elderly. *Ear and Hearing*, *7*(5), 295–299. doi:10.1097/00003446-198610000-00002 PMID:3770324

Chapter 8
Feasible Challenges and Applications of IoT in Healthcare:
Essential Architecture and Challenges in Various Fields of Internet of Healthcare Things

Seelam Vasavi Sai Viswanada Prabhu Deva Kumar
https://orcid.org/0000-0003-3304-888X
Pusan National University, South Korea

Shyam Akashe
ITM University, India

Hee-Je Kim
https://orcid.org/0000-0002-3620-0739
Pusan National University, South Korea

ABSTRACT

In this chapter, the major enhanced techniques of internet of healthcare things (IoHT) with wearable sensor technologies (WST), stationary medical devices (SMD), and integrated system technologies (IST) for heterogeneous healthcare professionals are explored. A detailed view of the system architecture for developing IoHT device and a lot of issues are also described. The latest innovative technologies are realistic to specific purposes in the field of healthcare assessment. Analysis, sensor, and data studies approach the opportunities to improve personal healthcare and benefits for the medical industry. The ultimate aim of succeeding superior healthcare practice is to competently combine with information from diverse bases, to allocate the accumulated data, to retrieve the collected data. Effective data analysis tools from data with initialed conception services are needed while maintaining their security and privacy. Healthcare professionals, patients, and clients can take benefit of the IoHT for giving personalized smart care guidelines or solutions for existing technologies.

DOI: 10.4018/978-1-7998-0261-7.ch008

INTRODUCTION

The first IoT was invented in 1990 by John Romkey. It's a device as the toaster with on and off features by the internet for INTEROP conference in October 1989. The president of interop Dan Lynch promised John that this toaster should be marketed. However, it is not popular at that time and not considered later. The device was communicated to the computer through TCP/IP protocols. In 1991, the first web page is developed by Tim Berners-Lee (Gubbi, Jayavardhana, Buyya, Marusic, & Palaniswami, 2013). In 1997, an article on sensors from the Next Wave of Infotech Innovation has released. Google is incorporated in 1998. In this duration, it slowly started callings as the Internet of Things (IoT) but not elaborated briefly. A project was developed by Scott Brave from MIT on InTouch in 1998. The year 1999 has a tremendous change in IoT and MIT. Kevin Ashton coined the term IoT. In addition to this started life of the IoT by the presentation made at Procter and Gamble by linking with a new idea of Radio Frequency Identification (RFID) that became a hot topic. Although it was still often misunderstood (Atzori, Luigi, Iera & Morabito, 2010). In the same year, a researcher Neil from MIT Media lab was speaking about the precipitous evolution of the World Wide Web (WWW) which is setting off the real explosion now on the internet. From 2003 to 2004, researchers started publications and developed few projects like the Cool town and the disappearing computer initiative and implementing new ideas.

In 2005 onwards, the other level of Information and Communication Technologies was added to IoT. Where the connections can be multiple and can be able to create their own dynamic networks. Similarly, little Wi-Fi enabled the systems. In 2008, the IPSO Alliance launched by the group of companies such as Ericsson, Intel, Bosch to motivation Internet Protocol (IP) networks in IoT (Kodali, Swamy & Lakshmi, 2015). The actual IoT was born in the years 2008 to 2009 whereas all the objects and things are connected at the point of time. The gradual usage of the IoT by people was started year by year. The no. of ways associated with the internet was carried about 12.6 billion by 2010. At this time the population of humans is about to 6.8 billion whereas the no. of systems a human beings connected to the internet is more than 1.6 billion that reaches to high expectations in the history of IoT. Later 2010 to till now, started developing various platforms as Thinkspeak and Pachube are interfaced to hardware and software (Subasi, Radhwan, Kurdi & Khateeb, 2018). Then IoT became a major industry in China and started plans to invest. Now the top MNC's like IBM, Intel manufacturing their own large in scale products for educational and marketing at this time. These companies launched basic static medical and healthcare products for pharma industries (Knicerkbocker, Budd, Dang, Chen, Colgan, Hung, Kumar et al., 2018). Till now, industries and companies have not invented the devices related to IoT with healthcare systems as compared to other IoT fields. Researchers are widely working on Data Base Management System, Sensor Networks, Security and Privacy issues on the IoHT.

LITERATURE SURVEY ON RECENT IOHT DEVICES

A survey that reveals the performance of several medical centers and their development for healthcare using information technology (Koppar & Sridhar, 2009). The scrutiny says that the patient registers were not properly managed. So they can't find the medical history of the patients in a defined manner. Hence there is a need for using information technology, especially using Electronic Health Records (EHRs).

The handling of EHR may have some malfunctioning problem associated with it. Hence, they propose a Web EHR to overcome this problem. This approach provides the web-based connectivity among various health care centers, simplifying the maintenance and sharing of the data.

Any person needs basic healthcare. For in-patients, there is a lack of medical facility to access his/her medical history for better diagnosis and treatment (Bhatia et al., 2013). Hence, there is a need to optimize the health care system to be more efficient. In this paper, a cloud computing methodology is proposed for assimilating all the hospital registers from all areas to preserve the patient's data in one place. This method decreases the monopoly of the corporate hospitals and better usage of the government sector services for all communities.

For in-patients in the hospital, this paper presents the better enactment and functioning of the wireless monitoring of in-patients inside and hospital vicinities (Chipata et al., 2010). The proposed wireless network works on the pulse and oxygen saturation measurements from patients on a regular basis. This gives a scope for the operation of the WSN in healthcare centers.

The stuffed medical staff makes the key strength of the Indian medical field. Certain efforts have been made to advance the healthcare system and the possible (Khambete & Murray, 2012). There are also some challenges like lack medical equipment safety processes and the preventive stages that need to be taken for better excellence of healthcare in India.

Tele-healthcare is in practice for the growing population of elder people and widespread of various chronic diseases (Hung, Zhang & Tai, 2004). It also gives an idea for the development of wearable technology in remote places. The idea to implement tele-home patient analysing by sourcing wearable devices to wireless communication along with multiple deployments of sensors.

The survey conducted recent times reveals the reason for the common of road accidents are occurred due to the driver's health disorders and cardiac problems and so on (Kavitha & Perumlraja, 2014). A smart healthcare monitoring system is proposed to provide instant access to the concerned authorities at the time of an accident. This system calibrates the temperature, pulse rate and transmitting the data from the smartphone to the Internet. If any abnormal assessments are detected from the driver, doctors and transport authorities are informed about the driver's location.

The wide use of the wireless sensor devices in healthcare because of the accurate data analysisat a low power operation of network systems and low power consumption of medical sensors (Ko, Lu, Srivastava & Stankovic, 2010). There are also some research challenges in WSNs with reverence to healthcare and enhances many security issues correlated to the privacy and access of the related medical data.

The mobile computing, medical sensors and communication technologies constitute M-Health (Istepanian, Jovanov & Zhang, 2004). The various wireless technologies used in M-health are GPRS, WLAN, ZigBee, Bluetooth, addresses pertain to the challenges, and potential performance concerns in the healthcare point of view.

The hierarchical model for elderly monitoring was introduced in Azimi et al. (2016). There are four layers in this architecture: Perception layer, Gateway layer, a cloud layer, and interfacing devices. Health monitoring, nutrition monitoring, safety, localization and navigation and social network monitoring makes ease of social life for elderly people.

The design and execution of the IoT built scrutinizing routine for emergency medical services are presented in Gupta et al. (2016). To demonstrate the collection, integration, and interoperation of data, they used INTEL GALILEO 2D. They also used a server linked to this board to upload and process data collected from sensors. Before analysis, the system changes data into numerical graphs.

The security and privacy are the major issues when data is transferred from the untrusted network. Moosavi (2016) intended an end to end security system comprising of verification using DTLS handshake, session management and renewal. It operates on a layered architecture and intends a mobility system based on smart ways such as to reduce communication overhead, energy. In this paper, they dealt with an all-embracing set of security reports and implement them.

The accessible IoT platforms and divergence evaluation by their inadequacies are assessed by Mineraud et al. (2016). The survey reveals that there is no de-facto communication protocol suite, and this sorts the assignment of interfacing heterogeneous devices more demanding and costly. There are also like IoT platforms do not assimilate enough security and privacy protocols for safety integration and management of data of the associated devices. The paper also studies IoT platforms like Xively, Open IoT, and IFTTT.

Future Scope of Healthcare Over Internet Platform

IoT has wide growth in upcoming generations in the field of Healthcare. According to the US IoT report in healthcare products usage will be increased by 15 billion in a couple of years. Industries and Researchers are gradually started new sophisticated ideas with monitoring the human being's health condition. Since data managing is majorly difficult to handle whereas big data is introduced to the raw data for useful medical relevant data by implementing various techniques such as data analytics and data extraction (Islam, Kwak, Kabir, Hossain & Kwak, 2015; Octav, Lu, Bailey & Roman, 2010). Whereas, the key elements of the IoT in healthcare and medical services systems are hitched by sensor networks. So microcontroller and source platform can measure sensor signals very accurately with monitoring the health status. This status can include various parameters like hypertension, pulse rate and oxygen levels. A few smart sensors can be instantly communicated to the network. In this case, it can generate alert notice at any uneven conditions occurring to the patient at any distant places. IoT is renovating medical services systems are being expended for the variety of smart applications (Sonune, Kalbande, Yeole & Oak, 2017). Although it has many concerns to overcome many inchoate technologies and the implementations in internet protocols. In addition, the computing systems have proficient communications among various devices leisurely than perpetually afore (Reyes-Ortiz, Oneto, Sama, Parra & Anguita, 2016). Furthermore, in upcoming technology Artificial Intelligence (AI) will be bounded with the IoHT. It performs automatic live health monitoring without any human effort.

This IoHT is a prerequisite gateway network over HTTP. Here is the aim of the compelled ways and no stabilization of protocols is ensured. To assimilate devices are fluently firm to IoT platforms depriving of openly exploiting the gateway, prevailing protocols similar to CoAP, MQTT (Sonune, Kalbande, Yeole & Oak, 2017). Likewise, the finest accessible privacy and security protocols would ensue instigated. The data is frequently distributed on a cloud server or local server. Data is constant by the intended users that are affable across by incredibly trouble-free access rules. Aimed at safe data storage, access control adequate, data prominence & the secure retrieve control request to stand afforded (Vasavi, Viswanada, Kumar, Akashe, 2017). For cross-platform amalgamation, there must be stabilized inward function communications. The accessible platforms utility application programming interface(API) service to retrieve data. Consequently, instability to advance a cross-platform method that preserves like an open platform for entire health allied facilities heterogeneous pragmatic furtherance. The accumulation, amputation of devices, amenities and use of API can communicate the devices certainly. The system architecture is obligatory phenomena taking keen on deliberation. The EveryAware platform lends the idea of enhanced data that escalates the potentials of allocating and processing data squabble. Sensors data unite to the cloud over Eurotech gateway in EveryAware. The data mining & machine learning have the two techniques of new data that achieved as a boundless involvement to develop beyond intelligent IoHT applications. The two techniques are consisting of the assortment of algorithms proper for special extents (Azimi et al, 2016). The data mining with data processing approaches includes major data types likewise velocity, volume and variety. The data paradigms like substantiated and unsubstantiated processes other operating effectual algorithms which remain expedient for the data attributes. While data is produced by altered mines with certain data categories like Artificial Neural Networks (ANN), Support Vector Machine (SVM), Decision Tree, Artificial Intelligence (AI), it is firm to embrace or progress algorithms which can be able to control the data attributes in future devices. Additionally, the results of the finest data prototype that uniforms the data arre one of the decisive stages for patient diagnosis data recognition and for restored consideration of data. Similarly, the Hardware compatibility also plays a keen role along with it whereas Intel developed a Galileo board. Moreover, the size of the hardware/device is efficient, reliable and cost-effective (Chung et al., 2008) in next generation systems.

ROLE OF INTERNET IN HEALTHCARE PRODUCTS

Healthcare characterizes one of the supreme smart relevance fields to the IoT. The IoT has a perspective to provide growth for several health functions such as inaccessible health monitoring, chronic diseases, and elderly care. Obedience by therapy and medicine by healthcare sources is the additionally essential application (Lomotey, Sofranko, & Orji, 2018; Kodali, Swamy & Lakshmi, 2015). Thus, numerous medical devices, sensors, diagnostic and imaging devices can be seen as smart strategies. IoT-based healthcare facilities are probable to decrease prices, intensification the quality of life and enhance the client's involvement. Since the perception of healthcare suppliers, the IoT has the possibility to decrease method interruption over remote condition (Alagar, Alsaig, & Wan, 2018). In addition, the IoT can appropriately recognize the finest intervals for reloading necessities for different devices for their efficient and uninterrupted process. Additionally, the IoT affords for the effectual development of regulated sources by confirming their superlative usage and provision to other patients. Therefore, this chapter was focusing on IoHT for the best substantial communicated things like sensors, healthcare professionals, medical and communication devices (Ullah, Kaleem, Shah, & Zhang, 2016). The regular of healthcare professionals involve physicians, nurses, caretakers, patients, pharmacologists, healthcare officials and health investigate authorities (Yuehong, Zeng, Chen & Fan, 2016). Respectively "thing" has a well-defined conventional of functions, whereas function is a medicament of the services consigned to that function. Individually patient could be linked to a determinate conventional of things through which the device transmit/receive the report.

The two types of essential sensors are body ware sensors and non-body ware sensors. Instances of body ware sensors involve implantation, wearable, hearing aids, and skin patches. Such kind of devices need to be chosen for imitating to persistent centric obligations and it has the capability to logical intelligence to connect with more devices. Their commitment is risk-free and harmless (Lee, Jeon & Kim, 2016). In specific, they should be cautious the patients in hypothetically serious health conditions. Illustrations of external sensors contain a thermometer, cameras, GPS and infrared sensors (Mineraud et al., 2016).

Figure 1. Overview diagram of Internet of Healthcare Things (IoHT)

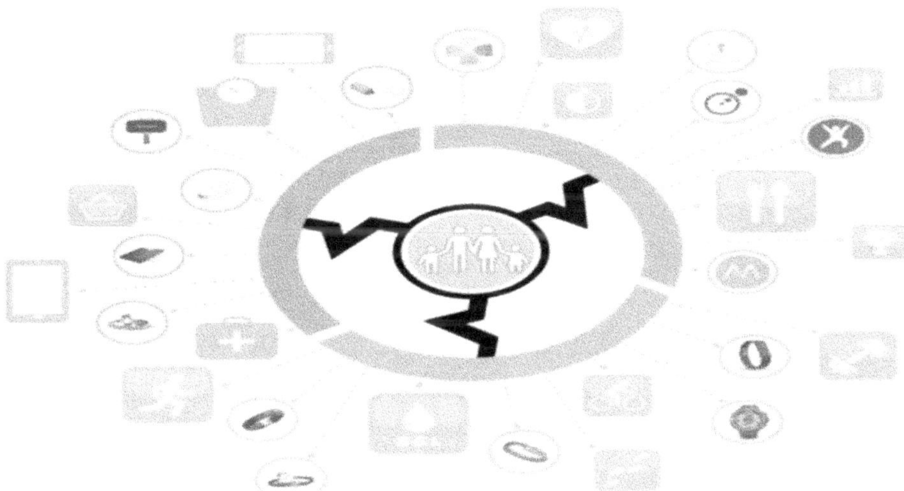

The non-body ware sensor technology might be efficiently used for patient supervising in home and warning providers when dangerous circumstances are sensed. Medical devices embrace normal human to wear, such as glucose and plasma stress monitors, mostly used for clinical analysis drives (Alagar, Alsaig, & Wan, 2018). They may be coded to continually sense, read, and communicate the dynamic signs of patients to accredited targets. Consistent medical devices in IoHT can be built functional by Embedded system programming sign ideologies (Vasavai et al., 2017). That is, assembly the chip robust with wellbeing and privacy features and embracing an element for natural consideration and authentication. In this chapter, we are not limiting to the existing technology, adequately innovate on potentially associated approaches. Certain this inform categories and functions in IoHT, that are classified in three types as shown in the figure and are discussed in the next section.

Wearable Sensor Technologies in IoHT

In addition to the IoHT technology, which allows the interaction between portable devices, human body sensors, integrated computing, and cloud servers lead to a new wearable technology called "Wearable Internet of Healthcare Things (W-IoHT)" (Haghi, Thurow, Habil, Stoll & Habil, 2017). This technology changes the human to monitor and to maintain good health. The determination of W-IoHT is easy to wear upon the human body surface, simplification of design and their Internet connection to allow people of the time to discreetly mimic many complex sensitive aspects of human realistic things and that is pointed at concentrations of unceasing monitoring of health, supervision of health inaccessible regulation, progress and actions specialist care, sport and provision for technology scrutinizing (Subasi, Radhwan, Kurdi & Khateeb, 2018; Luigi, Iera & Morabito, 2010). These W-IoHT devices achieve a specific goal in world healthcare organizations (WHO) and in the commercial region.

Few W-IoHT devices are developed by healthcare industries such as healthcare wrist watches, ECG & tilt modules, ankle or thigh bands, headbands, Earlobes, and Finger clips which has its own unique applications with multiple limitations (Lee, Jeon & Kim, 2016). These marked devices can be monitored

Figure 2. Connectivity diagram of Wearable Sensor Technologies (WST)

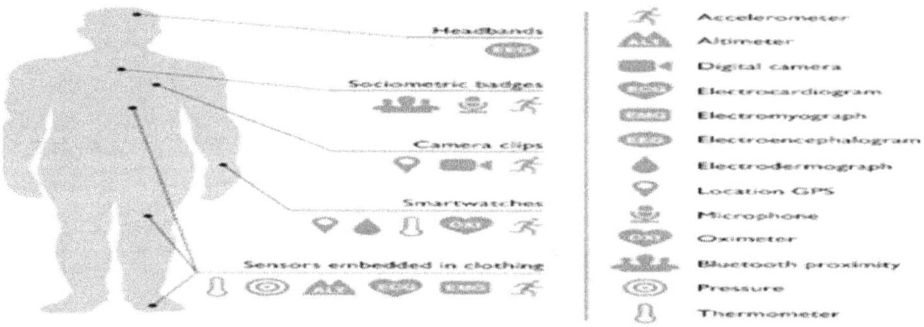

Figure 3. Overview of Wearable Sensor Technologies (WST)

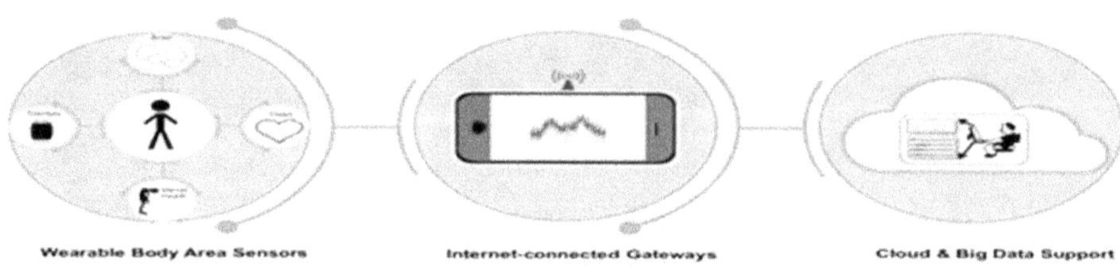

in a limited area by local area network which makes human to human interaction (Haghi, Thurow, Habil, Stoll & Habil, 2017). Such as user can receive the information about his personal health rather than the physician as shown in the figure. In the meantime, one of the under progressing advantages of W-IoHT in medical care allows us to provide personalized attention to medical professionals with the equipment that helps you to call patients for appointments automatically.

Various Wearable Sensing Devices

These smart wearable healthcare devices are the basic key elements of the IoT technologies and the elaboration from precise sensors that tolerate a softer ritual aspect for the effective occurrence of such an organism. These devices aim to proceed with the sensors that coexist non-prominent and non-offensive (Islam, Kwak, Kabir, Hossain & Kwak, 2015; Haghi, Thurow, Habil, Stoll & Habil, 2017). Three basic sensors are taken into consideration: pulse, respiration rate, and thermistor. Here the authors explained about basic sensors which are used commonly in the present scenario.

Pulse Sensor

Pulse can be used to identify the most importance sign to identify emergencies such as cardiac block, lung embolism and vasovagal syncope (Lomotey et al., 2016). Pulse sensors possess stood extensively deliberate, equally for medical principles and intended for checking the physical fitness state. The pulse is able to interpret from the chest, wrist, earlobe, fingers and few more. Sensing the ear-lobes and fingers offers high precision, but they are not consequently comfortable to wear (Lomotey, Sofranko, &

Figure 4. Devices of Wearable Sensor Technologies (WST)

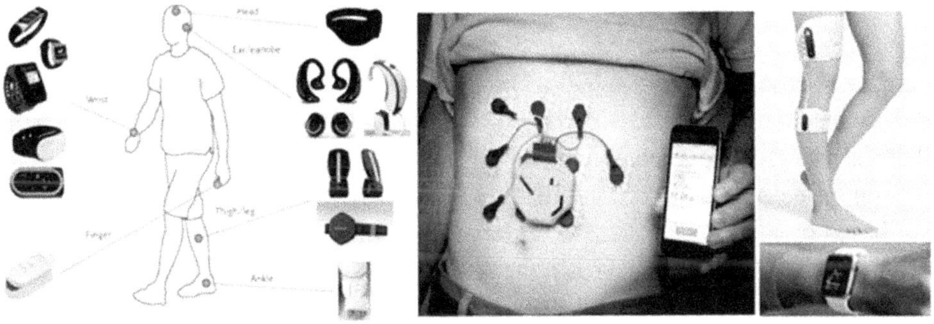

Orji, 2018). A system used in the chest is portable, but wrist systems are normally pondered as extreme comfy cheaper for an elongated wearing system. Various health tracking chest traps and wrist watches are commercially existing by the pulse measurement operation. These include HRM-Tri by Garmin, H7 by Polar, Fit Bit Pure Pulse and Tommeto Spark Cardio (Haghi, Thurow, Habil, Stoll & Habil, 2017). Though, these organizations totally unveil that systems are not intended for medical devices and should not rely on them toward identifying fitness circumstances (Mineraud et al., 2016).

There is a lot of research on the appropriate methods to identify the pulse. Recent work has developed, used and analyzed including pressure sensors photoplethysmographic (PPG), ultrasonic and radio frequency (RF). The PPG sensors work with a light emitting diode transmitting light, with a photodiode, which receives the amount of blood induced, as shown in Figure 2. Changes in the amount of light are recorded and therefore a pulse frequency can be detected.

Pressure sensors are intended to mimic a health profession, which reads the radial mental impulse by pressing it with the fingers. the most sensitive and flexible sensor is developed and tested for pulse recognition, which shows good results. This sensor is comfortable and requires more research to find out if the progress works well.

Figure 5. The Prototype of Pulse Sensing Devices in Wearable Sensor Technologies

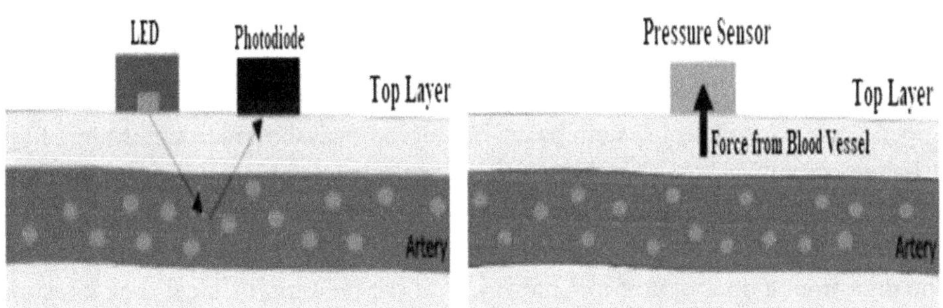

Respiration Rate Sensor

Another significant sign is the respiratory rate or the number of inhalations per minute a patient intake. Respiratory analysis senses illnesses such as asthma attacks, hyperventilation due to panic attacks, lung cancer, tuberculosis and many others. Because of the consequence of inhalation, various primary works have assimilated sensors to assess inhalation (Reyes-Ortiz, Oneto, Sama, Parra & Anguita, 2016). After groping preceding professions, there stand different kinds of respiratory rate sensors. One of them is a nasal sensor based on a thermistor. As the application of this sensor is based on warm air inhalation than the ambient temperature. In such a case, the sensor uses the inhalation and exhalation of the air to count the breath intake by the patient (Lee, Jeon & Kim, 2016). It shows a reasonably well, but the accuracy may be not much effective as compared to other sources of temperature fluctuations. Moreover, it is partially wearable because of an obstructive structure (Moosavi et al., 2016).

Echocardiogram (ECG) signals can correspondingly be expended to acquire the respiratory rate. It determines the respiratory patterns and detects apnea events. This application reads the respiratory rate well. Although it seems to effective as compared to nasal sensors it has limitations in wearing. Moreover, it is not reusable need to change regularly (Bhatia et al., 2013).

Thermistor Sensor

This thermistor sensor is used to detect heart stroke, fever, and some more. In all studies, the thermistor is shown to measure within the monitoring range of the human body temperature with acceptable levels. It is therefore recommended that future system designers continue to use these types of sensors (Rohokale, Prasad & Prasad, 2011). The accuracy of the temperature recognition limits the sensors to keep the sensor close to the human body. Therefore, many researchers developed flexible and flexible polymers sensors and adapted directly to human skin with sticky supports. Although it is an interesting development, performance is measured with relative accuracy using the temperature sensor assembly to the fabric (Gubbi, Jayavardhana, Buyya, Marusic, & Palaniswami, 2013). Therefore, Industries are developing this textile technique that contains temperature sensors, making it easier to manufacture electronic components printed in a flexible polymer.

Technical Aspect to Design a WST Device

To develop the real-time hardware system for IoHT-Wearable application it requires multiple sensors for different operations. The control system based on microprocessors/microcontrollers to perform the specific task, battery supply and the charging system to stabilize its long-term working conditions in on load and off-load. Low noise regulations for avoiding coupled signal form actual signal and filtering the weakens signal (Haghi, Thurow, Habil, Stoll & Habil, 2017) . The wireless system should be enabled to transmit the data from a control unit to Gateway with the medium of local area network (LAN) or wide area network (WAN) hence that can be a Bluetooth network or WiFi network (Kodali, Swamy & Lakshmi, 2015).

As it reads the analog data signal (ADS) from Multi-Channel Measurement Probes (sensors) with a wired connectivity to the control systems. This controller is programmed accordingly to the specific task to read the data from the sensors and it communicates to the Gateway/Host from the assigned server to upload the transmitted data from the microcontroller. In addition to this, a sufficient energy is supplied

Figure 6. Technically WST device can be developed by this block diagram

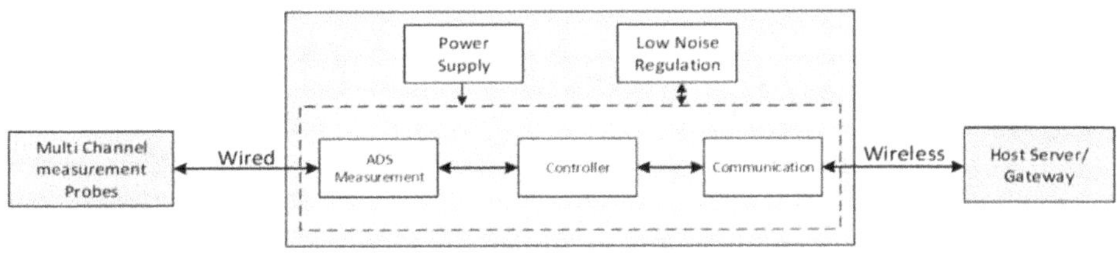

from the battery to every module to maintain standard communication (Lee, Jeon & Kim, 2016). To charge the battery a supplementary circuit with fast charging technique should be implemented. This all system is shown in the below figure.

In a basic development of wearable IoHT devices follow these steps. At first, select a sensor with the particular specification that reads analog data whereas digital read is not much accurate as analog read. Second, interface it with the control unit that should have an analog read port and must be enabled. Program it accordingly to our required rate. Third, transmit the data by enabling the USART (Universal Synchronous Asynchronous Receiver Transmitter) with the help of Wi-Fi module by its unique web server. Next, receive the data from the web server and upload to the web page or in a mobile application. Finally, maintain resourceful power supply to the developed device to work effectively and can observe the real-time monitoring of a specific task of the application developed for the patient.

STATIONARY MEDICAL DEVICES IN IOHT

The IoHT technology, which allows the interaction between physical devices, machines, integrated computing, and cloud servers lead to new stationary medical devices called "Stationary Medical Internet of Healthcare Things (SM-IoHT)". Here the authors explained about basic stationary devices which are used commonly in the present scenario (Kodali, Swamy & Lakshmi, 2015).

Intelligence Wheelchairs

Researchers are developing intelligence wheelchairs with complete computerization aimed to immobilized citizens. The IoT has the possible to hasten the speed of effort. A healthcare method developed for wheelchair handlers centered with the IoT technology is insinuated. This proposal approaches through WAN cohesive with several sensors whose purposes are custom-made to IoT desires (Islam, Kwak, Kabir, Hossain & Kwak, 2015). A medical care system making an allowance for peer to peer and the IoT technology is achieved (Atzori, Luigi, Iera & Morabito, 2010). This classification affords for chair vibration control and can find the status of the wheelchair user. Additionally, a significant model IoT based wheelchair development is associated to designed by Intel IoT department. This developed ultimately performances that usual "things" can progress into connected machines driven by data (Lee, Jeon & Kim, 2016). This machine can monitor vitals of the distinct assembling in the chair and accumulate data on the user's environments, permitting for the esteeming of a locality's convenience.

Figure 7. A Typical Model of Intelligence Wheelchair for Stationary Medical Devices (SMD)

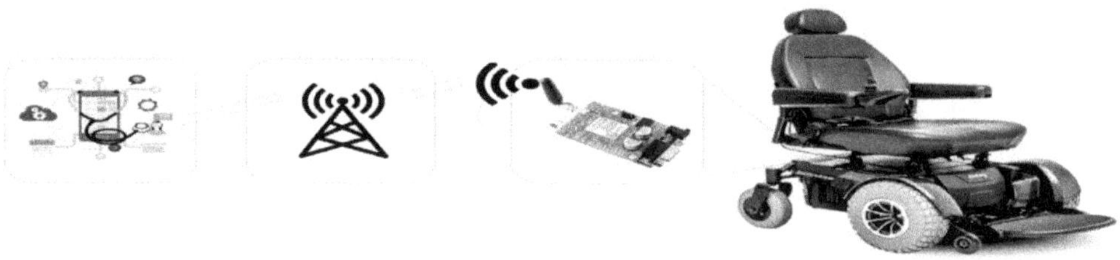

Mechanical Robots

The robot hands and legs parts are developed for the handicapped persons with inbuilt of tracking modules, like basic healthcare devices to monitor the patient pulse rate and blood pressure. These applications are connected wireless to a LAN/WAN via internet sources whereas the data is uploaded to the web server in a specific allocation of patients unique addressed in it. In addition to this, a new robot can be designed like a humanoid that notifies the patient to take the tablets within the time prescribed by the healthcare professional (Lee, Jeon & Kim, 2016). The humanoid robot can also monitor the patient health check-ups and it uploads the data of the patient's condition to the main server with its unique address. A new robot can be introduced to the world for pageant women, it is developed with artificial intelligence (AI) (Gwo-Jia & Gwo-Jiun, 2017). It helps the patient for maintaining food diet, physical fitness, health conditions, medicine to intake and surrounding hazardous effecting patients can be notified.

Mechanical Aspect to Design an SMD's

To develop the real-time hardware system for IoHT-Stationary application it requires multiple modules for different operations, control system based with microprocessors/microcontrollers to perform the specific task, battery supply and the charging system to stabilize its long-term working condition in on

Figure 8. A Model of Mechanical Robots for Stationary Medical Devices (SMD)

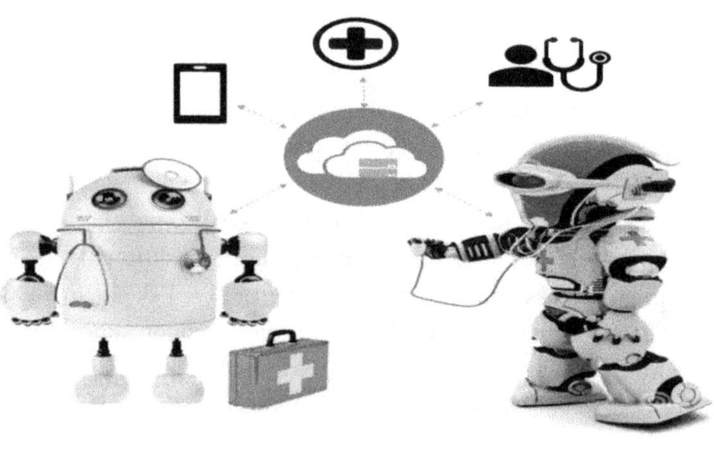

load and off-load, The wireless system should be enabled to transmit the data from the control unit to Gateway with the medium of local area network (LAN) or wide area network (WAN) hence it can be a GSM network or GPRS network (Lee, Jeon & Kim, 2016).

As it reads the information from GPRS/GSM with wired connectivity to the control systems. This controller is programmed accordingly to the specific test to collect the data from the modules and it communicates to the Gateway/Host from the assigned server to upload the transmitted data from the microcontroller. In addition to this, sufficient energy is supplied from the battery to every module to maintain standard communication (Kodali, Swamy & Lakshmi, 2015). To charge the battery a supplementary circuit with fast charging technique should be implemented. This all the nominal process is shown in the below figure 9.

In a basic development of Stationary IoHT devices follow these steps. At first select, a module with the particular specification that collects the information, interface it with the control unit that should have a USART (Universal Synchronous Asynchronous Receiver Transmitter) unit to receive the data from the modules and is transmitted the data to its unique web server as the program is developed. Next, receive the data from the web server and upload to the web page or in a mobile application. Finally, maintain the resourceful power supply to the developed device to work effectively and can observe the real-time monitoring of a specific task of the application is developed for the patient.

INTEGRATED SYSTEM TECHNOLOGIES IN IOHT

The IoHT technology, which allows the interaction between Nano-devices, machines, integrated computing and cloud servers, leads to a new integrated device called "Integrated System for the Internet of Healthcare Things (IS-IoHT)". Here the authors explained basic stationary devices which are used commonly in the present scenario (Lee, Jeon & Kim, 2016). The integrated systems are developed in very Nano-regions such as healthcare chips, sensors, flexible robots. It plays a major role in developing IoHT devices for wearable devices and stationary devices (Islam, Kwak, Kabir, Hossain & Kwak, 2015). In these integrated systems the communication and data transmission process is same as explained in the above topics (Istepanian, Jovanov & Zhang, 2004).

Figure 9. Technically SMD device can be developed by this block diagram

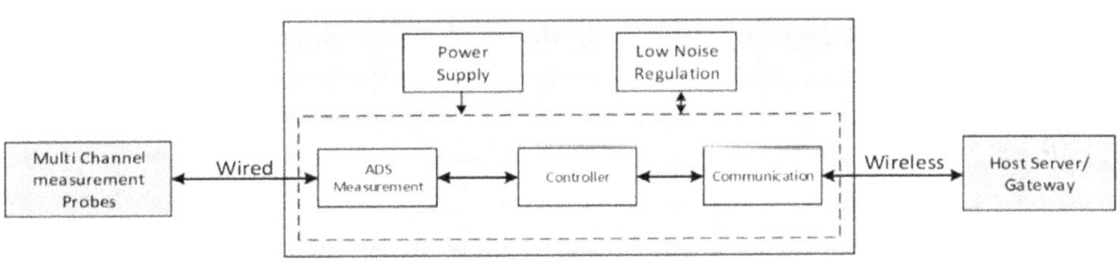

Healthcare Chips

The IoHT chips are designed in less than 45nm technology whereas it reduces the size of the portable devices, accuracy makes a system to work effectively without any misleads. The reliability defines the long life of the product, consuming the power should be very less and it helps the long back up the battery life and cost-effective. To develop these chips the material like silicon (Si) or germanium (Ge) is used. Most of all the specific task is developed inside the chip by integrating thousands of transistors (Knicerkbocker, Budd, Dang, Chen, Colgan, Hung, Kumar et al., 2018).

Healthcare Sensors

For any specific application like sensing any functionality of human physical structures mostly sensors are used. They are developed by using silicon materials because of good conductivity (Lee, Jeon & Kim, 2016). Its functionality depends upon the specific applications whereas it plays a key role in human and machine interface.

Flexible Robots

Researchers are still working on flexible robots. These robots are more advanced and it may use in an upcoming generation in medical regions. It operates a person without physician suggestions. In the future generation, if the patient is suffering for any mental issues (brain-off) a Nano-robot can operate a physical body as a normal human can be functioned (Mineraud et al., 2016). In the present generation few Nano-robots are developed for instance this is injected into a patient body whereas, it catches the tumor cells

Figure 10. A Kind of Healthcare Chips for Integrated System Technologies (IST)

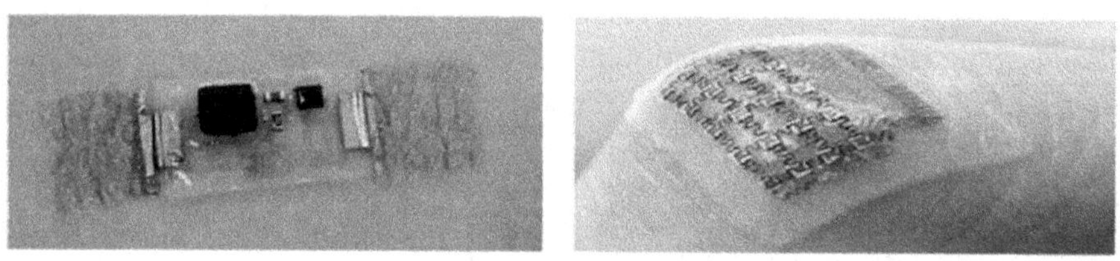

Figure 11. Basic Healthcare Sensors for Integrated System Technologies (IST)

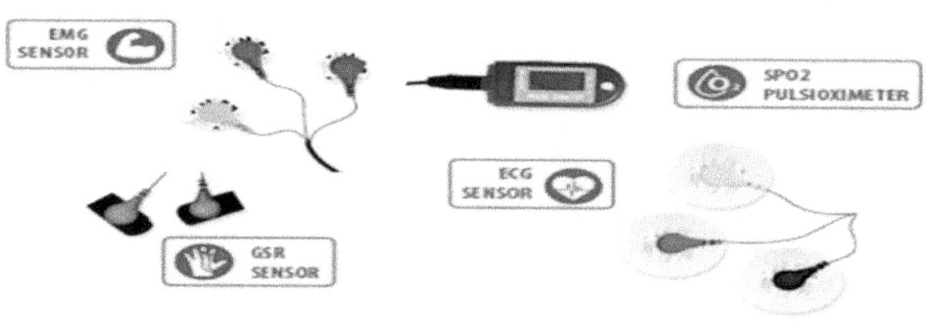

Figure 12. A Scientific View of Flexible Robots for Integrated System Technologies

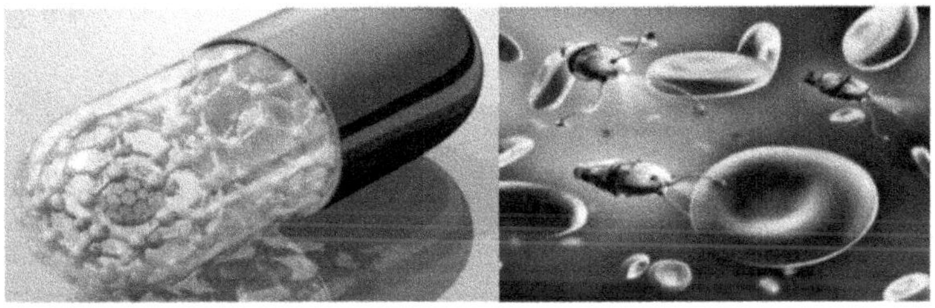

as shown in figure 12. It can't be seen by our naked eye although, it can be operated and self-operated. Insignificant to this it collects the data or information and transmits to the main organized device, from this it uploads to the main server with the same communication explained above.

IEEE SYSTEM ARCHITECTURE FOR INTERNET OF HEALTHCARE THINGS

This IEEE architecture is classified into four layers along with subsisting divisions. They are Data Layer, Network Layer, Data Processing Layer and Application Layer as shown in figure 13.

Layer A: Physical Layer

In this layer, it stores the medical information of various patients with their unique identity. Unlikely it collects the data from IoHT devices and physical upload from healthcare professionals. This data platform allocates through three leading categories of communication sources (Alagar, Alsaig, & Wan, 2018; Dridi, Sassi & Faiz, 2017).

Figure 13. IEEE System Architecture for the Internet of Healthcare Things (IoHT)

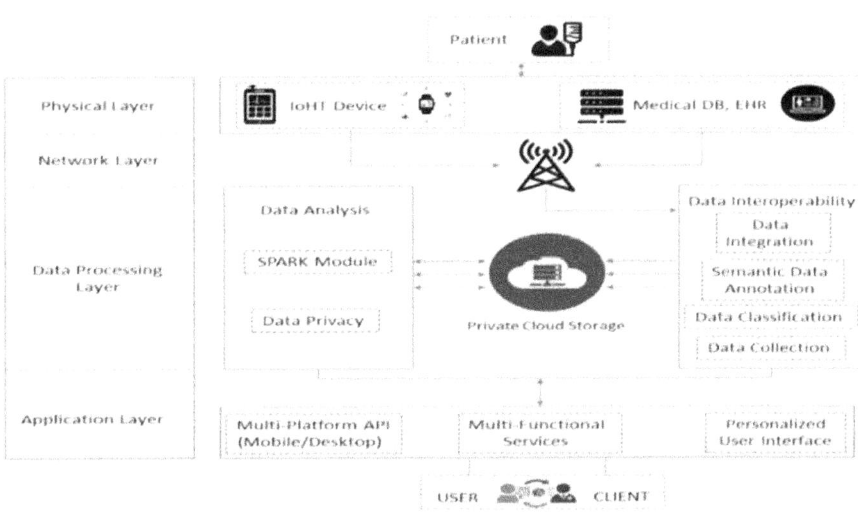

1. IoHT devices, such as smart devices like WST, SMD, IST used by patients to monitor the health conditions of heart rate, blood pressure, brain functioning, gaseous, internal operation region and various kinds of applications.
2. Non-IoHT devices, those specific devices commonly used by health professionals to diagnose and monitoring diseases such as ultrasound scanning and magnetic resonance imaging (MRI).
3. Supplementary sources, that involves electronic health records and other database sources of health information systems handled by different healthcare contributors.

Layer B: Network Layer

The network layer performances as gateway access on behalf of transmitting data/ information from different sources of the report to the next level i.e. data processing level (Dridi, Sassi & Faiz, 2017). Data produced by the IoHT devices are transmitted through wireless communication protocols (WCP), such as IPv4, IPv6, Wi-Fi and LTE (Islam, Kwak, Kabir, Hossain & Kwak, 2015). For now, IoHT devices and supplementary sources, these platform provides an instinctive Web access service that agrees healthcare specialists to clearly transfer/upload their data into the main server (Alagar, Alsaig, & Wan, 2018; Dridi, Sassi & Faiz, 2017).

Layer C: Data Processing Layer

Uneven data produced from distinctive sources, nodes of information, particularly the IoHT devices, and sensors cannot make sense. They cannot afford any practical communication. To make these utilized data, it needs to be cohesive, descriptive and relevant (Dridi, Sassi & Faiz, 2017). The main purpose of the data processing layer is

1. create a kind of schematic interoperability of the information sources to expedite data interpretation and integration.
2. Accumulation the received information/data in the cloud server.
3. Agrees to performprogressive analysis on these data like data compression and reduction techniques.
4. Confirm, the security and privacy of the stored data.

The data processing layer is classified into three elements:

1. **Data Interoperability Element:** this element agreement the interoperability of different data sources surrounded by our platform. It consists of four sections:
    a. **Data Collection Section:** It targets collecting data in real time from its sources, verification of safety and integrity. This section contains a file of data sources for respectively patient (Dridi, Sassi & Faiz, 2017). This file preference is updated repeatedly once a recognized data source is recorded on the platform.
    b. **Data Classification Section:** Which sorts the data concurring to their source into two classes. First class correspond the data from the sensors and IoHT devices. The second class involves medical documents and data from other healthcare professionals.
    c. **Schematic Annotation Section:** It presents schematic annotation and data interpretation based on an amenable schematic explication prototype.

   d. **Data Integration Section:** It establishes the path among acquired data and existing data in the real-time cloud.
2. **Data Storage Element:** Later the unification, annotation, transformation from raw data deprived of slight intellect into eloquent data and these data should be archived for advance dispensation and analysis. Due to security reasons, this information is stored in a private cloud (Dridi, Sassi & Faiz, 2017).
3. **Data Analysis Element:** This element agrees with theclient's function of progressive analysis of stored data. Additionally, it assurances the safekeeping and privacy of data. It·consists of two main units:
   a. **Spark Unit:** In this analysis, we used the Spark technique, an open source Big Data processing structure is designed to execute the advanced analysis. We choose this technique because of its advancement as associated with other Big Data techniques like Map Reduce and Hadoop (Dridi, Sassi & Faiz, 2017). In fact, sparks allow many types of data sets to work both on their nature and on the source code within the processing time. Along with considerable return during processing, the spark has dependence by its virtual accessibility.
   b. **Data Privacy Unit:**Our platform agrees with clients to have the proficiency to modify the privacy of the information they have created. It has the ability to select communicated and private information. This information can be access by all the main role in the healthcare of a patient without any restrictions (Dridi, Sassi & Faiz, 2017). In addition to this private information can be accessed by the patient and particular information maintainer. Having access to such private information mainly involves the agreement to the information maintained. In this case, we developed a contract based access protocol that permits only healthcare professionals to access privative information (Kavitha & Perumlraja, 2014). The contract has an agreement and permission to access the information of the patient for the information centers.

Layer D: Application Layer

This level specifies connectivity and access to the client to get the benefit of different qualities and facilities provided by this platform. This level contains a desktop/mobile application, which is mounted on a variety of platforms and in an application available from the web. The app agrees the client to network with custom GUIs to interact with platforms, which are also intuitive, unified, adaptable, and relevant (Islam, Kwak, Kabir, Hossain & Kwak, 2015; Alagar, Alsaig, Ormandjieva & Wan, 2018). Collection of patient health information generated from various resources and the benefit of other services, such as the user connected to our platform, to facilitate the integrity and transformation of this assistance:

1. **Physician and Patient Communication Assistance:** The patient will be able to communicate their state of health, side effects etc. This accepts the physician to communicate with the patient (when their updated health information is given in real time) and communicates with their family in emergency situations or patient communication, in any case of children, people in coma or individuals with incapacities (Dridi, Sassi & Faiz, 2017).
2. **Intelligent Emergency Assistance:** This service sends notifications when critical instances are identified and those require an emergency response. Indeed, these notifications occur if the value of sensitive physical parameters exceeds the predetermined threshold value. They are also directed to the patient, their relatives and guardians.

3. **Medical Text Assistance:** Medical text are difficult for the patient to understand often specific medical terms appear. Changing these critical words with the synonyms of easy terms to good reading and medical attention. By launching this application on medical devices, the user can have a basic awareness of healthcare terms rather than physician words (Dridi, Sassi & Faiz, 2017). In addition to this, an animated picture should define what actually this text mean whereas patients or users will never feel difficult to understand (Skeppstedt & Kvist, 2014).

OPEN ISSUES AND CHALLENGESIN THE INTERNET OF HEALTHCARE THINGS

Several scientific associate's efforts are continuously aiming and employing different IoHT aids besides on deciphering the architectural as well as technological crises to concomitant among those aids. Accessible accumulation toward research concerns in prose, there emerge more than a few additional impugns and open glitches that prerequisite to subsist wisely focused. This section pithily represents mutually surveyed and strange enveloping IoHT (Islam, Kwak, Kabir, Hossain & Kwak, 2015).

Calibration

In the trendy healthcare environment, there survive several merchants that fabricate a miscellaneous scope of designs and mechanisms, and more merchants maintain to join associate this auspicious industrial sprint. Conversely, they have not comprehended prevailing instructions and principles for attuned interfaces and protocols throughout the apparatus. These elevate the interoperability disputes. To focus device assortment, instantaneous exertions ensue elaborate. For instance, a consecrated company be able to regulate IoHT technologies. This calibration would ruminate an extensive scope of areas by way of communications layers, and protocol stacks, embracing physical, media access control (MAC) layers, device interfaces, data accumulation interfaces, and gateway interfaces. Managing of assorted consequence services equally to automated health reports is alternative stabilization concern (Reyes-Ortiz, Oneto, Sama, Parra & Anguita, 2016). This managing arises in many systems, containing access management and healthcare specialist chronicling. Different Healthcare bodies and IoT researchers can eager to effort jointly, to prevailing standardization federations like as the Information Technology (IT), Innovation Foundation (IF), the Internet Protocol for Smart Things (IPST) association, and the European Telecommunications Standards Institute (ETSI) can form IoT technology effective units for the calibration of IoHT service assistance.

Platforms for IoHT

The wide-ranging architecture of IoHT is based on hardware stands are much advanced than that of commonly used in IoT devices and entails a real-time functional technique by added strict prerequisites, here survives a requisite for a personalized processing platform by the run-time public library (Bhatia et al., 2013). To develop an appropriate platform, a service-oriented tactic (SOT) be able to acquire such that facilities can stand oppressed through exploiting unlike application package interfaces (APIs). Furthermore, to a specified platform, libraries and suitable frameworks must be developed so that software developers and designers of healthcare can be the considerate efficient practice of granted credentials, programs, classes, communication prototypes, besides additional valuable statistics. Additionally, the precise elegance of disease-oriented files can be worthwhile.

Cost Analysis of IoHT Device

Researchers might distinguish IoHT facilities as low-slung price equipment, although as per the author's comprehension, no relative analysis obtains posed any corroborative aimed at this. Here it looks, a cost analysis of a distinctive Internet provider on IoHT could be beneficial.

Faultless Data Transmission

Healthcare associations are able to transform their prevailing devices and sensors throughout the healthcare field aimed at smart sources with integrating IoT hooked on the prevailing system configuration. Consequently, a faultless transmission after the inheritance technique and framework to an IoHT centred configuration survives the foremost impugn. In other disputes, there is essential to confirm regressive compatibility and flexibility in the amalgamation of obtainable devices.

Low Energy Conservation Protocol

There remain several devices appearing in IoHT consequences, and such devices incline to persist heterogeneous in conditions of their rest, sleep, receive, transmit, and multiple conditions, including others. Accumulate to provisos of maintenance accessibility, apiece of communications layer aspects a surplus impugns in the duration of energy requisites. For instance, searching a suitable device detection protocol that commands low energy whereas ensuring service accessibility by the MAC layer subsists a hard task.

Network Model

In terminologies of the proposed method, an IoHT system can remain on these three essentially kinds: information, maintenance, and patient-centric architecture. In the information-centric system, the IoHT configuration is commonly divided into things centered continuously encapsulated health information Chung et al., 2008). In a maintenance centric system, the IoHT configuration is apportioned through the compilation of qualities that they essentially afford. In the patient-centric system, IoHT configuration is distributed rendering to the envelopment of patients along with the household fellows they deliberate for therapy. In this view, responding to the enquiry of a pardon system class attitudes the proper network for IoHT resolution improves an unrestricted glitch.

Long-Term Monitoring

Here various situations where the patient needs to monitor for long-term, in this case, IoHT data transmission should be accurate and challenge to develop noise cancellations in information to transmit & receive. Maintain a virtual login system to access for the long term.

Recognition

Healthcare bodies usually dispense through multiple patient upbringing accessible which manifold caregiver's excretion their obligations. After this assessment, the accurate recognition of patients and caregivers survives essentially.

Accurate of Service (AoS)

Healthcare assistance remains extremely phase perceptive and needs AoS assurances appearing in terminologies of significant constraints such as reliability, allowance, and the service quantity. In Concerning, the assessable extent of an individual factor inside the IoHT framework might be functional. In accumulation to routine accessibility and toughness are vital to contribution AoS secures for the reason that some kind of technique fiasco is able to abode endures the risk arrived in medical circumstances. Now the probability of other strategies inward the instance of a technique fiasco turns out to be a fascinating concern.

Security of Data

The fortification of encapsulated health fitness information as of different measuring device and sensors after illegitimate retrieve be present decisive. Consequently, rigorous strategies and methodological safety actions must come about familiarized to apportion health fitness information by certified clients, government bodies, and diligence. Now familiarizing the finest algorithm intended for collaboration concerning between security, recognition, and antiphon assistance to preclude many incidents, perils, and susceptibilities is an amenable impugns. Depends upon the dissertation proceeding in IoHT self-assurance, quite a lot of research glitches accessible to this extent subsist like source proficient security, tangible security, assure channeling and control of IoHT big data.

CONCLUSION

IoT is an assemblage of several skills that authorize various kind of applications, devices and things to interrelate and communicate through individual sourcing altered networking technologies. Therefore, abundant of the data located proceeding the Internet is equipped by human beings. In an instance of IoT smart things deliver the data. There exists an extensive diversity of functions established on IoT, embracing healthcare, which is the main effort of this chapter. Healthcare approaches formulate worth of unified smart devices to ascertain an IoT network for healthcare consideration, patient monitoring and repeatedly recognizing circumstances where a physician concern is desirable. IoHT has exposed immense approaching in several treatment areas, particularly in our day-to-day lifecycle that sorts it comfortable, easier and more satisfying. The custom of IoT in the healthcare procedures correspond several assistances such as diagnose and preclude illnesses, monitoring of vital signs, faster and more precise judgement making, and deliver a safer superiority of life for patients with less cost.

In this chapter, we explained the history from 1990 to 2010 and the gradual variation of the development of IoHT devices. Later, the present trend to future scope the researchers are enlarged with the flexibility of usage along with security and privacy methods. The IoHT systems are growing in various areas in medical fields such as wearable sensors. This is for the physical approach of monitoring the patient health conditions by reading the data from sensors and transmits to the web server. Stationary medical devices are co-relate with mechanical structures with supporting healthcare modules are assembled in it. Whereas, integrated systems are designing with advanced techniques to build flexible in Nano-regions. An architecture of IoHT Device has been proposed in this chapter, where it is classified into the physical layers, network layer, data processing layer and application layer. Here, the data received from heterogeneous information sources (containing sensors and IoHT devices) are transferred over a suitable gateway to the data interoperability element where this information is collected and described. The administered data are accumulated in a private cloud for progressive evaluation. Client requirements are achieved by the data processing element, which is built on the spark unit. This program assists the allocating of data among the various healthcare professionals affording to an up-to-date agreement established guarantee rules to safeguards the confidentiality of the records. The client is able to give access to the assorted functionality offered by the platform over personalized identification. Supplementary facilities offered by this platform for end to end clients such as physician-patient communication service, Intellectual emergency conditions recognition assistance, medical text explanation assistance into the IoHT devices. A literature review from a few pieces of research has been considered. Open issues and impugns of the IoHT are listed in detail.

In sum-up, after reading this chapter the developers get an idea to develop IoHT devices for a specific task. Furthermore, they are able to understand the communication between the client to a healthcare professional, data securing and maintaining data privacy.

REFERENCES

Alagar, V., Alsaig, A., Ormandjieva, O., & Wan, K. (2018), Context-based Security and Privacy for Healthcare IoT. *IEEE International Conference on Smart Internet of Things (SmartIoT)*, 122-128. 10.1109/SmartIoT.2018.00-14

Atzori, L., Iera, A., & Morabito, G. (2010). The Internet of Things: A Survey. *Computer Networks*, *54*(15), 2787–2805. doi:10.1016/j.comnet.2010.05.010

Azimi, I., Rahmani, A. M., Liljeberg, P., & Tenhunen, H. (2016). Internet of things for remote elderly monitoring: A study from user-centered perspective. *Journal of Ambient Intelligence and Humanized Computing*, *8*(2), 273–289. doi:10.100712652-016-0387-y

Bhatia, G., Lala, A., Chaurasia, A., & Rajpal, R. (2013), Implementation of Cloud computing technology for the improvement of entire healthcare services in India. *IEEE International Conference on Advances in Technology and Engineering (ICATE)*, 1–5. 10.1109/ICAdTE.2013.6524771

Chakraborty, Gupta, & Ghosh. (2013). A Review on Telemedicine-Based WBAN Framework for Patient Monitoring. *International Journal of Telemedicine and e-Health*, *19*(8), 619–626.

Chipara, O., Lu, C., Bailey, T. C., & Roman, G.-C. (2010), Reliable clinical monitoring using wireless sensor networks: experiences in a step-down hospital unit. *Proceedings of the 8th ACM Conference on Embedded Networked Sensor Systems*, 155–168. 10.1145/1869983.1869999

Chung, W.-Y., Lee, Y.-D., & Jung, S.-J. (2008). A wireless sensor network compatible wearable u-healthcare monitoring system using integrated ECG, accelerometer and SpO2. *IEEE 30th Annual International Conference on Engineering in Medicine and Biology Society (EMBS),* 1529–1532.

Derhamy, H., Eliasson, J., Delsing, J., & Priller, P. (2015). A Survey of Commercial Frameworks for the Internet of Things. *IEEE 20th Conference on Emerging Technologies & Factory Automation (ETFA),* 1-8.

Dridi, A., Sassi, S., & Faiz, S. (2017) A Smart IoT platform for personalized healthcare monitoring using semantic technologies. *IEEE International Conference on Tools with Artificial Intelligence (ICTAL),* 1198-1203. 10.1109/ICTAI.2017.00182

Gubbi, J., Buyya, R., Marusic, S., & Palaniswami, M. (2013). Internet of Things (IoT) A Vision, Architectural Elements, and Future Directions. *Future Generation Computer Systems*, *29*(7), 1645–1660. doi:10.1016/j.future.2013.01.010

Gwo-Jia, Aripriharta, & Gwo-Jiun. (2017). The PPG Physiological Signal for Heart Rate Variability Analysis. *Wireless Personal Communication, 97,* 5229–5276.

Haghi, M., Thurow, K., & Stoll, R. (2017). Wearable Devices in Medical Internet of Things. Scientific Research and Commercially Available Devices: Healthc Inform Res, 4-15.

Hung, K., Zhang, Y. T., & Tai, B. (2004). Wearable medical devices for tele-home healthcare. *IEEE 26th Annual International Conference on Engineering in Medicine and Biology Society,* 5384–5387.

Istepanian, Jovanov, & Zhang. (2004). Guest editorial introduction to the special section on m-health: Beyond seamless mobility and global wireless health-care connectivity. *IEEE Transactions on Information Technology in Biomedicine,* 405-414.

Kavitha, K. C., & Perumalraja, R. (2014), Smart wireless healthcare monitoring for drivers community. *IEEE International Conference on Communications and Signal Processing (ICCSP)*, 1105–1108 10.1109/ICCSP.2014.6950019

Khambete, N. D., & Murray, A. (2012), National efforts to improve healthcare technology management and medical device safety in India. *7th International Conference on Appropriate Healthcare Technologies for Developing Countries*, 1–5. 10.1049/cp.2012.1474

Knickerbocker, J. U., Budd, R., Dang, B., Chen, Q., Colgan, E., Hung, L. W., . . . Wen, B. (2018), Heterogeneous Integration Technology Demonstrations for Future Healthcare, IoT, and AI Computing Solutions. *IEEE 68th Conference Electronic Components and Technology (ECTC),* 1519-1528.

Ko, Lu, Srivastava, & Stankovic. (2010). Wireless sensor networks for healthcare. *Proceedings of the IEEE,* 1947–1960.

Kodali, R. K., Swamy, G., & Lakshmi, B. (2015). *An Implementation of IoT for Healthcare. In IEEE Recent Advances in Intelligent Computational Systems* (pp. 411–416). RAICS.

Koppar, A. R., & Sridhar, V. (2009), A workflow solution for electronic health records to improve healthcare delivery efficiency in rural India. *IEEE International Conference on eHealth, Telemedicine, and Social Medicine*, 227–232. 10.1109/eTELEMED.2009.30

Lee, J.-C., Jeon, J.-H., & Kim, S.-H. (2016), Design and Implementation of Healthcare Resource Model on IoTivity Platform. *IEEE International Conference on Information and Communication Technology Convergence (ICTC)*, 887-891. 10.1109/ICTC.2016.7763322

Li, X., Niu, J., Kumari, S., Liao, J., Liang, W., & Khan, M. K. (2016). A new authentication protocol for healthcare applications using wireless medical sensor networks with user anonymity. *Security and Communication Networks*, *9*(15), 2643–2655. doi:10.1002ec.1214

Lomotey, R. K., Nilson, J., Mulder, K., Wittmeier, K., Schachter, C., & Deters, R. (2016). Mobile Medical Data Synchronization on Cloud-Powered Middleware Platform. *IEEE Transactions on Services Computing*, *9*(5), 757–770. doi:10.1109/TSC.2016.2555313

Lomotey, R. K., Sofranko, K., & Orji, R. (2018). Enhancing Privacy in Wearable IoT through a Provenance Architecture. *Multimodal Technologies and Interaction*, *2*(2), 18. doi:10.3390/mti2020018

Mineraud Julien, O. (2016). A gap analysis of Internet-of-Things Platforms. *Computer Communications*, *89-90*, 5–16. doi:10.1016/j.comcom.2016.03.015

Moosavi, S. R., Gia, T. N., Nigussie, E., Rahmani, A. M., Virtanen, S., Tenhunen, H., & Isoaho, J. (2016). End-to-end security scheme for mobility enabled healthcare Internet of Things. *Future Generation Computer Systems*, *64*, 108–124. doi:10.1016/j.future.2016.02.020

Mora, H., Gil, D., Terol, R. M., Azorín, J., & Szymanski, J. (2017). An IoT-Based Computational Framework for Healthcare Monitoring in Mobile Environments. *MDPI Sensors*, *17*(10), 2302. doi:10.339017102302 PMID:28994743

Punit, Agrawal, Chhabra, & Dhir. (2016). IoT based smart healthcare kit. *IEEE International Conference on Computational Techniques in Information and Communication Technologies (ICCTICT)*, 237-242.

Reyes-Ortiz, J. L., Oneto, L., Sama, A., Parra, X., & Anguita, D. (2016). Transition-aware human activity recognition using smartphones. *Neurocomputing*, *171*, 754–767. doi:10.1016/j.neucom.2015.07.085

Riazul Islam, S. M., Daehan Kwak, M. D., Humaun Kabir, M., Hossain, M., & Kyung-Sup Kwak. (2015). The Internet of Things for Health Care: A Comprehensive Survey. *IEEE Access: Practical Innovations, Open Solutions*, *3*, 678–708. doi:10.1109/ACCESS.2015.2437951

Rohokale, V. M., Prasad, N. R., & Prasad, R. (2011), A cooperative internet of things (IoT) for rural healthcare monitoring and control. *IEEE 2nd International Conference on Wireless Communication, Vehicular Technology, Information Theory and Aerospace & Electronic Systems Technology (Wireless VITAE)*, 1–6.

Seelam, Vasavi Sai Viswanada Prabhu Deva Kumar, & Akashe, S. (2017). Implementation of GSM Based Security System with IOT Applications. *International Journal of Computer Network and Information Security*, *6*, 13–20.

Skeppstedt, E. A. T. F. M., & Kvist, M. (2014), Medical text simplification using synonym replacement: Adapting assessment of word difficulty to a compounding language. *Proceedings of the 3rd Workshop on Predicting and Improving Text Readability for Target Reader Populations*, 57–65.

Sonune, S., Kalbande, D., Yeole, A., & Oak, S. (2017), Issues in IoT Healthcare Platforms: A Critical Study and Review. *IEEE International Conference on Intelligent Computing and Control (I2C2)*, 1-5. 10.1109/I2C2.2017.8321898

Subasi, A., Radhwan, M., Kurdi, R., & Khateeb, K. (2018). IoT based Mobile Healthcare System for Human Activity Recognition. *IEEE 15th Learning and Technology Conference (L&T),* 29-34.

Ullah, K., Shah, M. A., & Zhang, S. (2016). Effective ways to use Internet of Things in the field of medical and smart health care. *IEEE International Conference on Intelligent Systems Engineering (ICISE)*, 372-379. 10.1109/INTELSE.2016.7475151

16. Yuehong, Y. I. N., Zeng, Y., Chen, X., & Fan, Y. (2016). The internet of things in healthcare: An overview. *Elsevier Journal of Industrial Information Integration*, *1*, 3–13. doi:10.1016/j.jii.2016.03.004

Chapter 9
Sensing and Monitoring of Epileptical Seizure Under IoT Platform

Akash Kumar Gupta
Birla Institute of Technology, Ranchi, India

Chinmay Chakraborty
https://orcid.org/0000-0002-4385-0975
Birla Institute of Technology, Ranchi, India

Bharat Gupta
National Institute of Technology, Patna, India

ABSTRACT

Epilepsy is a disorder that affects the life of the patient. In this neurological disorder, patients may suffer from different types of seizures. From epileptic patients, we may acquire electroencephalogram (EEG) data using various kinds of sensors and transmit them through the cloud. In this chapter, the authors have discussed various platforms related to IoT-enabled cloud for sharing the information and to get quick response in form suggestion. Use of smartphone applications for real-time monitoring of patients and for other applications is presented here. Various wearable devices may provide huge benefits for taking care of seizures and patients. The authors proposed a system model based on IoT-enabled cloud for sharing the information with various sensors and other devices to make a proper judgment about seizures, which will be able to provide improved e-health service. With the increasing rate of improvement in both IoT and e-health field, it is now a challenge to upgrade ourselves and work with the digital world to provide low cost, accurate, and quick solutions.

DOI: 10.4018/978-1-7998-0261-7.ch009

INTRODUCTION

Epilepsy is a neurological disorder by which a large volume of the population in this world is affected. Epilepsy seriously affects the life of human being with huge impact, which affects not only personal life but also professional and social too (M. Vergara et al., 2017). With the help of the Internet of things (IoT) platform sensing seizures and patient monitoring is reached at a great level of accuracy. IoT platform has basically consist of two different part which includes data sensing /collection with the help of wearable sensors and another one is the detection of epilepsy, with following various methods. At very first, the important thing is to a collection of data of epileptic patient before and after the seizure. Further using various features, analysis and detection seizure can be done. Initially, it was a very time-consuming task of prediction seizure by just visualizing the signals and it is getting tougher with a very small amount of information regarding the seizure. During the past few years, numbers of the algorithm have been proposed for signal classification /seizure detection.

IoT has a verity of the structure of interconnected networks of various types of sensors usually has limited capability of storing and processing the data. With clouds, IoT has a great range of applications which makes smart health system feasible (Yin et al., 2016). The requirement of cost optimization with the high quality of data transmission ability helps to grow IoT. The emergence of IoT with cloud technology is the result of this requirement, which makes real-time data processing possible for the remote patient too (Chen et al., 2018; Hou et al., 2016). Sometimes for the epileptic patient, it tends to impossible to move, in such cases a smart patient monitoring system is very much required to access the medical information between user end and hospital. In such an IoT network, smart sensors are very much required for biomedical (EEG) data. Smart sensors used to process the user-centric data to the cloud framework. This large volume of processed data is too complex to handle at the server end.

Figure 1. The basic structure of IoT-enabled epilepsy data management and monitoring system

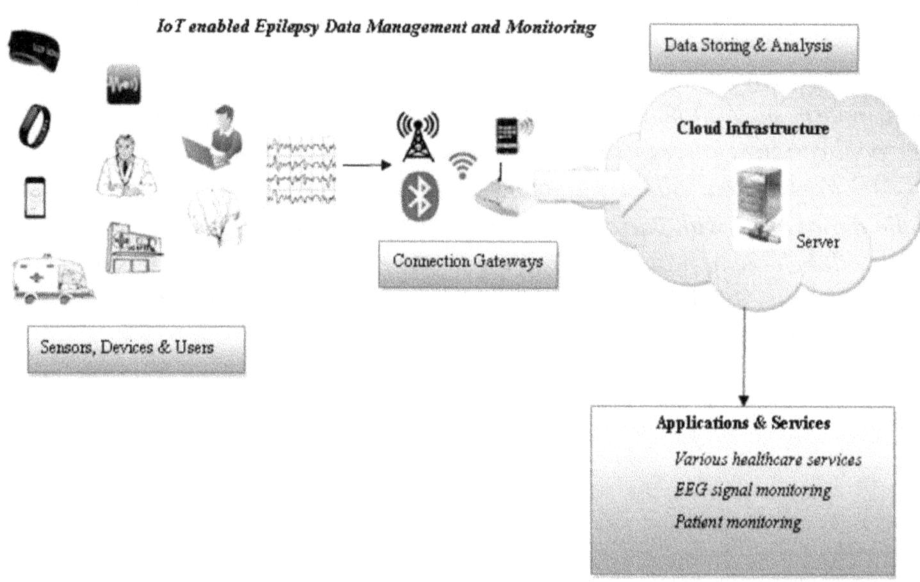

Besides providing medical information from patients, IoT industries help to grow a nation. Smart health service/IoT-cloud-based network is able to provide accurate service with the minimum service cost. With the amalgamation of IoT and cloud, real-time data processing of signals like EEG, ECG, etc becomes possible. For that, a standard and intelligent framework have been designed which one is able to make a proper decision. A particular framework based on cognitive computing has already been proposed which can also be treated as brain powered cognitive IoT (M Chen, Herrera, & Hwang, 2018). In this system, data with huge complexity like EEG or any health-related data, etc. can be processed with intelligence. In this cognitive IoT enabled cloud-based system; the patient is directly linked with special sensors or devices which are always with him. In this system, devices with patient body collect information and monitor signals like EEG. Cognitive IoT system is able to analyze the information and make a decision about patients, which are helpful for hospital /practitioner. IoT enabled cloud-based service with smart sensors along with real-time data processing for health service in a smart city is presented in (M Shamim Hossain & Muhammad, 2016b; Zanella, Bui, Castellani, Vangelista, & Zorzi, 2014). On the other hand, the IoT based health system incorporated with edge computing cognitive technology presented in (Min Chen, Li, Hao, Qian, & Humar, 2018). Such kind of system makes possible of transmission of sensor data in real-time. The patient's external expression and voice can be monitored under the IoT platform (M Shamim Hossain, 2016).

In reference (M S Hossain et al., 2015; M Shamim Hossain & Muhammad, 2016a), an emotion-based patient monitoring system, with the cloud has been proposed, which is a great application of IoT enabled cloud. It represents the basic structure of IoT enabled epilepsy data management and monitoring system that is shown in Figure 1, In which very first block contains various sensors and data collection devices. Through connection gateways information gathered in the cloud, which can be used for various purposes. IoT enabled cloud unit consist of data analytics, verification, processing included feature extraction and classification parts. This IoT enabled a cloud-based system is actually a machine to machine communication with cloud computation and analysis of real-time data collected from various sensors (M Chen, Wan, Gonzalez, Liao, & Leung, 2014). The dependency of this system follows cloud computation and data analysis. It provides the opportunity for evolving e-health, the decision-making ability of healthcare experts and helps patients to be active. IoT platforms for monitoring of epilepsy represent various features which are integrated (Ramgopal et al., 2014). These also include source problem regarding data collection, cost and mainly potential of the process. To simplify the above problem standard system has been proposed and using IoT platforms, mobile cloud computing presented in (Deshmukh & Shah, 2016). In this chapter further, we have discussed related work of sensing and monitoring of epilepsy and designing of various IoT platforms, which also describe cloud computation. Next, we have discussed the proposed system model and made a brief conclusion.

Regarding the basic information, we have got about epilepsy with various papers. Epilepsy is a kind of disorder that affects the whole human body by some king of jerks, contraction in the body resulting in loss of sensibility. Currently, a number of epileptic patients are too high whereas only a few of them are treated. Even very few of them get to know about this at the initial stage. If it is possible to detect during the early stage, it can be cured with proper medicines (Megiddo et al., 2016; Litt & Echauz, 2002). For epileptic patients, it is important to have quick service for care otherwise by seizures he may reach the critical condition. Hence IoT enabled cloud-based smart monitoring system is a fundamental need, which can be monitored by practitioners and may suggest to the patient. If the condition becomes crucial patient may avail the facility of the ambulance, mobile hospitals.

Motivation

Internet of things plays an important role in sensing the seizure and monitoring of epileptic patients. It allows small devices like sensors, actuators, etc to sense data, processing and for communication from source to hospital end. In this system, multiple numbers of devices are interlinked together through an environment. Cloud computing and the Internet of Things are two distinct domain. Their amalgamation and their application are increasing rapidly and becoming an important part of each other. Here, IoT-enabled cloud-based platform has been discussed for the above-mentioned purpose. The main advantage of using such a system is getting flexibility in computation. The IoT platform can be applied for the purpose of acquisition of real-time data and processing with higher accuracy. Another motivation behind using IoT enabled cloud-based platform is that the system will be able to make a decision in a quick and secure way and this data can apply for e-health applications and for observation of patients. With the help of this system optimization of various parameters can be done, which may help for cost-cutting and delay with respect to time. Presently, the cloud-based IoT platform is a topic of interest in information and communication technology. Another motivation is that IoT not only providing a wide range of application but also includes economic, social and technical growth.

Objectives

The main objective of this book chapter is to grasp the knowledge about the use of IoT for EEG signal monitoring over the cloud-based platform and represents, how the IoT-enabled cloud helps to monitor the epileptic patient. The system is purely focused on data collection and communication in a quick and secure way with accuracy. Use of cloud with IoT is a different concept for most of the application and objective is to grow e-health technology in a smarter way. IoT usually represents a real word with their limited capability, whereas the involvement of cloud enhances it by far superior way in regards to accuracy, security, and reliability (Jiehan Zhou et al., 2013). IoT-enabled cloud to give us a novel approach for finding the solution of any problem. In this chapter, we are going to introduce the usage of IoT-enabled cloud for monitoring of epileptic seizures of different patients, requirements, various platforms, etc. As IoT-enabled cloud reflects a variety of applications mentioned below in Figure 2, (Botta, de Donato, Persico, & Pescap, 2014), where e-health has been focused.

Figure 2. Various area of application of IoT enabled cloud

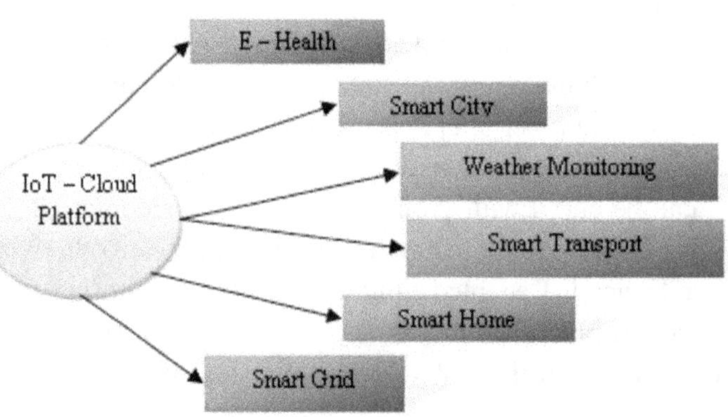

Organization of the Chapter

The organization of this chapter is mentioned in the given order: very first we have mentioned about brief introduction related to sensing and monitoring of epileptic patients under IoT-enabled cloud platform. We have gone through various literature about the use of IoT with the cloud in the e-health field. Then we described our motivation and objective of writing this book chapter. Further, using IoT-enabled cloud in the e-health field; we have proposed a system model for acquiring EEG signal, feature extraction, selection and classification for the purpose of monitoring epileptic patients. Then after we have briefly described the EEG signal and prepared the comparison table regarding types of data set and various noise removal techniques used in literature. The standard 10 – 20 system for acquiring EEG data has been considered. Then, we have mentioned about feature extraction, selection, and classification of various features of EEG data and presented a table for different types of classifier used with their achieved performance / accuracy. Later we have presented works related to epilepsy monitoring under the IoT platform and use of smartphone applications to achieve a better result. Using smartphone real-time monitoring of epileptic patients and their advantage is also presented here. Further, we have mentioned various factors and challenges related to sensing and mentoring issues. Finally, we have made some conclusion and presented the future scope of related work

IoT-ENABLED CLOUD IN E-HEALTH

IoT-enabled cloud to have a great impact on the healthcare field, which is growing continuously and supporting telemedicine facility (Q. Zhang, Cheng, & Boutaba, 2010). There are various smart devices, cloud services including internet may contribute to efficient health / medical services (Gachet, de Buenaga, Aparicio, & Padron, 2012). As we know that healthcare application like EEG analysis generates a very huge amount of sensor data and handling of data itself is a complicated task. Further data analysis, feature extraction, and classification require proper care of data too. Use of cloud with IoT solves this problem at a very satisfactory level (Doukas & Maglogiannis, 2012). Cloud service provides improved security for health data and provides accessibility and communication in a smooth way. Along with this, it may able to provide service for multimedia data and eliminates undesired issues (Nkosi & Mekuria, 2010).

System Model for Epilepsy Monitoring

System model presented here gives an idea about the basic elements of the epilepsy monitoring system of based on IoT-enabled cloud structure, which can also be preferable to pronounce as a smart healthcare monitoring system to cure seizures. Figure 3 presented here reflects that there is various type of sensor may use to collect data from the brain of patients on the basis of various types of activity (Alhussein, Muhammad, Hossain, & Amin, 2018). It is required to select a particular section of data to predict seizure; therefore in place of work with whole data, it will be suitable to reduce the size of data in a proper way. Further data will be transmitted or stored in the cloud with the use of various IoT devices for next steps of monitoring epileptic patients. These collected data may have noise due to various other sources like muscles movement, eye blinking, heart rate, etc., thus it is required to remove noise using different filtering methods. In the cloud environment itself filtering, segmentation of data, feature extraction and selection may be performed. Now further using various classifiers it will be suitable to predict the

Figure 3. IoT-enabled cloud-based epilepsy monitoring system

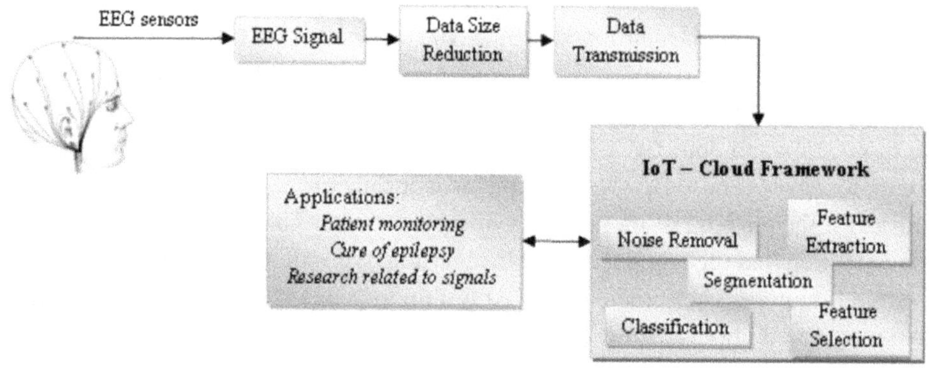

accuracy of prediction or detection of seizures. This will be helpful for monitoring of patients, epilepsy can be cured and most importantly research work can be carried out. Here IoT-enabled cloud provides connectivity to users for future applications of information. Here, IoT devices may play an important role in taking care of patients.

For sensing and monitoring of epileptic seizure based on IoT-enabled cloud platform, system or practitioner may use smart sensors to collect data. Internet of things technologies has the superior ability to access the information and that may be obtained with the help of wearable equipment. Through this end, users or patients can regularly monitor themselves by own. These systems are sufficiently able to perform necessary action in regards to patients. The data captured by sensors may send to the practitioner to get proper advice and assistance. In the present scenario, it is also required that patient should be able to monitor himself to grow smart health system to improve the efficiency, accuracy, cost reduction and majorly lifestyle. Currently, very comfortable and light-weighted wearable EEG sensors are present. Even epileptic may wear these for recording and monitoring of signals obtained from connected electrodes. Whenever the system recognizes that the patient feels any seizure activity in the body, these real-time epileptic data may be sent to the cloud for further diagnosis. From this IoT-enabled cloud, data may send to hospitals, where the practitioner can suggest the patients relatively. Along with this in case of any emergency, ambulance service or mobile hospital facility may send for patients. This IoT enabled cloud-based will be able to monitor remote patients and provide services to them.

In this IoT enabled cloud-based system different types of data like EEG signal collected directly through sensors, health-related multimedia data, etc. can be transferred to the cloud using a local/wide area network, which may be able for long or short distance communication. IoT device uses various protocols like Zigbee, Bluetooth, and LoWPAN, etc. for sharing information with the use of latest 4G /5G technologies. In the cloud, it is also required that data must be authenticated with the registered user. At present user may use different types of wearable devices which collect different sensor signals, like ECG, EEG, muscle movement, blood pressure, body temperature, etc. so it should be taken care that the required signal has been transmitted for the correct purpose. In a cloud network, it required for further processing of EEG data collected from epileptic patients. Cloud consists of various servers for feature extraction, classification and others like data handling unit, etc. Cloud will be able to manage data for transmission in a secure way. Data may include sensors data, multimedia data or data collected from patients by recognizing their facial expression and other activity, which overall may be termed as a cognitive system. Further data may be processed for feature extraction and classification purpose and may be transmitted to healthcare professional for further prediction /detection of seizures monitor the epileptic patient.

ELECTROENCEPHALOGRAM (EEG) SIGNALS

EEG signal represents the electrical activity occurs in the brain. With analyzing these signals, we are able to know, how the brain is functioning from time to time. Such signals are used by practitioners very frequently to recognize any kind of disorder in brain activity. It is important to predict or monitor epilepsy, any tumors in the brain, any kind of injury in the brain, a disorder in sleep, etc. EEG signals actually comprise different frequency range signals namely delta, theta, alpha, beta, and gamma. These are collected different states of patients like the patient is in a sleeping state or in an active state or doing some kind of work. Alpha waves having the frequency range around 8 – 13 Hz, whereas for beta wave, its frequency range is higher than 13 Hz. Delta and theta wave have the frequency range less than 4 Hz and 4 – 8 Hz respectively. Gamma wave has a frequency range of more than 30 Hz (Houssein, Hassanien, & Ismaeel, 2017). Now, it is very important to collect /acquire EEG data in a precise way, so we can detect any brain-related disease. To acquire EEG data from the brain, different ways of placement of electrodes are presented here. Along with this researcher, may use a primary or secondary type of EEG data. In the primary type of data, the researcher acquires them directly from the patient /person with concerned hospitals. Whereas, in some of the articles EEG data applied are gathered from, cited in reputed articles, collected by some standard institutions are secondary type data.

EEG Data Acquisition

EEG data can be collected directly from patients by placing the electrodes as per the requirement. The number of electrodes may be from 1 to 256 in parallel depending on use and signals are acquired from the channel by making pairs of electrodes presented in Table 1. For acquiring the data, 10 – 20 electrode placement system is the standard one and widely acceptable, presented in Figure 4 (Jasper, 1958).

In this electrode placement system, a specified region of the brain by Frontal, Temporal, Central, Parietal and Occipital are denoted by letter F, T, C, P, and O respectively, whereas middle line electrode point is represented by z. In the brain, left half region electrode points are represented by odd numbers, whereas the right half points are represented by even numbers. EEG data collected by making channels using a pair of electrodes, consecutive to each other are known as Bipolar Montage like pair of F4 – C4, Fz – F4, etc. EEG data acquired by making a particular electrode as a reference electrode then data collected by making a pair of the electrode using this reference is known as reference montage. In another case, when all signals collected from the different electrode are sum together are taken the average, this one can be used as a reference and making pair with other electrodes, the collected signal is known as Average reference montage. Here we are presenting a recent list of few articles with EEG data, they have used to carry out their research.

Figure 4. The International 10–20 electrode placement system

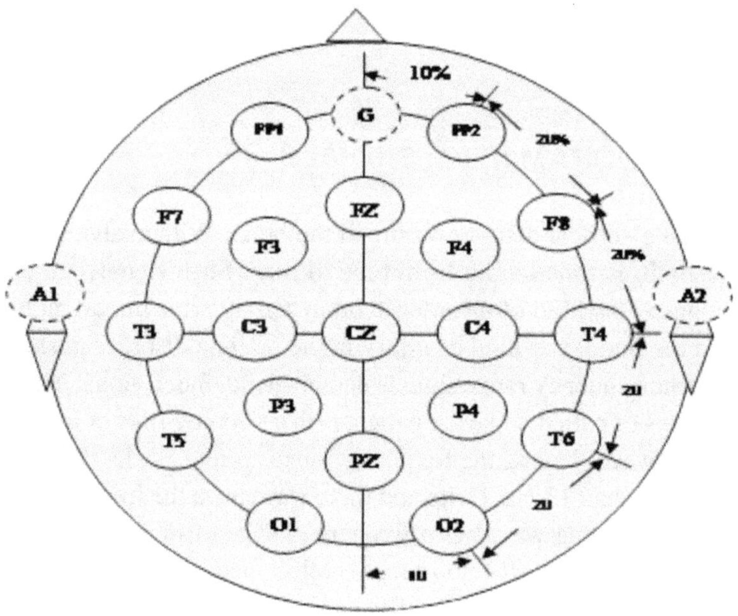

Noise removal from EEG data

EEG data contains various types of noise elements and artifacts for example muscle movement, heart rate, eye blinking, etc. Thus, it is required to eliminate such noises for the proper prediction of epilepsy and monitoring of patients. Removal of noise itself is a tedious job; we have to take care of any loss of data. There are various filtering or noise removal methods, which are able to remove these at a particular level. In Table 2, we are listing here various noise removal method used in presented references.

FEATURE EXTRACTION AND SELECTION FROM EEG DATA

After the noise removal from EEG data, it is required to pick some sort of features with maintaining appropriate information. For feature extraction, various methods have already been presented in various articles, which will be helpful for the detection of any diseases. Features are classified itself in two groups; one is time-domain features and the other one is frequency-domain features. Within the time domain, various features like – mean, variance, absolute mean, standard deviation, absolute deviation, skewness, energy of signal, entropy, maximum value, numbers of local maxima, minimum value, number of local minima, zero-crossing rate etc. whereas in the frequency domain features comes like frequency component having maximum and minimum value of amplitude, power spectral density, autoregressive coefficients, etc. These features may helpful for describing discrete /continuous wavelet transform, empirical mode decomposition, independent component analysis, principal component analysis, etc. By extracting various features, it is required to select some required features to built proper classifier, which can give a superior performance with an accuracy of detection of seizures and monitoring of patients. With a higher number of features, classifiers should also have the capacity to give better classification

Table 1. List of references with various EEG dataset

Authors	Electrode Placement System (International Standard)	Data Acquisition (Database)	Number of channels
Mahmoodian et al. (2019)	10–20	Freiburg iEEG	128
Emami et al. (2019)	10–20	24 patients from age (8-62 years)	19
Zhang et al. (2019)	10–20	Bonn University CHB-MIT EEG scalp	100 23
Vicnesh et al. (2019)	10–20	Bonn University	100
Sharma et al. (2019	10–20	Bonn University 10 patients collected at Neurology & Sleep Center, Sir Ganga Ram Hospital, New Delhi	100 -
Tzimourta et al. (2018)	10–20	University of Freiburg	6
Harpale et al. (2018)	10–20	CHB-MIT EEG scalp	23
Paul et al. (2018)	10–20	CHB-MIT EEG scalp	23
Ullah et al. (2018)	10–20	Bonn University	100
Sharma, Pachori (2018)	10–20	Bonn University	100
Chen et al. (2017)	10–20	CHB-MIT EEG scalp	23
Redelico et al. (2017)	10–20	2 data set taken - Bonn University	200
Mukherjee et al. (2017)	10–20	10 subjects collected - Bonn University	100
Gao et al. (2017)	10–20	online - Bonn University	100
Sharma et al. (2018)	10–20	Bonn University Database B available Neurology & Sleep center, New Delhi	100 -
Nanthini et al. (2017)	10–20	Data were taken directly from 10 normal and 10 abnormal (seizure) patients Bonn University	16 100
Bhattacharyya et al. (2017)	10–20	Bonn University	100
Zhang et al. (2017)	10–20	Bonn University	100
Olejarczyk et al. (2017)	10–20	Data were taken directly from 19 healthy people (10 males, age:22.8 $\pm$ 3.9 years)	128 electrodes
Keller et al. (2017)	10–20	Data set 1 was taken from an age of eight years child Data set 2 was taken from an age of eleven years, fours month child	19 19

accuracy with a huge amount of data or some new testing data. In literature, there are various features have been selected with the various algorithm of feature selection (Mahmoodian, Boese, Friebe, & Haddadnia, 2019; S.-L. Zhang, Zhang, Su, & Song, 2019; Nanthini & Santhi, 2017; Rahman, Bhuiyan, & Das, 2019).

Feature Classification

After extracting and selection of various features, the main objective is to train the classifier by using some set of data for the prediction /detection of epileptic seizures (Giannakakis, Sakkalis, Pediaditis, & Tsiknakis, 2015). After training the classifier we can allow passing the data for testing so that we can

Table 2. List of references with various noise removal methods

Authors	Noise removal Method	Filter Output
Mahmoodian et al. (2019)	Infinite Impulse Response Forward-Backward Notch filter	AC power supply noise of frequency approx 50 Hz removed
Zhang et al. (2019)	4th Order Chebyshev Band Pass Filter	Removes the artifacts of frequency range less than 0.5 Hz and greater than 30 Hz
Sharma et al. (2019)	Band Pass Filter	Removes power line noise of frequency range less than 0.5 Hz and greater than 40 Hz
Alhussein et al. (2018)	Ignored	–
Tzimourta et al. (2018)	Visual Inspection	Removes noise due to muscle activity and eye blinking
Harpale et al. (2018)	Independent Component Analysis	Removes noise due to muscle activity and eye blinking
Redelico et al. (2017)	Visual Inspection	Noise due to muscle activity and eye blinking removed
Mukherjee et al. (2017)	Butterworth Low Pass Filter or order 10 and FIR Band Pass Filter of order 9	Low pass filter removed electrooculography (EOG) artifact, then bandpass filtered of frequency range 1Hz to 500 Hz
Gao et al. (2017)	Visual Inspection	Noise due to muscle activity and eye blinking removed
Nanthini et al. (2017)	Band Pass Filter	Removes noise of frequency range less than 0.1 Hz and greater than 60 Hz
Olejarczyk et al. (2017)	Independent Component Analysis	Removes noises due to eye movement, cardiac activity, & muscle movement

obtain better prediction accuracy. In previous articles numbers of classifiers have already been proposed, which can be applied depending on the choice of selected features. Few of the classifiers are like Artificial Neural Network (ANN), Decision trees (DT) (Vicnesh & Hagiwara, 2019), Fuzzy Logic System (FLS) (Harpale & Bairagi, 2018; Krishnamurthi & Goyal, 2019), Linear Discriminant Analysis (LDA), Support Vector Machine (SVM) (Tzimourta et al., 2019; D. Chen, Wan, Xiang, & Bao, 2017; Gao, Cai, Yang, Dong, & Zhang, 2017; Bhattacharyya, Pachori, Upadhyay, & Acharya, 2017) etc. In some of the articles, researchers have used the combination of classifiers to improve the accuracy (Michielli, Acharya, & Molinari, 2019; Sun, Lo, & Lo, 2019), whereas, in some of the articles instead of using classifiers, they differentiated between ictal and non–ictal periods. Here in Table 3, we are presenting a list of references which uses various types of classifiers.

Table 4, shows performance comparison of RF classifier used by different researchers with various combinations of features of data, whereas Table 5 represents comparison of SVM classifier.

EXISTING WORK ON EPILEPSY MONITORING UNDER THE IoT PLATFORM

For epileptic seizure detection and real-time monitoring of patients, various IoT platforms have been introduced already. For this purpose, numbers of wireless body sensor and wearable equipment have been designed, which work on data collection basis and transmit them through the cloud. Data may be processed through the use of cloud computing or mobile cloud computing. The maximum amount of

Table 3. List of references with various classifiers with their performance

Authors	Classifiers	Performance
Bhati et al. (2019)	The two-band bi-orthogonal wavelet filter	A - 98.20%
Krishnamurthi et al. (2019)	Hybrid neuro-fuzzy system	A - 97%
Rahman et al. (2019)	ensemble stacking approach	A - 95.2% S - 96.1% Sp - 94.4%
Michielli et al. (2019)	Cascaded LSTM	A - 86.7%
Sun et al (2019)	Convolutional-Long Short-term Memory Neural Network (1D-Convolutional LSTM)	A - 99.58%
Mahmoodian et al. (2019)	Support Vector Machine (SVM)	A - 96.8% S - 95.8% Sp - 96.7%
Zhang et al. (2019)	Extreme Learning Machine (ELM) Support Vector Machine (SVM)	A - 99.68% (ELM) A - 99.56% (SVM)
Vicnesh et al. (2019)	Decision Tree (DT)	A - 93% S - 97% Sp - 88%
Sharma et al. (2019)	Support Vector Machine (SVM)	A - 100%
Fasil et al. (2018) [52]	Exponential energy feature used for classification	A - 89% (Bern-Barcelona EEG dataset) A - 99.5% (Ralph Andrzejak EEG dataset)
Hussein et al. (2019)	Deep neural network	A - 100% S - 100% Sp - 100%
Harpale et al. (2018)	Fuzzy Classifier	A - 96.48%
Ullah et al. (2018)	Convolutional Neural Network (CNN)	A - 99.1 ± 0.9%
Tzimourta et al. (2018)	Random Forest (RF)	A - 97.74 S - 99.74% Sp - 97.30%
Keller et al. (2017)	Random Forest (RF)	A - 70.6%
Nanthini et al. (2017)	Support Vector Machine (SVM)	A - 85 – 100%
Bhattacharyya et al. (2017)	Support Vector Machine (SVM)	A - 99%
Gao et al. (2017)	Support Vector Machine (SVM)	A - 100% S - 100% Sp - 100%
Mursalin et al. (2017)	Random forest (RF)	A - 98.45%
Chen et al. (2017)	Nearest Neighbour SVM classifier	A - 100% A - 93.6%

Notation: Accuracy – A, Sensitivity – S, Specificity - Sp

data, which stored in the cloud, will be helpful for training the model and achieving test accuracy. Cloud computing will also provide assistance or signaling to the patient, practitioner regarding the seizure. In references, various methods for finding electrical activity in the brain and detecting seizures already have been mentioned along with the use of various IoT based EEG equipment. One of them is an Epi-Care, performs mobile cloud computing based prediction of epilepsy, even monitoring is possible from home (Callegari et al., 2014). In this movable EEG devices helps to predict seizures, with the help of the

Table 4. Performance comparison based on RF classifier

Authors	Classifier	Performance	Remarks
Tzimourta et al. (2018)	Random Forest	Average A - 97.74% S - 99.74% Sp - 97.30%	-10-fold cross-validation Accuracy with different class ZONF-S A - 95.23% S - 99.74% Sp - 97.42% Z-S A - 99.95%, S - 100% Sp - 91.66% NF-S A - 98.15%, S - 98.64%, Sp - 97.18%
Keller et al. (2017)	Random Forest	A - 70.6%	Classification based on entropy
Mursalin et al. (2017)	Random forest	Average A - 98.45%	Accuracy with a different class A-E 100 B-E 98.0 C-E 99.0 D-E 98.5 ACD-E 98.5 BCD-E 97.5 CD-E 98.67 ABCD-E 97.4
Wang et al. (2018)	Random forest	A - 96.7% S - 95.6% Sp - 96.4%	10 fold cross-validation Dataset class ZO-FN-S
Tautan et al. (2018)	Random forest	A - 94%	EEG Database collected from 23 channels, 24 patients; For patient ID24

Notation: Accuracy – A, Sensitivity – S, Specificity - Sp

mobile cloud, it transmits information to the required destination. After mobile cloud computing, cloud computing also has been mentioned (Sareen, Sood, & Gupta, 2016). Further, body sensor networks have been used with the mobile cloud for seizure prediction (Lokhande & Mote, 2016).

During epilepsy, digital care has been proposed in (Page, Shankar, McLean, Hanna, & Newman, 2018). In this technological therapies as a solution have been mentioned. It works on the basis of mobile-based application, in which recorded data can be used for further taken care. For the real-time prediction of epileptic seizures, wearable devices (e-Glass) have been proposed (Sopic, Aminifar, & Atienza, 2018), which is based on four electrodes. It helps to early notify the seizures. An automatic epilepsy seizure detection method with wearable devices based on the cloud has been mentioned in (Escobar Cruz, Solarte, & Gonzalez-Vargas, 2018). In this paper, the proposed system is able to predict a tonic-clonic seizure and helps to alert member related to patients. An adaptive method for feature selection, extraction, and prediction of epilepsy has been mentioned in (Harpale & Bairagi, 2018). A cognitive system based on IoT-enabled cloud-related health platform for patient's monitoring and epilepsy detection (Alhussein et al., 2018) has been presented. This system is able to communicate with sensors, IoT devices and able to make a conclusion regarding the patient's health. In this proposed system, it also includes, obtaining information on a patient's condition using facial expression and patient movement, gestures, etc. In the cognitive system, IoT devices like sensors, etc. are linked with each other to store the information, process them. From the acquired information, drawing proper information and trained /adapt the system, cognitive system are itself capable.

Table 5. Performance comparison based on the SVM classifier

Authors	Classifier	Performance	Remarks
Mahmoodian et al. (2019)	Support Vector Machine (SVM)	Average A - 96.84% S - 95.83% Sp - 96.7%	Performance determined for 21 patients individually and out of 78 seizures, 75 detected correctly
Zhang et al. (2019)	Support Vector Machine (SVM)	A - 99.56% (SVM)	Accuracy measured with class F and S only
Sharma et al. (2019)	Support Vector Machine (SVM)	Average A - 96.4%	-10-fold cross-validation Accuracy with a different class of private database X-Y-Z 90.67 X-Z 97 Y-Z 100 XY-Z 98
Nanthini et al. (2017)	Support Vector Machine (SVM)	A - 85 – 100%	-10-fold cross validation
Bhattacharyya et al. (2017)	Support Vector Machine (SVM)	Average A - 99%	-10-fold cross-validation S-Z 100 S-O 100 S-N 99.50 S-F 98 S-FNZO 99 S-FN-ZO 98.60
Gao et al. (2017)	Support Vector Machine (SVM)	A - 100% S - 100% Sp - 100%	Leave one out and 10-fold cross-validation of set A, B, E
Chen et al. (2017)	SVM classifier	A - 93.6%	Dataset class {A, B, C, D}–{E}

Notation: Accuracy – A, Sensitivity – S, Specificity - Sp

For EEG analysis, a cloud-based mobile platform has been presented in (Dzaferovic et al., 2016). In this reference, for predicting seizures and transmitting information to nearby, wireless closed-loop system has been designed. The system consists of devices to collect the EEG data and Android-based applications are there for transmitting the information. These mobile-based applications are able to store the real-time information for a while and send them to cloud for further application. In this reference, the Neurosky Mind Wave device has been used and connected with application in android based Smartphone. Later, a number of mobile applications based on sensors have been developed for epilepsy care. There is a huge number of such apps based on android, windows, and iOS are available. With proper use of these applications benefited both epileptic patients and care providers too.

SMARTPHONE APPLICATIONS FOR THE CARE OF EPILEPTIC PATIENTS

The use of smartphone applications by epileptic patients gives them the freedom to take care of himself and is also beneficial for the practitioner to continuously monitor the patients and give them feedback on time. In Figure 5, various mobile apps presented for the care of epileptic patients like other bio-medical applications (Chinmay Chakraborty, 2017; Ranganathan, Aadhimoolam Chinnadurai, Samivel, Kesavamurthy, & Mehndiratta, 2015). Smartphone application like My Seizure Diary provides self-management structure for the care of epilepsy. This application helps to track seizures and related evidence and provide required therapies with proper communication to patient caretakers. It allows for capturing the timing of seizure, duration, etc. Such kind of information may send to the practitioner for suggesting further treatment. Using some other apps direct contact to the practitioner is also possible. These applications provide not only proper care but also their rectification too by suggesting the use of medicines, their dosage, etc.

Seizure Tracker is another such kind of application, which is based on a smartphone. This app can be effectively useful to manage epilepsy by maintaining the record of the seizure of timing, length, type of seizure, etc. the main aim of this app is to collect and share information in seizure library that can be accessible by practitioners. Another such type app is Seizure First Aide, which is developed by Epilepsy Foundation of Minnesota. As we know, a very huge amount of the population is affected by some kind of seizure. This application page provides real-time monitoring of seizure, which is able to capture video and can help in case of emergency. myChildren's is another app created by Nationwide Children's Hospital, it helps parents to track their children health. This app has an inbuilt epilepsy monitoring kit. By providing details of the child, parents will be able to monitor child epilepsy by adding this kit. This app is able to maintain record like the type of epilepsy, time, date duration, etc. and in case of emergency, it is useful too.

SeizAlarmis is also an epilepsy-related application, which is able to track seizure abnormality and helpful for contacting a practitioner in case of emergency. This application page is able to monitor abnormal activity /motion of the patient, heart rate abnormality, etc. along with, this app also provides help during an emergency by sending a help request. Another application, Epilepsy Heart Storylines provides a different kind of features to maintain patients. The app is able to keep record about indications of seizures, types, timings, a reminder of taking medicines, the behavior of patients, etc. it is able

Figure 5. Smartphone applications for the care of epileptic patients

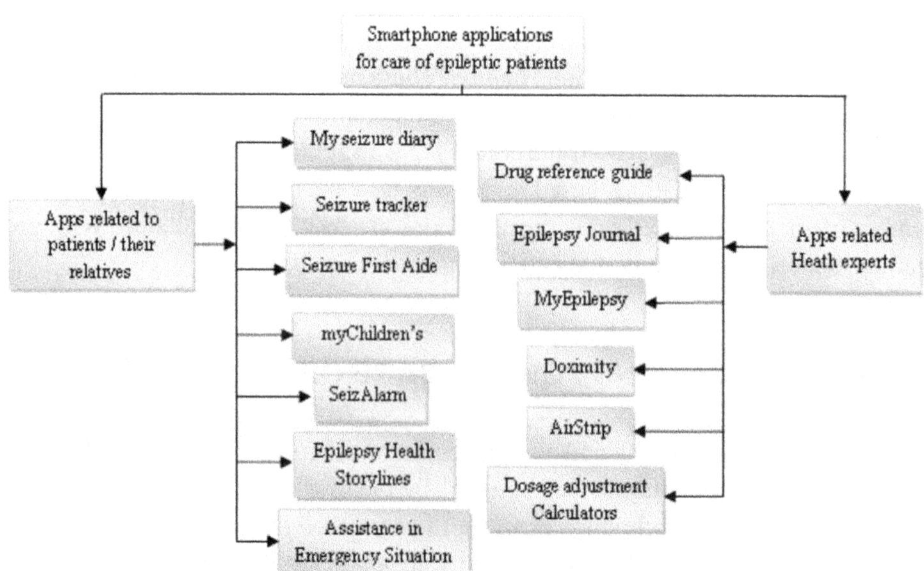

to display the daily report on the graphical pattern, which can be analyzed by the practitioner. Above all mentioned apps work for tracking and maintaining epileptic patients. Some other apps also available which are able to record data in form video clipping of seizure. Along with these clipping also have the description regarding the date, timings, length, location, etc. these recorded data are directly available for access to the practitioner for giving suggestion to patients and helps to investigate epilepsy.

There are some epilepsy care applications, which are particularly developed for experts /practitioner. These apps have quicker access to data related to epilepsy and their management. Some of the apps like drug reference guide can are adopted by the practitioner, so he will be able to get the information related to a particular medicine and respond to patient earliest. There are several apps already designed for the purpose of finding the required dosage for the cure of epilepsy on the basis of a particular patient. Various other applications are available, which makes this job easier for the practitioner. Currently, for practitioner searching for information through a mobile browser is become a tedious job, instead of it various apps are there which are able to access each type of such information very easily. Accessing all such kind information related to medical treatment given huge advantage to expert also. MyEpilepsy is another application, which provides all educational information related to epilepsy to practitioners as well as patients. It provides a base for keeping the record of seizure on a daily basis, helps to make an appointment with doctors, help to track information regard medicine, and health improvement, etc. Another few applications like Doximity, AirStrip, etc. basically provide a connection with different medical experts, practitioner, and patients. The main aim of AirStrip is to provide delivery of medicines to concern person suggesting via experts.

REAL-TIME EPILEPSY DETECTION AND PATIENT MONITORING USING SMARTPHONE

For monitoring of epileptic patients and detection of seizures, wireless monitoring devices are now available. Now it is possible for 24×7 monitoring of patients and getting easier. For this purpose wireless EEG headset connected with a smartphone is already developed, which works based on various applications. These apps provide a more accurate and reliable way to monitor seizures and patients. Along with these mobile apps other devices like a smartwatches are suitable for the prediction of seizures. During Seizure, information like timings, types of seizure, duration, location, etc. collected by different applications using a smartphone can be transmitted to patient caretakers/practitioners/medicine delivery system. In case of emergency help may be provided to the patients. Sometimes it is very difficult for patients to memories the occurrence of an event. Then this type of apps provides accurate information regarding epilepsy.

In Figure 6, the mobile base application has been presented, shows the different application of epilepsy monitoring and response from users, etc (Escoffery et al., 2018).

IoT BASED PATIENT MONITORING: VARIOUS FACTORS

With regards to seizure detection and monitoring of epileptic patients, some of the factors are there which should be taken care or we can say these factors are the area of concern. The very first is a real-time monitoring of patients and their response regarding epilepsy. Whenever the patient /caretaker feels any abnormal activity, such kind of facility or mobile application or environment must be there,

Figure 6. Elements for mobile applications for epilepsy and patient monitoring

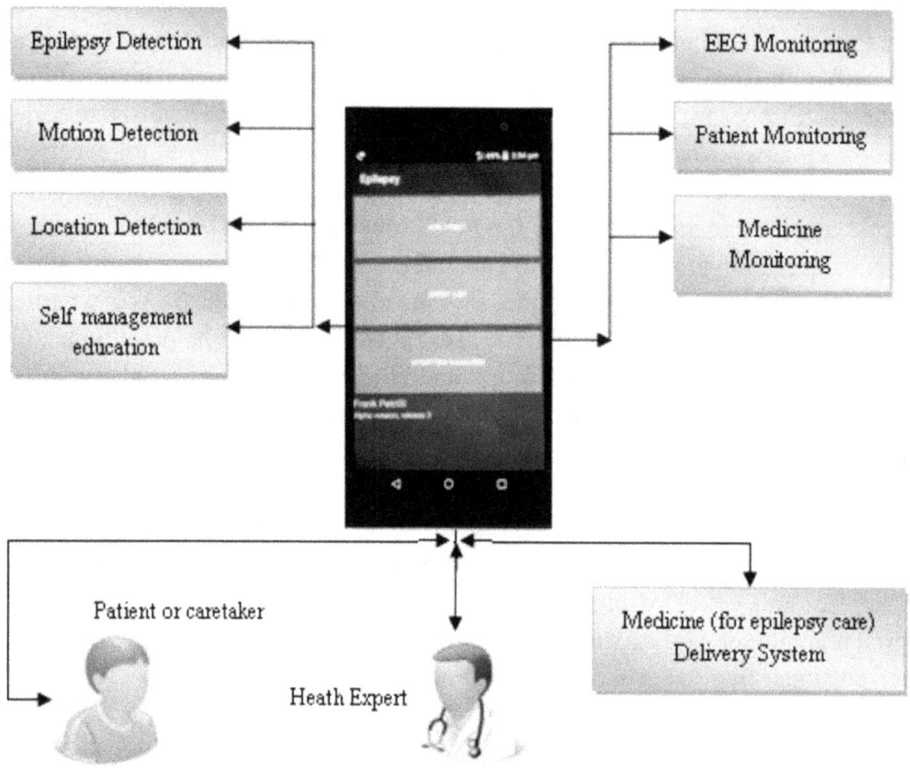

which can alert the caretaker or hospital staff and related real-time information needed to send to the practitioner. In other words, the gap between any abnormal activity and information transmission and response /health service from practitioner should be as lower as possible. Presently, a smartphone with proper applications should be that much capable so that they can keep the record and able to perform sufficient computation (C Chakraborty, Gupta, & Ghosh, 2014). Along with this batter, life is also an issue that cannot be ignored.

The requirement of wireless wearable devices is another small but important factor. For good success rate of monitoring of patient under the IoT platform, such devices are very much necessary with longer battery life. The implementation cost of the IoT platform is another factor which creates some obstruction for improvement in technology. Along with cost, how IoT related devices, sensors, etc. performing is the cause of concern. Service provided by the cloud is another factor, actually whatever the data collected by sensors or mobile-based applications are being transmitted in the cloud, where they stored. As these data required a very huge amount of storing capacity and managerial skill, henceforth cloud service is very much required and this information must be accessible by the practitioner for proper health related service. The amalgamation of a smartphone with cloud computation will be an added advantage. The smartphone can detect seizures and monitor the epileptic patient very efficiently with the use of various applications and able to provide medical delivery services, able to control the dosage of medicine, able to provide time to time expert service, able to cure disease in a smarter way. But all this could happen with proper service of internet, the speed of smartphone, battery life, etc.

EPILEPSY MANAGEMENT USING SMARTPHONE

Epilepsy is a disease caused due to disorder in the brain and its data management like signal recording, a record of seizure occurrence, types, issuing related medicine is a tough task. Smartphone plays a very important role for this purpose and can help practitioners regarding monitoring and treatment for epileptic patients. Proper use of smartphone applications related to epilepsy by patients /caretaker of patients as well as a health service provider, gives huge benefits. These applications can also help for epilepsy prediction, seizure detection and regarding their treatment. Smartphone applications like SeizAlarm, Assistance in an emergency situation can help to alert caretaker of patients quickly, helps to monitor patient and may help in case of an emergency. These applications are able to keep records regarding medicines, their effect. These applications help to remind epileptic patient for dosage in proper time. Usually, the epileptic patient is not able to recall the previous history of seizures. These smartphone applications help them to keep data and access them wherever they want. Another very useful point regarding these applications is an effective use of prediction and detection, which helps patients for medicines and self-care. These applications also help for automatic monitoring and delivery of medicine.

SENSING AND MONITORING OF EPILEPTIC SEIZURES: CHALLENGES

Prediction of epileptic seizures is a tedious job, henceforth identifying seizures and providing exerts them as early as possible is very challenging. Although the prediction rate is improving, the cure is not up to the mark. There is always a scope of improvement in reducing the seizures in epileptic patients. With the use of the smartphone-based application, it provides very good chances to monitor epilepsy and able to get proper suggestions from the practitioner. There are various apps, which provide the solution for the same. The main challenge is to monitor these data and provide suggestion and help very much requirement of hospital staffs. So their hiring, training regarding particular disease is the necessary and challenging job (Ranganathan et al., 2015). As technology is growing very rapidly, the main area of interest in real-time detection of seizures and monitoring of patients. There is a need for wireless wearable devices or such kind of equipment that can be implanted within the body, to improve the rate of successful cure.

Another challenge that presents the era if facing is a technical issue. As the staff of hospitals is very much trend in working manually, it is quite challenging to change their habit and forced to work them with the present smartphone-based application. For them maintaining patient health record electronically is getting tough. Maintaining huge epileptic data like seizures, rate, timing, etc. manually is tough, even though the acceptance rate for the digital form of hospital /patient record is very slow. As we know technology is growing very faster way with IoT and at present, there is a very huge number of the population is using a smartphone. It is very much accepted that the user should use any digital facility. But many of us avoid this facility or we fear using them. There is also another issue that most of the places are not properly connected with the internet or Wi-Fi facility. So, it is getting tougher the proper communication or transmission of information between patients and hospitals very frequently (Chinmay Chakraborty, Gupta, & Ghosh, 2014).

CONCLUSION

In the last few decades, IoT is growing very rapidly and also adaptation rate of this technology by patients and health experts is continuously increasing. In this chapter, we have discussed the use of IoT platform for seizure detection and monitoring of epileptic patients. We have seen how the use of smartphone completely changes the scenario of the diagnosis of patients. Along with cloud computation, the use of mobile under the IoT platform, we have discussed here. We have gone through a literature survey and find the works going on and already happened in the current situation. We have mentioned the role of IoT-enabled cloud in the e-health field. In this chapter, our main focus was seizure detection and for this, we have mention way of acquiring EEG data, feature extraction, selection, and classification. We have analyzed some of the recent work in this field. In this chapter, we also discussed various smartphone-based applications for analyzing the epileptic data, sharing of information with practitioner through the cloud and for providing better care of epileptic patients. As we know, presently real-time monitoring of patients is a tedious job. We have gone through some of the references and mentioned in this chapter about the applications based solution for this problem and improvement for quality of life standard. The provided solution may change the future prospects of analyzing patients. In this chapter, we also introduced in short about cognitive health monitoring system related with the cloud, which is able to monitor epileptic patients by using facial expression, gestures of patients, etc. and making a real-time decision. We have proposed a system model for prediction of seizure and monitoring of patients under the IoT platform and discussed how acquired data will be processed to experts through the cloud.

FUTURE SCOPE

As IoT evolving day by day, it is necessary to upgrade technologies in the e-health field too. Smartphone playing a very important role to evolve IoT and other services, so it required to upgrade the speed of internet, availability in the remote area too. For predicting epileptic seizures and monitoring of patients, providing them a quick service as a response, delivery of medicine, required dosage, quicker expert advice, taking care of epileptic patients each sector needs an up-gradation, so proper care of patients became possible. IoT enabled cloud-based technologies, platforms, various structures of network, topology, use of the protocol, etc. continuously upgrading and able to provide quality of service, the requirement of information transmission and reception speed. The main issue related to these, need to work for security and scalability of data during transmission and reception. Along with the security aspect, quality of data, the privacy of data should maintain and it is required to work in this field. With the transmission of a huge amount of medical data through IoT enabled cloud, there is a need for a smart home-based solution. Transmission of multiple patients' data will be an added advantage. In future work, we can analyze the cognitive structure to deal with EEG.

REFERENCES

Alhussein, M., Muhammad, G., Hossain, M. S., & Amin, S. U. (2018). Cognitive IoT-Cloud Integration for Smart Healthcare: Case Study for Epileptic Seizure Detection and Monitoring. *Mobile Networks and Applications*, *23*(6), 1624–1635. doi:10.100711036-018-1113-0

Bhattacharyya, A., Pachori, R. B., Upadhyay, A., & Acharya, U. R. (2017). Tunable-Q Wavelet Transform Based Multiscale Entropy Measure for Automated Classification of Epileptic EEG Signals. *Applied Sciences*, *7*(4), 385. doi:10.3390/app7040385

Botta, A., de Donato, W., Persico, V., & Pescape, A. (2014). On the Integration of Cloud Computing and Internet of Things. In *2014 International Conference on Future Internet of Things and Cloud* (pp. 23–30). Academic Press. 10.1109/FiCloud.2014.14

Callegari, D., Conte, E., Ferreto, T., Fernandes, D., Moraes, F., Burmeister, F., & Severino, R. (2014). EpiCare: A home care platform based on mobile cloud computing to assist epilepsy diagnosis. In *2014 4th International Conference on Wireless Mobile Communication and Healthcare - Transforming Healthcare Through Innovations in Mobile and Wireless Technologies (MOBIHEALTH)* (pp. 148–151). Academic Press. 10.4108/icst.mobihealth.2014.257379

Chakraborty, C. (2017). Chronic Wound Image Analysis by Particle Swarm Optimization Technique for Tele-Wound Network. *Wireless Personal Communications*, *96*(3), 3655–3671. doi:10.100711277-017-4281-5

Chakraborty, C., Gupta, B., & Ghosh, S. K. (2014). Tele-wound monitoring through smartphone. In *2014 International Conference on Medical Imaging, m-Health and Emerging Communication Systems (MedCom)* (pp. 197–201). Academic Press. 10.1109/MedCom.2014.7006003

Chakraborty, C., Gupta, B., & Ghosh, S. K. (2014). Mobile metadata assisted community database of chronic wound images. *Wound Medicine*, *6*, 34–42. doi:10.1016/j.wndm.2014.09.002

Chen, D., Wan, S., Xiang, J., & Bao, F. S. (2017). A high-performance seizure detection algorithm based on Discrete Wavelet Transform (DWT) and EEG. *PLoS One*, *12*(3), 1–21. doi:10.1371/journal.pone.0173138 PMID:28278203

Chen, M., Li, W., Hao, Y., Qian, Y., & Humar, I. (2018). Edge cognitive computing based smart healthcare system. *Future Generation Computer Systems, 86*, 403–411.

Chen, M., Hao, Y., Hu, L., Hossain, M. S., & Ghoneim, A. (2018). Edge-CoCaCo: Toward Joint Optimization of Computation, Caching, and Communication on Edge Cloud. *IEEE Wireless Communications*, *25*(3), 21–27. doi:10.1109/MWC.2018.1700308

Chen, M., Herrera, F., & Hwang, K. (2018). Cognitive Computing: Architecture, Technologies and Intelligent Applications. *IEEE Access: Practical Innovations, Open Solutions*, *6*, 19774–19783. doi:10.1109/ACCESS.2018.2791469

Chen, M., Wan, J., Gonzalez, S., Liao, X., & Leung, V. C. M. (2014). A Survey of Recent Developments in Home M2M Networks. *IEEE Communications Surveys and Tutorials*, *16*(1), 98–114. doi:10.1109/SURV.2013.110113.00249

Deshmukh, S., & Shah, R. (2016). Computation offloading frameworks in mobile cloud computing : a survey. In *2016 IEEE International Conference on Current Trends in Advanced Computing (ICCTAC)* (pp. 1–5). IEEE. 10.1109/ICCTAC.2016.7567332

Doukas, C., & Maglogiannis, I. (2012). Bringing IoT and Cloud Computing towards Pervasive Healthcare. In *2012 Sixth International Conference on Innovative Mobile and Internet Services in Ubiquitous Computing* (pp. 922–926). Academic Press. 10.1109/IMIS.2012.26

Dzaferovic, E., Vrtagic, S., Bandic, L., Kevric, J., Subasi, A., & Qaisar, S. M. (2016). Cloud-based mobile platform for EEG signal analysis. In *2016 5th International Conference on Electronic Devices, Systems and Applications (ICEDSA)* (pp. 1–4). Academic Press. 10.1109/ICEDSA.2016.7818497

Escobar Cruz, N., Solarte, J., & Gonzalez-Vargas, A. (2018). Automated Epileptic Seizure Detection System Based on a Wearable Prototype and Cloud Computing to Assist People with Epilepsy. In J. C. Figueroa-García, J. G. Villegas, J. R. Orozco-Arroyave, & P. A. Maya Duque (Eds.), *Applied Computer Sciences in Engineering* (pp. 204–213). Cham: Springer International Publishing. doi:10.1007/978-3-030-00353-1_18

Escoffery, C., McGee, R., Bidwell, J., Sims, C., Thropp, E. K., Frazier, C., & Mynatt, E. D. (2018). A review of mobile apps for epilepsy self-management. *Epilepsy & Behavior*, *81*, 62–69. doi:10.1016/j.yebeh.2017.12.010 PMID:29494935

Gachet, D., de Buenaga, M., Aparicio, F., & Padron, V. (2012). Integrating Internet of Things and Cloud Computing for Health Services Provisioning: The Virtual Cloud Carer Project. In *2012 Sixth International Conference on Innovative Mobile and Internet Services in Ubiquitous Computing* (pp. 918–921). Academic Press. 10.1109/IMIS.2012.25

Gao, Z.-K., Cai, Q., Yang, Y.-X., Dong, N., & Zhang, S.-S. (2017). Visibility Graph from Adaptive Optimal Kernel Time-Frequency Representation for Classification of Epileptiform EEG. *International Journal of Neural Systems*, *27*(04), 1750005. doi:10.1142/S0129065717500058 PMID:27832712

Giannakakis, G., Sakkalis, V., Pediaditis, M., & Tsiknakis, M. (2015). Methods for Seizure Detection and Prediction: An Overview. In V. Sakkalis (Ed.), *Modern Electroencephalographic Assessment Techniques: Theory and Applications* (pp. 131–157). New York, NY: Springer New York. doi:10.1007/7657_2014_68

Harpale, V., & Bairagi, V. (2018). An adaptive method for feature selection and extraction for classification of epileptic EEG signal in significant states. *Journal of King Saud University - Computer and Information Sciences*.

Hossain, M. (2016). Patient State Recognition System for Healthcare Using Speech and Facial Expressions. *Journal of Medical Systems*, *40*(12), 272. doi:10.100710916-016-0627-x PMID:27757715

Hossain, M., & Muhammad, G. (2016a). Audio-visual emotion recognition using multi-directional regression and Ridgelet transform. *Journal on Multimodal User Interfaces*, *10*(4), 325–333. doi:10.100712193-015-0207-2

Hossain, M., & Muhammad, G. (2016b). Cloud-assisted Industrial Internet of Things (IIoT) – Enabled framework for health monitoring. *Computer Networks*, *101*, 192–202. doi:10.1016/j.comnet.2016.01.009

Hossain, M. S., Muhammad, G., Song, B., Hassan, M. M., Alelaiwi, A., & Alamri, A. (2015). Audio-Visual Emotion-Aware Cloud Gaming Framework. *IEEE Transactions on Circuits and Systems for Video Technology*, *25*(12), 2105–2118. doi:10.1109/TCSVT.2015.2444731

Hou, L., Zhao, S., Xiong, X., Zheng, K., Chatzimisios, P., Hossain, M. S., & Xiang, W. (2016). Internet of Things Cloud: Architecture and Implementation. *IEEE Communications Magazine*, *54*(12), 32–39. doi:10.1109/MCOM.2016.1600398CM

Houssein, E. H., Hassanien, A. E., & Ismaeel, A. A. K. (2017). EEG Signals Classification for Epileptic Detection: A Review. In *Proceedings of the Second International Conference on Internet of Things, Data and Cloud Computing* (pp. 70:1--70:9). New York: ACM. 10.1145/3018896.3018970

Jasper, H. H. (1958). The ten twenty electrode system of the international federation. *Electroencephalography and Clinical Neurophysiology*, *10*, 371–375. Retrieved from https://ci.nii.ac.jp/naid/10020218106/en/

Krishnamurthi, R., & Goyal, M. (2019). Hybrid Neuro-fuzzy Method for Data Analysis of Brain Activity Using EEG Signals. In J. Wang, G. R. M. Reddy, V. K. Prasad, & V. S. Reddy (Eds.), *Soft Computing and Signal Processing* (pp. 165–173). Singapore: Springer Singapore. doi:10.1007/978-981-13-3600-3_16

Litt, B., & Echauz, J. (2002). Prediction of epileptic seizures. *Lancet Neurology*, *1*(1), 22–30. doi:10.1016/S1474-4422(02)00003-0 PMID:12849542

Lokhande, P. P., & Mote, T. S. (2016). *Epilepsy Monitoring and Analysis System using Android Platform*. Academic Press.

Mahmoodian, N., Boese, A., Friebe, M., & Haddadnia, J. (2019). Epileptic seizure detection using cross-bispectrum of electroencephalogram signal. *Seizure*, *66*, 4–11. doi:10.1016/j.seizure.2019.02.001 PMID:30769009

Megiddo, I., Colson, A., Chisholm, D., Dua, T., Nandi, A., & Laxminarayan, R. (2016). Health and economic benefits of public financing of epilepsy treatment in India: An agent-based simulation model. *Epilepsia*, *57*(3), 464–474. doi:10.1111/epi.13294 PMID:26765291

Michielli, N., Acharya, U. R., & Molinari, F. (2019). Cascaded LSTM recurrent neural network for automated sleep stage classification using single-channel EEG signals. *Computers in Biology and Medicine*, *106*, 71–81. doi:10.1016/j.compbiomed.2019.01.013 PMID:30685634

Nanthini, B., & Santhi, B. (2017). Electroencephalogram signal classification for automated epileptic seizure detection using genetic algorithm. *Journal of Natural Science, Biology, and Medicine*, *8*(2), 159–166. doi:10.4103/jnsbm.JNSBM_285_16 PMID:28781480

Nkosi, M. T., & Mekuria, F. (2010). Cloud Computing for Enhanced Mobile Health Applications. In *2010 IEEE Second International Conference on Cloud Computing Technology and Science* (pp. 629–633). IEEE. 10.1109/CloudCom.2010.31

Page, R., Shankar, R., McLean, B. N., Hanna, J., & Newman, C. (2018). Digital Care in Epilepsy: A Conceptual Framework for Technological Therapies. *Frontiers in Neurology*, *9*, 99. doi:10.3389/fneur.2018.00099 PMID:29551988

Rahman, M. M., Bhuiyan, M. I. H., & Das, A. B. (2019). Classification of focal and non-focal EEG signals in VMD-DWT domain using ensemble stacking. *Biomedical Signal Processing and Control*, *50*, 72–82. doi:10.1016/j.bspc.2019.01.012

Ramgopal, S., Thome-Souza, S., Jackson, M., Kadish, N. E., Fernández, I. S., Klehm, J., … Loddenkemper, T. (2014). Seizure detection, seizure prediction, and closed-loop warning systems in epilepsy. *Epilepsy & Behavior, 37*, 291–307.

Ranganathan, L. N., Aadhimoolam Chinnadurai, S., Samivel, B., Kesavamurthy, B., & Mehndiratta, M. M. (2015). Application of mobile phones in epilepsy care. *International Journal of Epilepsy, 02*(01), 28–37. doi:10.1016/j.ijep.2015.02.002

Sareen, S., Sood, S. K., & Gupta, S. K. (2016). An Automatic Prediction of Epileptic Seizures Using Cloud Computing and Wireless Sensor Networks. *Journal of Medical Systems, 40*(11), 226. doi:10.100710916-016-0579-1 PMID:27628727

Sharma, M., Shah, S., & Achuth, P. V. (2019). A Novel Approach for Epilepsy Detection Using Time–Frequency Localized Bi-orthogonal Wavelet Filter. *Journal of Mechanics in Medicine and Biology, 19*(01), 1940007. doi:10.1142/S0219519419400074

Sharma, R. R., & Pachori, R. B. (2017). Time–frequency representation using IEVDHM–HT with application to classification of epileptic EEG signals. *IET Science, Measurement & Technology*. doi:10.1049/iet-smt.2017.0058

Sopic, D., Aminifar, A., & Atienza, D. (2018). e-Glass: A Wearable System for Real-Time Detection of Epileptic Seizures. In *2018 IEEE International Symposium on Circuits and Systems (ISCAS)* (pp. 1–5). IEEE. 10.1109/ISCAS.2018.8351728

Sun, Y., Lo, F. P.-W., & Lo, B. (2019). EEG-based user identification system using 1D-convolutional long short-term memory neural networks. *Expert Systems with Applications, 125*, 259–267. doi:10.1016/j.eswa.2019.01.080

Tzimourta, K. D., Tzallas, A. T., Giannakeas, N., Astrakas, L. G., Tsalikakis, D. G., Angelidis, P., & Tsipouras, M. G. (2019). A robust methodology for classification of epileptic seizures in EEG signals. *Health and Technology, 9*(2), 135–142. doi:10.100712553-018-0265-z

Vergara, M., de la Cal, E., Villar, J. R., González, V. M., & Sedano, J. (2017). An IoT Platform for Epilepsy Monitoring and Supervising. *Journal of Sensors, 2017*, 1–18. doi:10.1155/2017/6043069

Vicnesh, J., & Hagiwara, Y. (2019). Accurate Detection of Seizure using Nonlinear Parameters Extracted from EEG Signals. *Journal of Mechanics in Medicine and Biology, 19*(01), 1940004. doi:10.1142/S0219519419400049

Yin, Y., Zeng, Y., Chen, X., & Fan, Y. (2016). Journal of Industrial Information Integration The internet of things in healthcare : An overview. *Journal of Industrial Information Integration, 1*, 3–13. doi:10.1016/j.jii.2016.03.004

Zanella, A., Bui, N., Castellani, A., Vangelista, L., & Zorzi, M. (2014). Internet of Things for Smart Cities. *IEEE Internet of Things Journal, 1*(1), 22–32. doi:10.1109/JIOT.2014.2306328

Zhang, Q., Cheng, L., & Boutaba, R. (2010). Cloud computing: State-of-the-art and research challenges. *Journal of Internet Services and Applications, 1*(1), 7–18. doi:10.100713174-010-0007-6

Zhang, S.-L., Zhang, B., Su, Y.-L., & Song, J.-L. (2019). A novel EEG-complexity-based feature and its application on the epileptic seizure detection. *International Journal of Machine Learning and Cybernetics*. doi:10.100713042-019-00921-w

Zhou, J., Leppanen, T., Harjula, E., Ylianttila, M., Ojala, T., & Yu, C., … Yang, L. T. (2013). CloudThings: A common architecture for integrating the Internet of Things with Cloud Computing. In *Proceedings of the 2013 IEEE 17th International Conference on Computer Supported Cooperative Work in Design (CSCWD)* (pp. 651–657). IEEE. 10.1109/CSCWD.2013.6581037

Chapter 10
Smart ECG Monitoring Through IoT

Ibtihel Nouira
Technology and Medical Imaging Laboratory, Medicine Faculty of Monastir, University of Monastir, Tunisia

Mohamed Hadj Said
https://orcid.org/0000-0003-4510-544X
Higher Institute of Computer Science and Mathematics, University of Monastir, Tunisia

ABSTRACT

The emergence of internet of things allows the integration of health systems by enabling real-time monitoring with a low cost. Therefore, one of the essential targets in this work is the realization of a new smart real-time electrocardiogram remote monitoring system based on cloud networks. This health wireless system allows the acquisition of electrocardiogram signal with the temperature and acceleration measurement of the patient's body using the inertial measurement unit module sensor. A strong access schemes is employed to transfer the data from sensors to cloud environment by keeping the protection of e-health information. The second objective in this chapter is designing a flexible and stretchable health circuit basing on design considerations, aiming the combination of flexible, elastic, and rigid materials around minimal constraints and maximum mechanical dependability in the structures. The flexible fabrication part was inspired from the biocompatible process technology.

INTRODUCTION

The electrical activity of organs is increasingly used in medicine to guide a diagnosis or to follow a therapy. These activities provide information on the physiological behavior of the person's body. The measurement of physiological signals allowed a better understanding of the electrical activities of certain organs, for example the heart's activity measured by the electrocardiogram (ECG).

DOI: 10.4018/978-1-7998-0261-7.ch010

In this area, the rise of new technologies as well as the progress made in the areas of microelectronics, telecommunications, networks and information processing have led to the emergence of new tools and communicating objects, and more particularly the systems of medical applications.

In fact, the arrival of such communication technologies has made it possible to acceede another dimension in order to improve the quality of the individual's life. Actually, the electronic transfer of medical data promotes control at distance and health care provision of any patient. This ensures not only a rapid exchange of medical information but also a real-time diagnosis of the physiological and medical state of the patient. In this context, the designers of medical applications are constantly competing to satisfy the user's needs by providing solutions to various daily problems.

BACKGROUND

Recently, several studies have been interested in developing systems for remote monitoring of cardiac signals (Yang et al, 2016; Xia et al, 2013; Manikandan et al, 2019). In fact, the arrival of the Internet of Things (IoT) allows driving the development of large advanced information services, which requires the treatment in real-time and the storage of data centers with a great capacity and computing power (Chakraborty et al, 2016). In addition to that, the rapid growth of the (IoT) has led to the development of a multitude of new access technologies targeted at low power- wide area networks (LP-WANs). For example, sensors and monitoring solutions can exchange very small data rate and very little energy consumption can be considered as the typical applications for the LPWAN (Qadir et al, 2018; Rashid et al, 2016). In addition, the arrival of new processing technologies in the field of biomedical engineering allows for a considerable development. More specifically, the emergence of the field of artificial intelligence and its integration with IoT applications makes it possible to innovate automatic tools that help real-time medical diagnosis in the development of therapeutic strategies and follow-up care (Rashid et al, 2016; Rashid et al, 2018).

However, despite the fact that these systems are undergoing a great technological evolution, they suffer from several major problems. The most critical problem is the lack of a rigorous system design. Often, the ECG monitoring systems are based on conventional rigid and flat printed circuits. Nevertheless, portable and implantable cardiac monitoring circuits require non-flat assemblies for an easy deployment because this type of systems must follow their regular shapes on which the circuit is integrated. An option to achieve a significant degree of comfort is the deep miniaturization of the circuit using fine pitch circuits, small components, 3D integration, etc. By applying this strategy, the circuit can be realized on a sufficiently small surface (Sterken et al, 2011). In fact, many techniques were introduced to make the medical devices comfortable and unobtrusive. Among these techniques, many works have proposed to improve the type of electrodes using bio potential electrodes, which can acquire the ECG signals better than the normal Ag/AgCl ones (Thap et al, 2016; Chlaihawia et al, 2018). Other research works have explored dry ECG electrodes by establishing conductive materials (Zhou et al, 2014; Wang et al, 2013) and developing microelectro-mechanical systems (MEMS) based on microelectrodes (Wang et al, 2013). However, most of those techniques used different integrated components onto a flex polymer substrate that can be stretched, bendable and twistable, depending on the application. One way to create this device can be made by placing rigid or flex components over the polymer surface and interconnect them by a stretchable connection (Wang et al, 2013). This method can increase the conformability of the circuitry and the ability to deform in the same irregular way as the surface (skin) onto which it is applied. Several works have been interested in applying these techniques for manufacturing ECG signal recording circuits. For example; R.Carta et all (Carta et al, 2009) were designed by resorting to a flexible-stretchable platform for biomedical application using two islands, both of them contain different components interconnected by a stretched bridge with a meander motif. This platform was fabricated using a biocompatible process, which is described in (Brosteaux et al, 2007). Other works have used the fast prototyping technology process (Kim et al, 2006). This method as described in (Axisa et al, 2008), used different rigid or flexible electronic components interconnected with the stretchable shaped meander. The latter was created by using the Yttrium Aluminum Garnet (YAG) laser and molded in silicone rubber afterwards (Axisa et al, 2008). Many other works have studied the different stretchable shaped meander using Finite Element Methods (FEM) analysis, for improving the performance of such circuitry or platform (Gonzalez et al, 2008; Nordine t al, 2019).

MAIN FOCUS OF THE CHAPTER

The major contribution of this work is the designing of a stretchable and elastic ECG system of remote monitoring, which is supplied by tiny batteries. In fact, this work provides and realizes, firstly, a portable system that simultaneously measures the heart rate, body temperature and acceleration rate of the patient. This system allows the analysis and characterization of the ECG signal in relation to the temperature and the movement of the patient in order to properly analyze and detect cardiac pathologies if there is any. This makes it possible to establish an accurate, reliable and effective diagnosis for an application of remote monitoring. In this case and to facilitate the treatment, this system also allows the transmission of recorded data (ECG, temperature and acceleration) to a medical center to monitor the patient's condition. The main advantage of such IoT (Internet of Things) system is the provision of remote monitoring in real time (Chakraborty et al, 2014; Akash et al, 2019. With such a monitoring, the identification of emergencies like heart attacks or sudden falls for at-risk patients will become easier. In addition, people with cognitive and physical disabilities can have a more independent and easier life. In addition, this work proposes the study of the biocompatible process fabrication for the stretchable flexible board; this process will be implemented for the circuitry design of this work. The implementation of flex-rigid technology for the developed ECG system can make the device wearable and unobtrusive, this can make the systems more efficient. Therefore, this chapter touches upon important topics in the healthcare technology field: Internet of medical things, remote patient monitoring, telemedicine, eHealth… It proposes an effective and secure solution in order to transmit medical data from patients to doctor by offering a flexible design of the wearable ECG circuit.

This manuscript is organized as follow: Firstly, the different blocs of ECG remote monitoring system are presented by detailing the components and the operating principle of each block and exposing the different results of the ECG system. Next, the design of the stretchable IoT ECG system is described. Finally, this chapter will elicit the given conclusion.

ECG Remote Monitoring System

This chapter consists in creating an ECG remote monitoring system to facilitate and improve the quality of care and remote medical surveillance. This system is characterized by its adaptability to tele-monitor the medical condition of the patient by highlighting the relationship between, on the one hand, its cardiac

Figure 1. General architecture of the ECG remote monitoring system

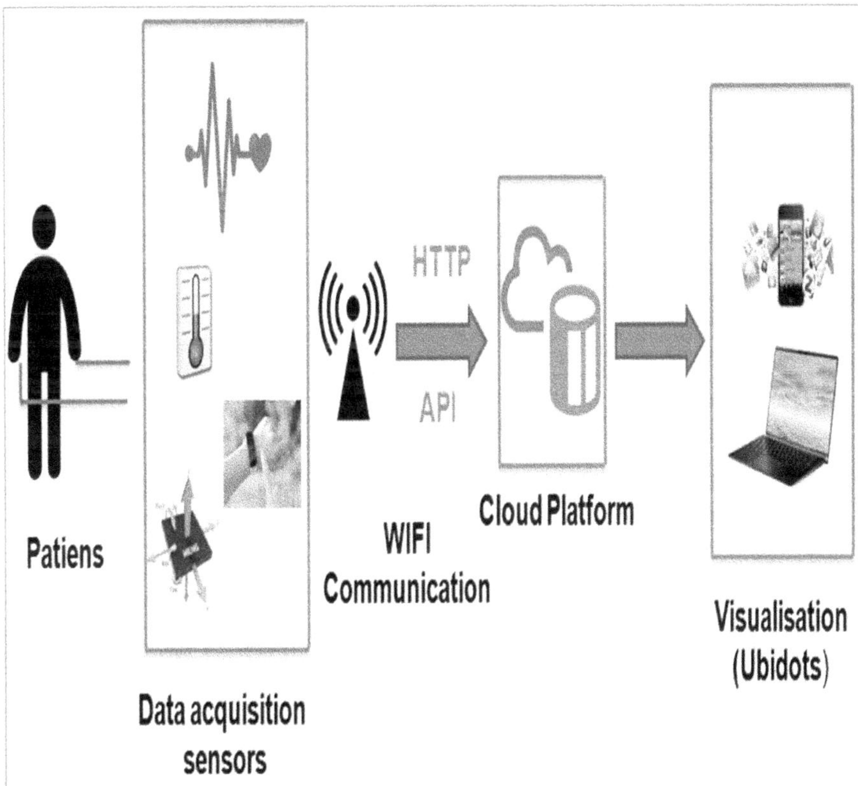

activity and on the other hand, the temperature and movement of the patient's body. This solution will be able to send data information to a storage server for remote medical monitoring by allowing the doctor have cardiac activities by means of a wireless link. Further, an IoT Cloud platform (Ubidots) will then be developed to collect this information and present it in a simple way to the user. This chapter has an important advantageous point for monitoring elderly people, persons with reduced mobility, people at risk and patients with heart disease. In addition, this system allows the monitoring of their living environment and overcome their disabilities while ensuring efficiency, cost reduction and analysis in real time. The general architecture of this ECG remote monitoring system is described in Figure 1:

This chapter puts into evidence the manufacturing of the data monitoring circuit of ECG, temperature and acceleration of patients. This block is composed of two floors; the first is a data acquisition and transmission stage that includes an ECG acquisition circuit with a gyroscope and accelerometer Gy-521 module for temperature and acceleration measurement. In addition, this block is responsible for the analog/ digital conversion of the ECG signals and the transmission of different measured data to the server. This function is provided by a module called Node MCU. The second stage allows sending the data on the Cloud Ubidots, where the patient can consult his data.

Data Acquisition and Transmission Stage

In fact, this chapter focuses on the block of ECG data acquisition and processing. This block consists of three important parts (Figure 2):

- ECG signal acquisition unit
- Gyroscoe-accelerometer sensor
- Gateway unit

ECG Signal Acquisition Unit

Preamplifier

The amplitude of the signal coming from the electrodes is very weak. Consequently, in order to suppress the Common Mode Noise (CMN) and to supply the essential differential amplification, this work uses an amplifier characterized by a high input impedance and a high common mode rejection ratio (CMRR) (Akash Et al, 2019).

Figure 2. Synoptic scheme of data acquisition and processing for the ECG monitoring system

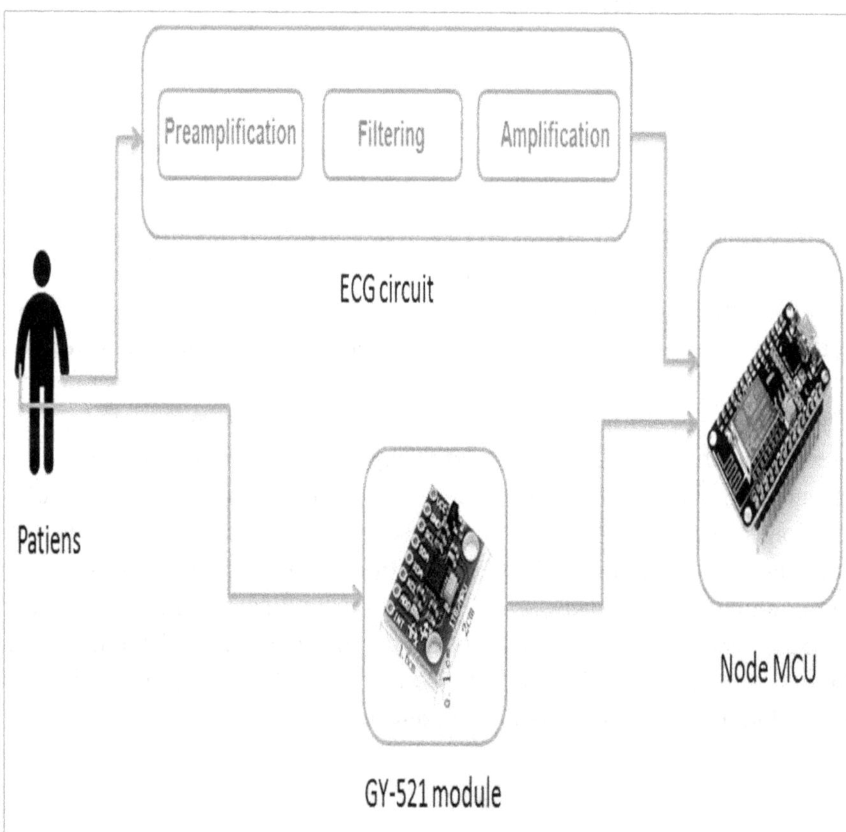

In this context, the amplifier AD620AN is chosen to ensure the amplification of the ECG signal.The AD620AN is a high precision instrumentation amplifier with a very large input impedance and a large common mode rejection rate, which implies noise reduction at the input. The amplitude of the signal at the output of the sensor is between 1mV and 3mV. In this case, the resistance RG is equal to 560Ω, which corresponds to a gain in voltage G of 89.21. The gain of the AD620 is given by Eq. 1 (Sun et al, 2012).

$$G = \frac{49.4K\Omega}{RG} + 1. \qquad (1)$$

Filter Blocks

The low nature of the ECG signal and the large noise that affects it requires the implementation of several stages of filters. In this chapter, three types of low-pass, high-pass, and rejector filters are used.

Low-Pass Filter

The signal obtained at the output of the pre-amplification phase is completely embedded in the noise. For this purpose, a low-pass filter is necessary in order to suppress all the high-frequency noises. It is known that the frequency content of an ECG signal (pathological or normal) is less than 150Hz (Abdol et al, 2014). Therefore, a first order low-pass filter of type RC is chosen. For a resistance R=1KΩ and capacitor C=1µf, the cutoff frequency f_{c1} is calculated by Eq. 2:

$$f_{c1} = \frac{1}{2\Pi RC} = 150Hz. \qquad (2)$$

High Pass Filter

This RC first order filter removes low frequency (<0.03Hz) noise due to breathing and electrode movement resulting in a drift of the ECG signal baseline.

For a resistance R=5.6KΩ and capacitor C=1000µf, the cutoff frequency f_{c2} is calculated by the Eq. 3:

$$f_{c2} = \frac{1}{2\Pi RC} = 0.03Hz. \qquad (3)$$

Notch 50Hz Filter

This filter is used to suppress the 50Hz sector noise. The structure of this filter is shown in Figure 3 A.

In this structure, the different components must be taken as follows:

C1 = C3; C2 = 2C1; R1 = R2; R3=R1/2.

So for resistance R1=100KΩ and capacitor C1=33nF, the cutoff frequency fc3 is given by Eq. 4:

$$f_{c3} = \frac{1}{2\Pi R1C1} = 49Hz\,. \tag{4}$$

Amplification

After the filtering operation using passive components, a second amplification operation with the lm833D amplifier is recommended. A simple non-inverting amplifier is realized with an adjusted gain of six (figure 3 B).

The resistors R1 and R2 are used to adjust the gain. The latter is given as follows:

$$G = \frac{R1 + R2}{R2}. \tag{5}$$

If R1= 50KΩ and R2=10KΩ, the gain G is equal to six.

Figure 3. A) Structure of a notch filter, B) A non-inverting amplifier mounting

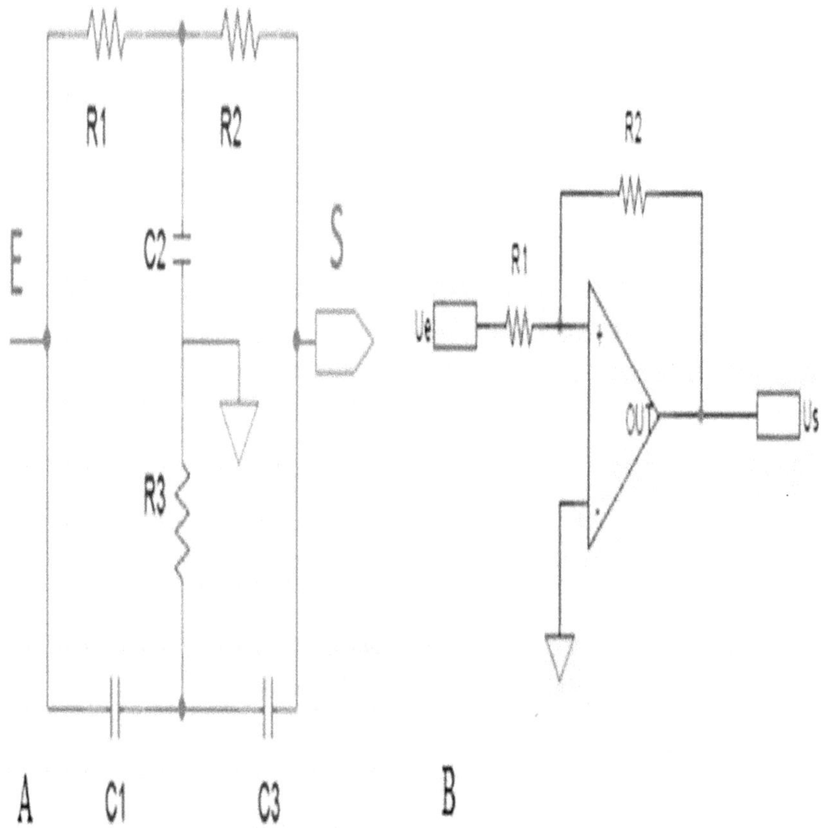

Global ECG Acquisition Circuit

The basic steps in detecting and conditioning the ECG signal are the following:

- Signal detection.
- Preamplifier (instrumentation amplification "AD620AN").
- Filtering (low pass filter / high pass filter / 50Hz notch filters).
- amplification (lm833D).

In order to assemble all the blocks mentioned above, Figure 4 is a representation of the final circuit of acquisition. In fact, the signal is detected by means of three electrodes. The electrodes are selected gelled so as to ensure a good connectivity between the electrodes, cables and mounting to limit noise. The detected signal by the electrodes reaches an instrumentation amplifier (AD620) that will amplify the difference. The exit of the AD620 is then filtered by a high-pass filter, which attenuates frequencies below its cutoff frequency fc, and retains only the high frequencies. Then, the ECG signal is filtered by a low-pass filter that attenuates the frequencies higher than its cut-off frequency fc, and keeps only the frequency bases. Finally, the 50Hz sector noise is suppressed with the notch filter. Once the signal is filtered, it will be amplified by a non-inverting amplifier (lm833D).

Figure 4. Overall electrical scheme of the ECG signal acquisition system

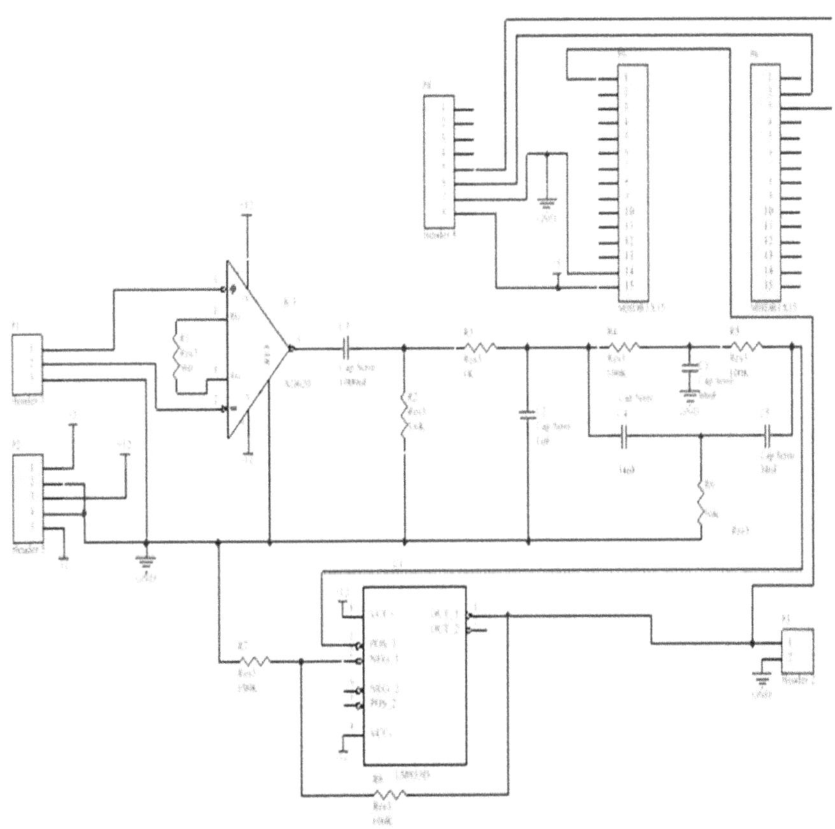

Gyroscoe-Accelerometer Sensor

The GY-521 module is a branching board for MEMS MPU-6050 (microelectro-mechanical systems) that includes a three-axis gyroscope, a three-axis accelerometer, a digital motion processor (DMP), and a sensor temperature. The three -axis gyroscope can spot rotational swiftness along the x,y and z axis with the Micro-Electro Mechanical System technology (MEMS). Once the sensor is rotated around any axis, a vibration is generated due to the Coriolis Effect that is detected by the MEMS.

The three-axis accelerometer detect tilt or inclination angle along the x, y and z axis with MEMS.

The acceleration along the three axes deviates the moving mass that unbalances the differential capacitor detected by the MEMS.

The digital motion processor can be used to process complex algorithms directly on the map. Usually, the DMP processes the algorithms that convert the raw values of the sensors into stable position data. The values of sensors are recovered using the I2C serial data bus (Inter-Integrated Circuit), which only requires two SCL (Serial Clock Line) and SDA (Serial Data Line) wires.

With this inertial sensor positioned on the human body, the desired parameters (acceleration and temperature) can be measured to follow patients: walking, activity and falling. Besides, the use of Gy-521 allows calculating the temperature of the patient in relation to time by using the following equation:

$$Temperature(°C) = \frac{temperature(GY)}{340} + 36,53. \tag{6}$$

The values of sensors are recovered using the I2C (Inter-Integrated Circuit) serial data bus, which requires only two SCL (Serial Clock Line) and SDA (Serial Data Line) wires. In fact, whenever the SCL line is in the high state, a bit is available on SDA. A frame starts with a start condition and ends with a stop condition and a master can string multiple frames by returning a restart condition to the following a first frame.

Each I2C component has an address. When a master sends a message, it starts with transmitting the address of the component to which it wants to address and the direction of transmission (writing or reading). In this case, when the slave is connected to the bus, there is a detection of its address.

The connection of this module with the gateway is given by Figure 5.

Gateway Unit

In this chapter, the project requires a central part capable of receiving the data from the acquisition card and sending them to an emergency server via a mobile internet connection.

The choice of the NodeMCU card as a gateway is justified by the qualification of its price (30 dollars)-performance ratio and the compatibility of its size with the developed system. In addition, the NodeMCU IoT platform supports analog inputs and digital outputs. It integrates its own analog / digital converter and an integrated wifi card.

In fact, the gateway card is connected with the acquisition card and the accelerometer. An interface of the ECG acquisition card with the analog input of NodeMCU is performed. Therefore, the analog / digital converter of NodeMCU will convert the acquired data into a digital signal. However, the NodeMCU is connected through its digital input with the GY-521 by I2C serial data bus.

Figure 5. Connection between the Gateway board and the accelerometer sensor – gyroscopes Gy-521 through I2C bus

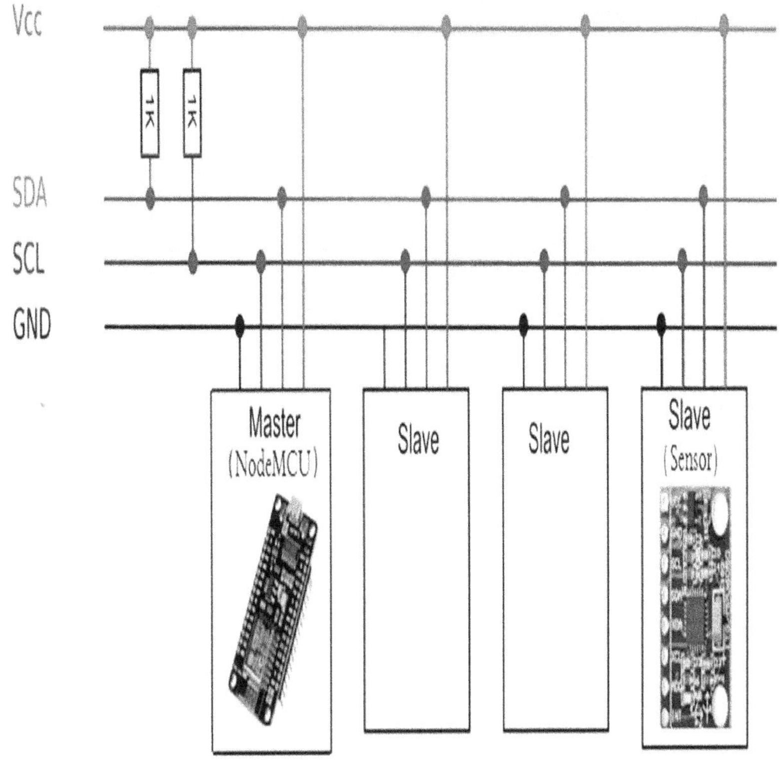

The SCL and SDA of the Gy-521 were connected to the ESP Node configured by default; SDA line on pin D2 and the SCL line on pin D1. The I2C bus can move from the default pin by adding the library: Wire.h. In Figure 6, the package of the Sensor and the Node was substituted by the Header connector.

Remote Monitoring

The Internet of Things exploits the network of objects and sensors. In fact, the integration of IoT with Cloud Computing technology adduces not only the high computational power and the large storage capacity, but they permit to IoT services to be invasive, cost-effective, and accessible from anywhere in the world using whatever device (stationary or mobile) (Pacheco et al, 2018). Therefore, the unfolding of Cloud system is very beneficial to achieve intelligent and smart healthcare conditions (Gravina et al, 2017).

In this work, after connecting the sensor, the data will send on the Cloud, where the patient can view his data. Raw sensor data and recognized activity are sent from the Cloud using protocol HTTP (Hypertext Transfer Protocol) and processed in real time to make a diagnosis of the current situation and propose actions. The data are exchanges with all the actors concerned: the doctor, administrator and the patient.Figure7 shows the IoT architecture developed in this work. This architecture is composed of three layers, which are IoT end-nodes, communications and the third layer is services and applications.

Figure 6. Connection between the Gy-521 and Gateway

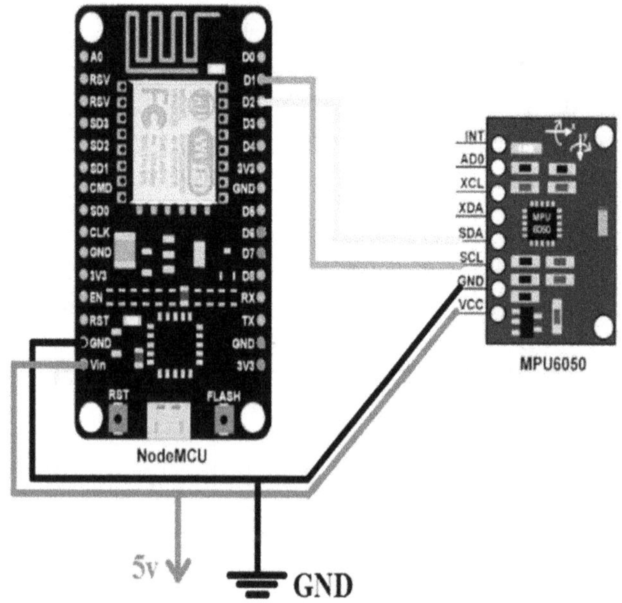

Figure 7. Hierarchical architecture for IoT ECG system

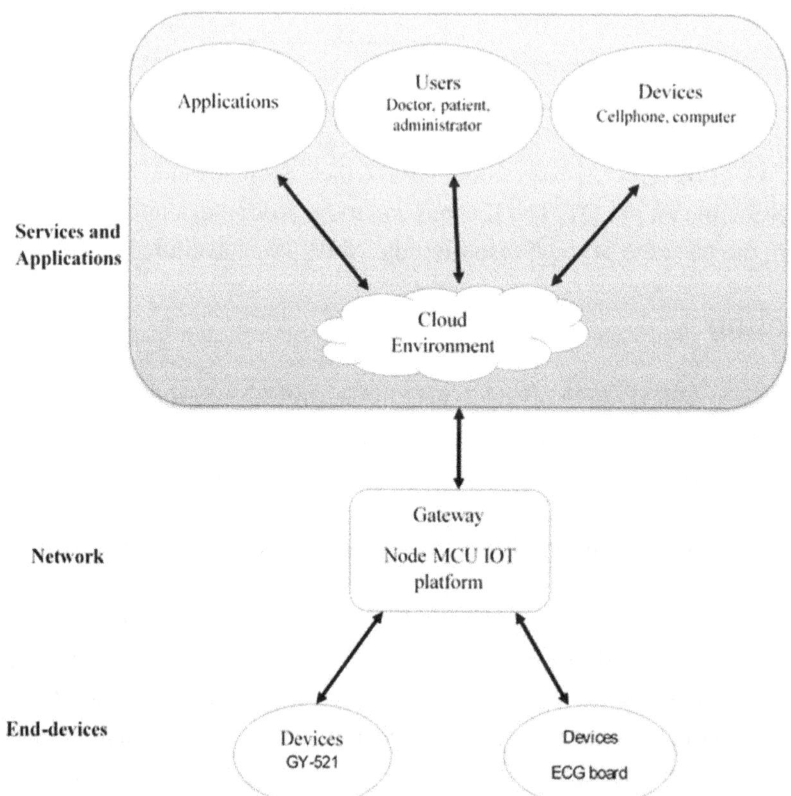

The layer of end-nodes encompasses components. These components can be sensors for receiving and converting the physical measurements to the digital domain. Furthermore, they can be an actuator whose role is the modification of the environment to a desired condition or state (Sun et al, 2012) In this work, the end-nodes layer includes the body sensors that are the ECG acquisition board and the GY-521 module.

The network layer is in charge of the transmission of reliable information from and to end-nodes. This layer integrates communication protocols, mobile communication and wireless sensor networks, etc (Hossain et al, 2015). In the developed ECG system, the network layer comports the Gateway unit, which is the NodeMCU IoT platform. The layer of application affords personalized services depending on user needs (Manadhata et al, 2011). The access to these services is achievable across mobile technology such as cellphone and mobile applications, smart devices and appliances (Pacheco et al, 2018).

For the Cloud environment, a platform called Ubidots has been selected. It is about an integrated solution that covers all the services needed to successfully implement small to medium sized solutions at an affordable cost.

The developed application must ensure the acquisition and display of data (temperature, ECG signal and acceleration). However, to guarantee a great security against the important growth in the attack surface and heterogeneity, this work integrates a special identification process. In fact, being different from a traditional identification process basing on username/password authentication, IoT Ubidots adopts the HTTP token-based authentication. This authentication process assures a high level of security by transmitting a token in the HTTP headers, more particularly by using the HTTP header field of 'X-Auth-Token'.

The developed IoT application allows each user to token authenticate and access his workspace. In this work, the administrator allows to manage the list of doctors and medical staff (add, update, deletion). However, each doctor allows authorizing the management of the list of his patients only (add, update, select, delete).

In fact, in order to connect to the application, the system checks the submitted data. If the transmitted token authentication is correct, the authentication succeeds. Otherwise, the authentication fails and the user can not acceed the application.

A display of the history of acquired signals for each patient using the capabilities offered by Cloud technology is provided. In addition, this platform calculates the heart rate frequency by using the time intervals between each peak and counting the number of beats in 60 seconds. In case of heart malfunction, an alarm message is sent to the doctor and patient with minimum and maximum level alerts. Figure 8 shows the data transmission scenario from the acquisition card to the user (doctor or patient). As a first step, after a validated establishment of an HTTPS connection using WIFI, the user asks to accede the health Cloud services in order to receive and get the resource data.

Then, this interface sends a request to the database, which in turn asks to recover the values of the processing unit. This unit uses the sensor to capture the data. In this case and after the acquisition of data, the sensor sends the acquired information to the processing unit (NodeMCU IoT) to transmit it to Ubidots REST (Representational State Transfer)API (Application Programming Interface) via HTTPS and saves it in the database. Finally, the latter sends this information to the acquisition interface (Ubidots platform) to allow the display to the doctor.

Figure 8. Acquisition scenario of the IoT ECG system

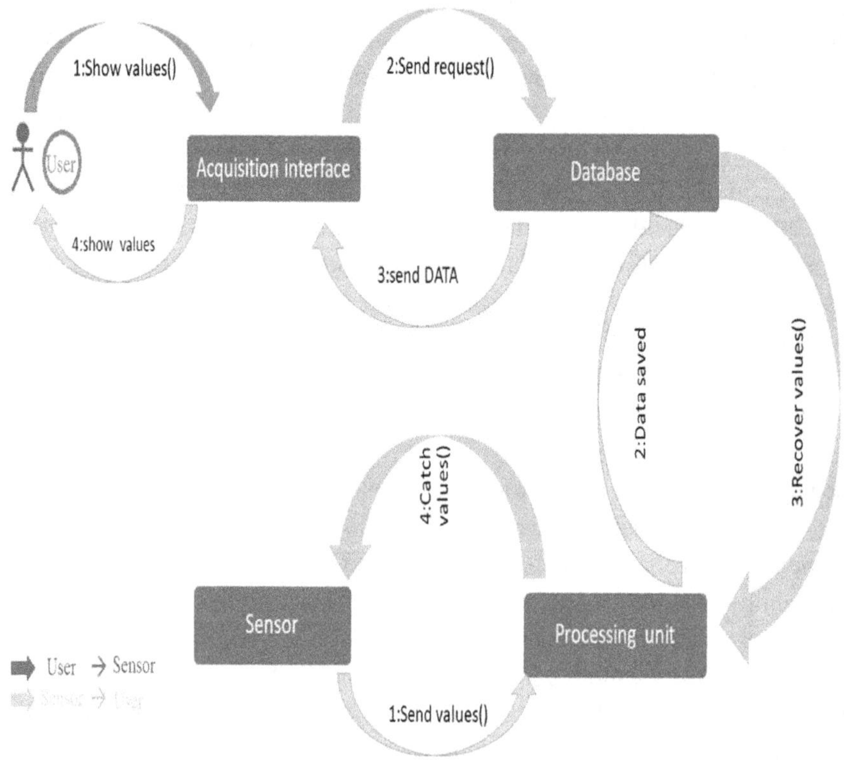

In fact, the principal objective of this application of wearable ECG system in Cloud technology is to guarantee to the users a secured access control in real time to the health data (ECG, temperature, acceleration) and services. Thus, the developed IoT ECG system must meet the following needs:

- **Authenticity and Security:** The application will have to be highly secure; the information need not be accessible to everyone. In order to ensure a high level of security, the authenticity is required by validating the process of HTTP header token used by the various actors who request to accede the ECG system.
- **Extensibility:** As part of this work, the application will have to be extensible, which allows add new features or change features already developed.
- **Availability:** The data availability exposes serious problems for the online health process. Hence, the high and easy accessibility of the e-health services by healthcare providers will be an urgent necessity. The availability of ECG resources is assured by the rapid and easy accessing to ECG health Cloud system.

Evaluation of IoT ECG System

After the completion of the ECG analog circuit, the results obtained are shown in Figure9:

Figure 9 shows that the ECG signal is well detected. The different waves such as the P wave, the QRS complex and the T wave are clearly visible; Also the rhythm heart can be easily determined.

After creating an account on Ubidots, a "data source", which will contain the variables where the data is stored, is created (Figure 10).

Then, the geo-location of the patient is used by the Google map application (Figure 10). The result on Ubidots shows the storage of data in real time. It is a representation that shows the details of sending the data as (date, variables ...). A dashboard that displays variable data is created.

Figure 11A shows the displayed GY-521 parameters, which are the three values x, y, z for the acceleration and the temperature value of a patient. The event part on Ubidots makes it possible to exploit the data to inform someone with an SMS or email. For example, an SMS is sent to a doctor or patient to indicate the condition of a patient if the temperature exceeds 39 ° C (Figure 11B).

An example of the ECG signal from a healthy subject volunteer is displayed through a wirelessly transmission to a receiving computer. Figure 12 shows the good quality of displayed digital ECG signal.

Figure 9. Display of the ECG signal on the oscilloscope

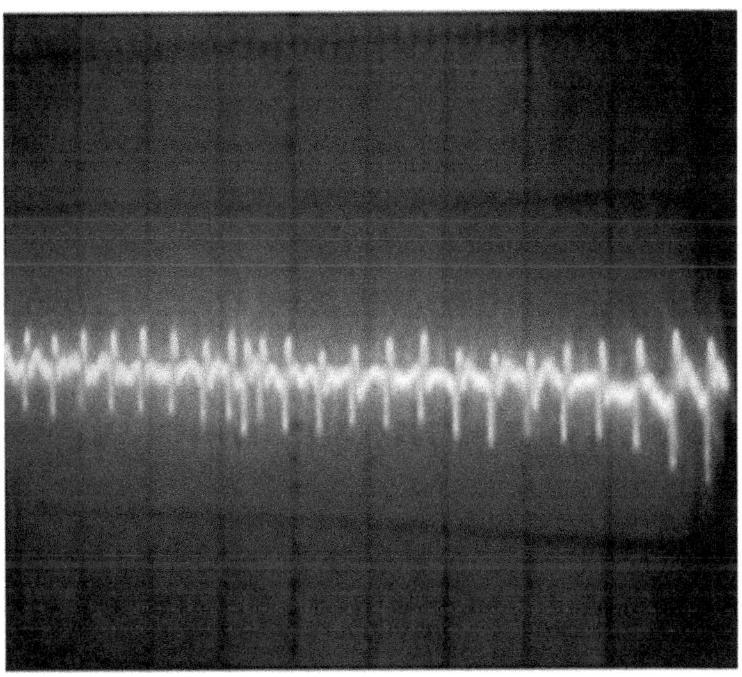

Figure 10. Storage of data on "Ubidots"

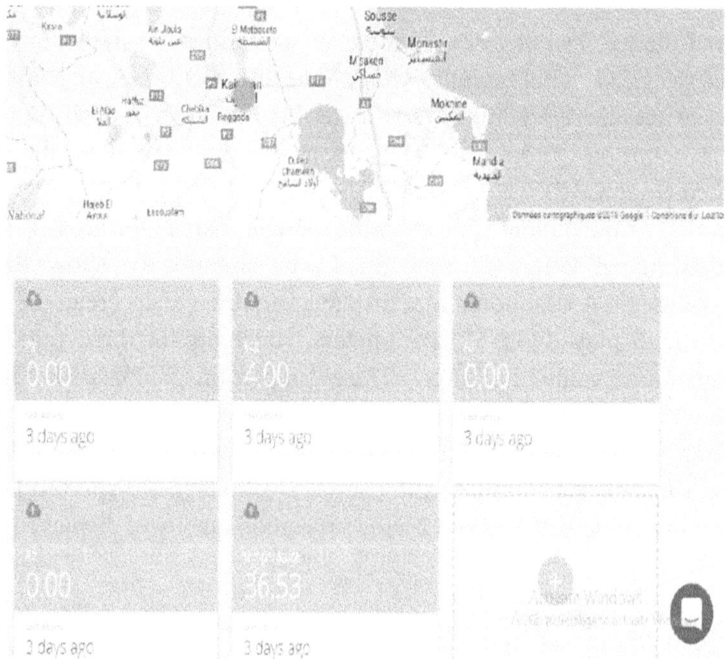

Figure 11. A) Temperature and acceleration display on the dashboard, B)event part in Ubidots

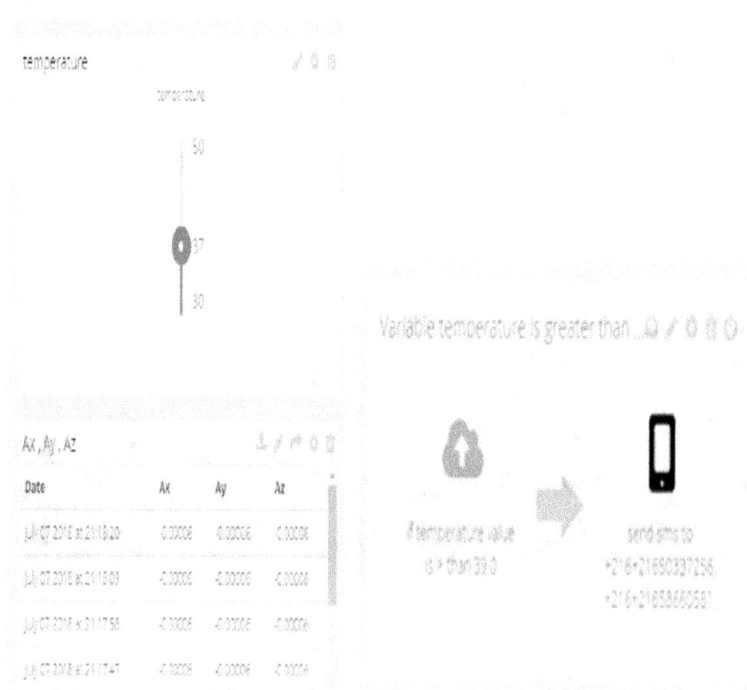

A B

Figure 12. ECG signal display

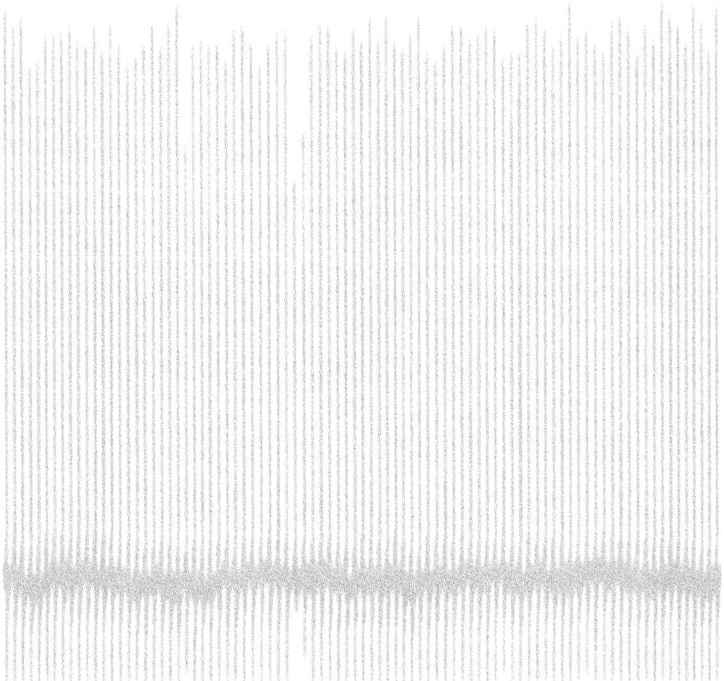

STRETCHABLE ECG REMOTE MONITORING SYSTEM

Stretchable IOT ECG Circuit Design

In this section, the realization possibility of stretchable electronic systems is presented for the ECG detection. In this way, an overall flexible-stretchable electronic circuit will combine the miniaturization of such devices with the desired comfort. The approach of this work consists of the use of non-stretchable functional units placed on islands board, connected by a stretchable joint with a meander shape, for the power supplies and the ECG output signal. The different block described above was designed using Altium designer software, which can identify the flex and rigid part of the circuitry. Surface-mount device (SMD) component was the most common component incorporated in the design instead of the through-hole component (Figure13).

The flex part was inspired from the biocompatible process using a U shape meander motif. This process as mentioned in Figure14 generally started by spin coating of photo resist materiel in top of copper foil, then patterned to make the conductor with the meandering shape. After that, the metal layer will be deposited composed of the gold, platinum and nickel in the copper. The platinum and nickel layers were added to electroplates the gold with the copper and improve solderability. Following that, the photo resistability will be removed and the sample will be encapsulated in the polymer materiel (generally PDMS). Finally, the copper foil removed, and the sample reversed and molded. The rigid part was designed by an island with a component part. These latter are designed to host and protect the traditional and rigid electronic components upon deformation. To include some degree of flexibility in these islands some pioneering works to thin down the Si chips were performed (Dahiya et al, 2013).

Figure 13. Layout of the ECG circuitry board

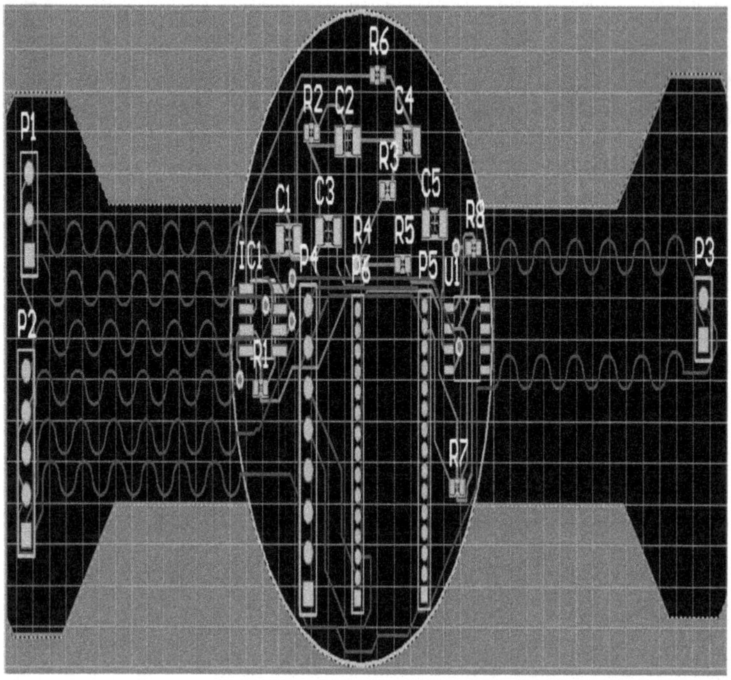

In Altium software, the design of the meander flexible part can be inspired from the process described below, where the island part (used component) designed with the preexisting standard PCB fabrication process (photolithography, development, wet etching, stripping, screen-printing of solder mask and component soldering) on a FR4 board. After that, both circuits (rigid and flex part) can be encapsulated and connected into the PDMS polymer flexible layer, using two-step injection molding processes. The different materials used for the design illustrated in Table 1 and Figure15 shows the ECG circuitry board layout.

Results of 3D ECG Rigid-Flexible Board

Figure 15 shows the ECG rigid-flexible board in 3D visualization. From this latter, the flex part located in the left and in the right, for the alimentation and circuitry visualization, when the rigid part located in the center with the different components. This circuit records the ECG signal from the body by using measurement Ag/AgCl electrodes (p1, p2 and p3). These electrodes take contact with the skin through the PDMS molding.

This circuit records the ECG signal from the body by using measurement Ag/AgCl electrodes (p1, p2 and p3). These electrodes take contact with the skin through the PDMS molding. This design uses the H0 meander shape design of the conductor in order to allow high deformations of the conductor, without a permanent damage. This example of shape was used because it has a very low increase of resistivity (<2%) during the mid-elongation and because of the 57% ability of elongation (Carta et al, 2009).

The design can improve performance by studying the different meander shape presented in the literature based in the Finite Element Method (FEM) (Gonzalez et al, 2008).

Figure 14. Fabrication process of flexible stretchable part

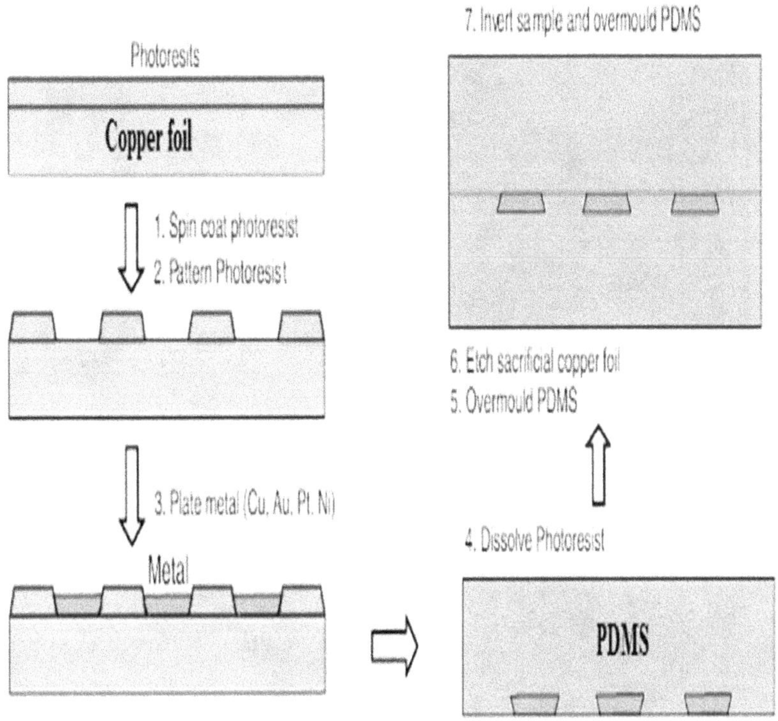

Table 1. Different materials used for the wearable ECG design

Part	Layer name	Layer Type	Thickness (mm)	Dielectric constant
Flex Part	Flex top cover layer Flex top over layer Conductor Flex Bottom over layer Flex Bottom cover layer	Polymide (PDMS) Polymide (PDMS) Signal (Gold) Polymide (PDMS) Polymide (PDMS)	0.102 0.102 0.035 0.102 0.102	4.2 4.2 - 4.2 4.2
Rigid Part (Island)	Top solder Top Layer Dielectric1 Bottom Layer Bottom solder	Resist Signal (copper) Dielectric (FR4) Signal (copper) Resist	0.0201 0.035 0.254 0.035 0.0201	3.5 - 3.4 - 3.5

Discussion

Wearable ECG monitoring systems by using body sensors are very important for patients with cardiovascular diseases, which are the main mortality cause worldwide. However, several works are interested in developing ECG remote monitoring systems that can be more reliable, efficient, secure and energy efficient especially for wireless healthcare applications. However, the lack of the easy and flexible design in such medical systems make these applications not enabled to obtain and oversight ECG signals over long periods.

Figure15. 3D visualization of the ECG circuitry board

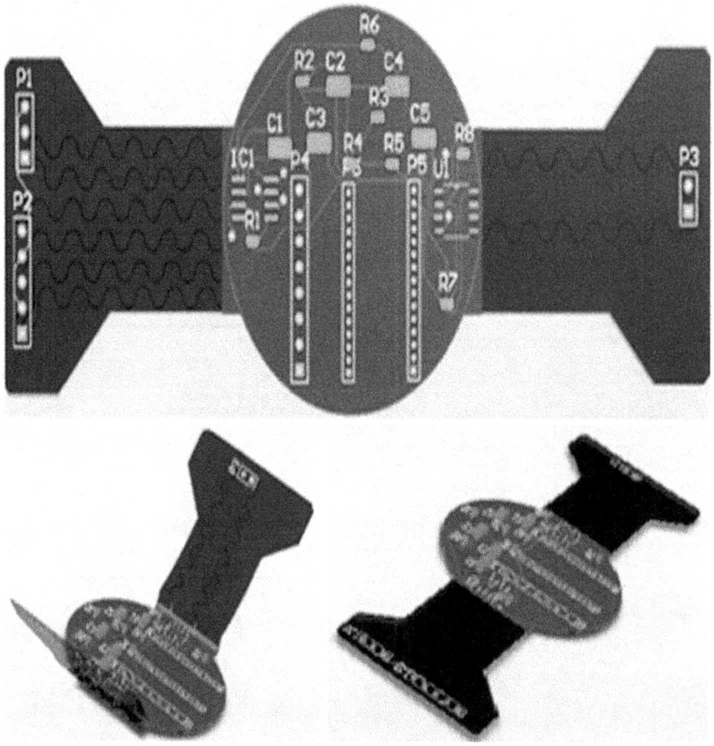

The ECG system developed in this chapter consists in creating an ECG remote monitoring system to facilitate and improve the quality of care and remote medical supervision. This system is characterized by its ease of deployment and its self-organization. This is an advantageous point for the monitoring of the elderly, persons with reduced mobility, people at risk and people with heart disease. In addition, this system allows the monitoring of their living environment and level their disabilities while ensuring efficiency, reducing costs and real-time analysis.

The main goal of this chapter is to realize an IoT solution. This solution allows on the one hand the detection of the signal electrocardiogram (ECG) and measuring the temperature and the acceleration of the patient's body using different electronic devices. First, the ECG signal collected by the electrodes requires an electronic circuit for its shaping. The chain of acquisition and of treatment chosen in this work consists of several stages essential for the formatting of the ECG tracing: pre-amplification, filtering and amplification. The result shows a good clear signal that can help ECG signal processing and detection of arrhythmias. The result shows a good clear signal that can be used for ECG signal processing and detection of arrhythmias.

In fact, various existing ECG measurement system detects the heartbeat by measuring the frequency heart rate in the fingers. Most of those types of sensors record only the higher impulse heart (peaks R) without displaying the global signal as the PPG Sensing Unit [35]. Therefore, the actual solutions cannot detect the other waveform of the ECG signal (wave P and wave T). The proposed solution has the advantage to detect the maximum of heart wave's pulses (P, Q, R, S and T waves), which makes the diagnosis more reliable and effective for an application of remote monitoring.

Secondly, to characterize the patient's movement and activity, a Gy-521 gyro is used to measure or maintain the patient's orientation. This module can calculate the temperature of the foot with respect to time.

On the other hand, this solution will be able to send the data information using the NodeMCU to a storage server for remote medical monitoring by allowing the doctor to have cardiac activities by means of a wireless link. In addition, an Ubidots platform is developed to collect this information and present it in a simple way to the user. This platform was used to view the history of recognized activities, heart rate, posture and acceleration values. The alarms have been configured for heart rate, temperature and maximum acceleration (behavior that indicates a fall) with minimum and maximum level alerts.

In addition to that, this ECG prototype has a low cost design with easily processed fabrication. In fact, this work offers a design of developed ECG circuit respecting a very specific manufacturing process. The prototype was successfully designed with a rigid-flexible process and our next work will include the fabrication and characterization steps. This stretchable circuit is a trend for the integrated circuit manufacturing technology and for the medical application.

FUTURE RESEARCH DIRECTIONS

The system developed in this work is very successful in recording the ECG signals. These signals should be sent to the doctor for treatment using the Ubidots platform. However, the improvement of this system could relate first, to the addition of an application that makes it possible to analyze and to treat the ECG signals by integrating automated methods in order to detect and localize the cardiac anomalies. These automated methods are emerging as a major new medical technology, with the goal of performing real-time analysis of ECG physiological signal traces and monitoring over long periods. This will make it possible to validate system performance in terms of efficiency, accuracy and reliability by offering the doctor the ability to better analyze information for a proper diagnosis. Secondly, to make this application more accessible, a mobile application development is proposed for people who use smartphones (Android and IOS).

Finally, the manufacturing of elastic circuit design studied in this chapter is required to facilitate the use of wireless wearable ECG monitoring system. In addition, the transfer to a biomedical industrial environment offers flexibility and allows a large production mass.

CONCLUSION

This chapter realizes an IoT system of cardiac remote monitoring which allows the detection of electrocardiogram (ECG) signal. In addition, the system can measure the temperature and the acceleration of the patient's body. Besides, this solution will be able to send the information data to an IoT Cloud platform for remote medical monitoring by allowing the doctor to have cardiac activities through a wireless link. The major contribution of this chapter is the conception of a stretchable circuit that combines both miniaturizations and conformability for the patient's body. This circuit is designed using Altium software with a rigid part for the component and flexible parts for the connection, the flexible part includes the manufacturing of the stretchable meander was inspired from the biocompatible technology process. A future implementation of this work will involve the integration of other medical sensors and the fabrication of this circuit with a given characterization.

REFERENCES

Abdol Aziz, M. A. F., Salleh, A. F., Sudin, S., Aziz, F., Shakaff, A. Y. M., Shahril Salim, M., & Abdul Rahim, N. (2014). Athlete Overtraining Monitoring System. In R. Adnan, S. Ismail, & N. Sulaiman (Eds.), Effects of Eccentric Training Using Theraband on Hamstring Flexibility in Elderly (pp. 209–217). Academic Press.

Akash, G., Chakraborty, C., & Bharat, G. (2019). Medical Information Processing Using Smartphone Under IoT Framework, Springer: Energy Conservation for IoT Devices, *Studies in Systems. Decision and Control*, *206*, 283–308.

Axisa, F., Bossuyt, F., Vervust, T., & Vanfleteren, J. (2008). Laser based fast prototyping methodology of producing stretchable and conformable electronic systems. *Proc. 2nd Electronics System-Integration Technology Conference ESTC*, 1387–1390. 10.1109/ESTC.2008.4684558

Brosteaux, D., Axisa, F., Gonzalez, M., & Vanfleteren, J. (2007). Design and Fabrication of Elastic Interconnections for Stretchable Electronic Circuits. *IEEE Electron Device Letters*, *28*(7), 552–554. doi:10.1109/LED.2007.897887

Carta, R., Jourand, P., Hermans, B., Thoné, J., Brosteaux, D., Vervust, T., ... Puers, R. (2009). Design and implementation of advanced systems in a flexible-stretchable technology for biomedical applications. *Sensors and Actuators. A, Physical*, *156*(1), 79–87. doi:10.1016/j.sna.2009.03.012

Celik, N., Manivannan, N., & Balachandran, W. (2016). Evaluation of a Behind-the-Ear ECG Device for Smartphone based Integrated Multiple Smart Sensor System in Health Applications. *International Journal of Advanced Computer Science and Applications*, *7*(7), 409–418. doi:10.14569/IJACSA.2016.070757

Chakraborty, C., Gupta, B., & Ghosh, S. K. (2014). Mobile metadata assisted community database of chronic wound. *Elsevier Int. Journal of Wound Medicine*, *6*, 34–42. doi:10.1016/j.wndm.2014.09.002

Chakraborty, C., Gupta, B., & Ghosh, S. K. (2016). *Mobile Telemedicine Systems for Remote Patient's Chronic Wound Monitoring. M-Health Innovations for Patient-Centered Care, 11*, 217–243.

Chlaihawia, A. A., Narakathua, B. B., Emamiana, S., Bazuina, B. J., & Atashbar, M. Z. (2018). Development of printed and flexible dry ECG electrodes. *Sensing and Bio-Sensing Research*, *20*, 9–15. doi:10.1016/j.sbsr.2018.05.001

Chtioui, I., Bossuyt, F., Vanfleteren, J., & Bedoui, M. H. (2017). 2.5/3D dynamically stretchable and permanently shaped electronic circuits. *Microsystem Technologies*, *24*(2), 831–853. doi:10.100700542-017-3582-7

Dahiya, R. S., & Gennaro, S. (2013). Bendable Ultra-Thin Chips on Flexible Foils. *IEEE Sensors Journal*, *13*(10), 4030–4037. doi:10.1109/JSEN.2013.2269028

Gonzalez, M., Axisa, F., Bulcke, M. V., Brosteaux, D., Vandevelde, B., & Vanfleteren, J. (2008). Design of metal interconnects for stretchable electronic circuits. *Microelectronics and Reliability*, *48*(6), 825–832. doi:10.1016/j.microrel.2008.03.025

Gravina, R., Alinia, P., Ghasemzadeh, H., & Fortino, G. (2017). Multi-Sensor Fusion in Body Sensor Networks: State-of-the-art and research challenges. *Information Fusion*, *35*, 68–80. doi:10.1016/j.inffus.2016.09.005

Hossain, M. M., Fotouhi, M., & Hasan, R. (2015). Towards an analysis of security issues, challenges, and open problems in the internet of things. In *Proc. 2015 IEEE World Congress on Services (SERVICES)*, (pp. 21-28). New York: IEEE. 10.1109/SERVICES.2015.12

Jung, H., Moon, J., Baek, D., Lee, J., Choi, J., Hong, J., & Lee, S. (2012). CNT/PDMS composite flexible dry electrodes for long-term ECG monitoring. *IEEE Transactions on Biomedical Engineering*, *59*(5), 1472–1479. doi:10.1109/TBME.2012.2190288 PMID:22410324

Kim, G., Son, J., Park, S., & Kim, W. (2008). Hybrid Process for Fabricating 3D Hierarchical Scaffolds Combining Rapid Prototyping and Electrospinning. *Macromolecular Rapid Communications*, *29*(19), 1577–1581. doi:10.1002/marc.200800277

Landers, R., Hubner, U., Schmelzeisen, R., & Mulhaupt, R. (2002). Rapid prototyping of scaffolds derived from thermoreversible hydrogels and tailored for applications in tissue engineering. *Biomaterials*, *23*(23), 4437–4447. doi:10.1016/S0142-9612(02)00139-4 PMID:12322962

Manadhata, P. K., & Wing, J. M. (2011). An Attack Surface Metric. *IEEE Transactions on Software Engineering*, *37*(3), 371–386. doi:10.1109/TSE.2010.60

Manikandan, S., & Kulkarni, A. S. (2019). IoT based Low Power Wearable ECG Monitoring System. *Current Signal Transduction Therapy*, *14*(1), 68–74. doi:10.2174/1574362413666180622105447

Megalingam, R. K., Veliyara, P. S., Prabhu, R., Krishna, R. R., & Katoch, R. (2014), Wheeled Patient Monitoring System. In L.C. Jain, S. Patnaik, & N. Ichalkaranje (Ed.), *Intelligent Computing, Communication and Devices: Proceedings of ICCD* (vol. 1, pp. 779-786). New Delhi: Academic Press.

Nordin, A. N., & Ramli, N. (2019). Flexible and Stretchable Circuits for Smart Wearables. *Journal of Telecommunication*, *9*(3-8), 117–122.

Pacheco, J., Tunc, C., & Hariri, S. (2018). Security Framework for IoT Cloud Services. *Proc. IEEE/ACS 15th International Conference on Computer Systems and Applications (AICCSA).*

Qadir, Q. M., Rashid, T. A., Al-Salihi, N. K., Ismael, B., Kist, A. A., & Zhang, Z. (2018). Low Power Wide Area Networks: A Survey of Enabling Technologies, Applications and Interoperability Needs. *IEEE Access: Practical Innovations, Open Solutions*, *6*, 77454–77473. doi:10.1109/ACCESS.2018.2883151

Rashid, T.A., &Abdulla, S. A. (2018). A Hybrid of Artificial Bee Colony, Genetic Algorithm, and Neural Network for Diabetic Mellitus Diagnosing, *ARO-The Scientific Journal of Koya University, 6*(1), 55-64.

Rashid, T. A., Abdulla, S. M., & Abdulla, R. M. (2016). Decision Support System for Diabetes Mellitus through Machine Learning Techniques. *International Journal of Advanced Computer Science and Applications*, *7*(7), 170–178.

Rashid, T. A., Abdullah, S. M., & Abdullah, R. M. (2016). An Intelligent Approach for Diabetes Classification, Prediction, and Description. In V. Snášel, A. Abraham, P. Krömer, M. Pant, & A. Muda (Eds.), *Innovations in Bio-Inspired Computing and Applications* (Vol. 424, pp. 323–335). Cham: Springer. doi:10.1007/978-3-319-28031-8_28

Rashid, T. A., Fattah, P., & Awlaa, D. K. (2018). Using Accuracy Measure for Improving the Training of LSTM with Metaheuristic Algorithms. *Procedia Computer Science*, *140*, 324–333. doi:10.1016/j.procs.2018.10.307

Sterken, T., Vanfleteren, J., Torfs, T., de Beeck, M. O., Bossuyt, F., & Van Hoof, C. (2011). Ultra-Thin Chip Package (UTCP) and Stretchable Circuit Technologies for Wearable ECG System. *Proc. Annual International Conference of the IEEE Engineering in Medicine and Biology Society*. 10.1109/IEMBS.2011.6091734

Sun, B., Chen, W., & Zheng, X. (2012). The System Design for the Extraction and Pre-processing of Surface EMG. *Proc. World Congress on Medical Physics and Biomedical Engineering*, 33, 8 – 13. 10.1016/j.phpro.2012.05.023

Suo, H., Wan, J., Zou, C., & Liu, J. (2012). Security in the internet of things: a review. In *Proc. 2012 IEEE International Conference on Computer Science and Electronics Engineering (ICCSEE)*, (Vol. 3, pp. 648-665). Hangzhou, China: IEEE. 10.1109/ICCSEE.2012.373

Thap, T., Yoon, K. H., & Lee, J. (2016). Graphite based electrode for ecg monitoring: Evaluation under freshwater and saltwater conditions. *Sensors (Basel)*, *16*(4), 542. doi:10.339016040542 PMID:27092502

Wang, L. F., Liu, J. Q., Yan, X. X., Yang, B., & Yang, C. S. (2013). A MEMS-based pyramid micro-needle electrode for long-term EEG measurement. *Microsystem Technologies*, *19*(2), 269–276. doi:10.100700542-012-1638-2

Xia, H., Asif, I., & Zhao, X. (2013). Cloud-ECG for real time ECG monitoring and analysis. *Computer Methods and Programs in Biomedicine*, *110*(3), 253–259. doi:10.1016/j.cmpb.2012.11.008 PMID:23261079

Yang, Z., Zhou, Q., Lei, L., Zheng, K., & Xiang, W. (2016). An IoT-cloud Based Wearable ECG Monitoring System for Smart Healthcare. *Journal of Medical Systems*, *40*(286), 1–11. PMID:27796840

Zhou, Y., Ding, X., Zhang, J., Duan, Y., Hu, J., & Yang, X. (2014). Fabrication of conductive fabric as textile electrode for ECG monitoring. *Fibers and Polymers*, *15*(11), 2260–2264. doi:10.100712221-014-2260-y

Compilation of References

16. Yuehong, Y. I. N., Zeng, Y., Chen, X., & Fan, Y. (2016). The internet of things in healthcare: An overview. *Elsevier Journal of Industrial Information Integration*, *1*, 3–13. doi:10.1016/j.jii.2016.03.004

Abbate, S., Avvenuti, M., Corsini, P., Light, J., & Vecchio, A. (2010). Monitoring of human movements for fall detection and activities recognition in elderly care using wireless sensor network: a survey. *Wireless Sensor Networks: Application-Centric Design.*

Abbate, S., Avvenuti, M., Bonatesta, F., Cola, G., Corsini, P., & Vecchio, A. (2012). A smartphone-based fall detection system. *Pervasive and Mobile Computing*, *8*(6), 883–899. doi:10.1016/j.pmcj.2012.08.003

Abdmouleh, M. K., Khalfallah, A., & Bouhlel, M. S. (2017). A Novel Selective Encryption Scheme for Medical Images Transmission based-on JPEG Compression Algorithm. *Procedia Computer Science*, *112*, 369–376. doi:10.1016/j.procs.2017.08.026

Abdol Aziz, M. A. F., Salleh, A. F., Sudin, S., Aziz, F., Shakaff, A. Y. M., Shahril Salim, M., & Abdul Rahim, N. (2014). Athlete Overtraining Monitoring System. In R. Adnan, S. Ismail, & N. Sulaiman (Eds.), Effects of Eccentric Training Using Theraband on Hamstring Flexibility in Elderly (pp. 209–217). Academic Press.

Abdullah, W. A. N., Yaakob, N., & Elobaid, M. E. (2016). Energy efficient remote healthcare monitoring using IoT: a review of trends and challenges. In *Proceedings of the international conference on the Internet of Things and cloud computing*. New York: ACM. 10.1145/2896387.2896414

Abelson, J. S., Symer, M., Peters, A., Charlson, M., & Yeo, H. (2017). Mobile health apps and recovery after surgery: What are patients willing to do? *American Journal of Surgery*, *214*(4), 616–622. doi:10.1016/j.amjsurg.2017.06.009 PMID:28666581

Abiola, S. O., Portman, E., Kautz, H., & Dorsey, E. (2015). *Node view: a mHealth real-time infectious disease interface disease interface-2014 Ebola outbreak case study*. Paper presented at the International Joint Conference on Pervasive and Ubiquitous Computing and International Symposium on Wearable Computers, Osaka, Japan. 10.1145/2800835.2800851

Abowd, G. D., Dey, A. K., Brown, P. J., Davies, N., Smith, M., & Steggles, P. (1999). Towards a better understanding of context and context-awareness. In *International symposium on handheld and ubiquitous computing* (pp. 304-307). Springer. 10.1007/3-540-48157-5_29

Adnan, S. F. S., Hashim, H., & Pasya, I. (2011). *Implementation of MIDlet application on probability of Alzheimer's disease via mobile phone*. Paper presented at the IEEE International Conference on Computer Applications and Industrial Electronics, Penang, Malaysia. 10.1109/ICCAIE.2011.6162115

Afolayan, T., Aiterebhe, E. F., & Mejabi, V. (2015). Mobile phone usage in rural communities in Kwara state, Nigeria. *Inform Technolt, 12*(2), 1–15.

Agarwal, P., Mukerji, G., Desveaux, L., Ivers, N. M., Bhattacharyya, O., Hensel, J. M., ... Cooper, M. (2019). Mobile app for improved self-management of type 2 diabetes: Multicenter pragmatic randomized controlled trial. *JMIR mHealth and uHealth, 7*(1), e10321. doi:10.2196/10321 PMID:30632972

Aggarwal, C. C. (2014). *Data Classification: Algorithms and Applications* (1st ed.). Chapman & Hall/CRC. doi:10.1201/b17320

Ahanathapillai, V., Amor, J. D., Goodwin, Z., & James, C. J. (2015). Preliminary study on activity monitoring using an android smart-watch. *Healthcare Technology Letters, 7*, 4456–4462. PMID:26609402

Akash,, G., Chakraborty, C., & Bharat, G. (2019). Medical Information Processing Using Smartphone Under IoT Framework. *Springer: Energy Conservation for IoT Devices, Studies in Systems. Decision and Control, 206*, 1–26.

Akash, G., Chakraborty, C., & Bharat, G. (2019). Medical Information Processing Using Smartphone Under IoT Framework, Springer: Energy Conservation for IoT Devices, *Studies in Systems. Decision and Control, 206*, 283–308.

Alagar, V., Alsaig, A., Ormandjieva, O., & Wan, K. (2018), Context-based Security and Privacy for Healthcare IoT. *IEEE International Conference on Smart Internet of Things (SmartIoT)*, 122-128. 10.1109/SmartIoT.2018.00-14

Albert, J., Aliu, E., Anderhub, H., Antoranz, P., Armada, A., Asensio, M., ... Zapatero, J. (2008). Implementation of the random forest method for the imaging atmospheric Cherenkov telescope MAGIC. *Nuclear Instruments & Methods in Physics Research. Section A, Accelerators, Spectrometers, Detectors and Associated Equipment, 588*(3), 424–432. doi:10.1016/j.nima.2007.11.068

Al-Dowaihi, D., Al-Ajlan, M., Al-Zahrani, N., Al-Quwayfili, N., al-Jwiser, N., & Kanjo, E. (2013). *Mbreath: Asthma monitoring system on the go*. Paper presented at the International Conference on Computer Medical Applications, San Francisco, CA. 10.1109/ICCMA.2013.6506169

Alhussein, M., Muhammad, G., Hossain, M. S., & Amin, S. U. (2018). Cognitive IoT-Cloud Integration for Smart Healthcare: Case Study for Epileptic Seizure Detection and Monitoring. *Mobile Networks and Applications, 23*(6), 1624–1635. doi:10.100711036-018-1113-0

Aliev, T., Babayev, T., Sabziev, E., Pashayev, A., & Alizada, T. (2012). *Monitoring of condition of the cardiovascular system by means of mobile phones using ECG noise variance*. Paper presented at the 4th International Conference of Problems of Cybernetics and Informatics, Baku, Azerbaijan. 10.1109/ICPCI.2012.6486303

Ali, M., Ahn, C. W., & Pant, M. (2014). A robust image watermarking technique using SVD and differential evolution in the DCT domain. *Optik-Int. J. Light Electron Opt, 125*(1), 428–434. doi:10.1016/j.ijleo.2013.06.082

Ali, Z. H., Ali, H. A., & Badawy, M. M. (2015). Internet of Things (IoT): Definitions, challenges and recent research directions. *International Journal of Computers and Applications, 128*(1), 37–47. doi:10.5120/ijca2015906430

Alloghani, M., Hussain, A., Al-Jumeily, D., Fergus, P., Abuelma'Atti, O., & Hamden, H. (2016). *A mobile health monitoring application for obesity management and control using the internet-of-things*. Paper presented at the Sixth International Conference on Digital Information Processing and Communications, Piscataway, NJ. 10.1109/ICDIPC.2016.7470785

Almeida, A., Fiore, A., Mainetti, L., Mulero, R., Patrono, L., & Rametta, P. (2017). An IoT-Aware Architecture for Collecting and Managing Data Related to Elderly Behavior. *Wireless Communications and Mobile Computing, 2017*, 1–18. doi:10.1155/2017/5051915

Almeida, R. F., Sousa, T. J., Couto, A. S., Marques, A. J., Queirós, C. M., & Martins, C. L. (2019). Development of weCope, a mobile app for illness self-management in schizophrenia. *Archives of Clinical Psychiatry (São Paulo)*, *46*(1), 1–4. doi:10.1590/0101-60830000000182

Almotiri, S. H., Khan, M. A., & Alghamdi, M. A. (2016). *Mobile health (m-health) system in the context of IoT*. Paper presented at the 4th International Conference on Future Internet of Things and Cloud Workshops, Vienna, Austria.

Amin, N. U., & Asad, M. C. (2013). An authenticated key management with rekeying for secured body sensor networks based on Hybrid cryptography. *ICNC, 9th IEEE international conference*.

Amor, J. D. (2011). *Detecting and monitoring behavioral change through personalized ambient monitoring* (Ph.D. Doctoral Thesis). Institute of Sound and Vibration Research, University of Southampton.

Amor, J. D., & James, C. J. (2009). *Personalised ambient monitoring: accelerometry for activity level classification*. 4th European Conf. Int. Federation for Medical and Biological Engineering, Antwerp, Belgium.

Amor, J. D., & James, C. J. (2015). Setting the scene: Mobile and a wearable technology for managing healthcare and wellbeing. *37th Annual International Conference in IEEE Engineering in Medicine and Biology Society*, *5*, 3752–3755. 10.1109/EMBC.2015.7320189

Amor, J. D., Hattersley, J. G., Barber, T. M., & James, C. J. (2015). Characterization of wrist-a wearable activity measurement using whole-body calorimetry in semi-free-living conditions. *37th Annual International Conference in IEEE Engineering in Medicine and Biology Society*, *5*, 2735–2738. 10.1109/EMBC.2015.7319205

Amor, J. D., Ahanathapillai, V., & James, C. J. (2014). Detecting and analyzing activity levels for the wrist a wearable unit in the USEFIL project. *Proc. XIII Mediterranean Conf. Medical and Biological Engineering and Computing*, 1201–1204. 10.1007/978-3-319-00846-2_297

Anand, A., Chamberlain, D., Kodgule, R., & Fletcher, R. R. (2018). *Pulmonary screener: A mobile phone screening tool for pulmonary and respiratory disease*. Paper presented at the IEEE Global Humanitarian Technology Conference, San Jose, CA. 10.1109/GHTC.2018.8601821

Anava, O., & Levy, K. Y. (2016). k*-Nearest Neighbors: From Global to Local. *Proceedings of 30th Conference on Neural Information Processing Systems (NIPS)*.

Ani, R., Krishna, S., Anju, N., Aslam, M. S., & Deepa, O. S. (2017). Iot based patient monitoring and diagnostic prediction tool using ensemble classifier. In *International Conference on Advances in Computing, Communications and Informatics (ICACCI)* (pp. 1588-1593). Udupi, India: IEEE. 10.1109/ICACCI.2017.8126068

Arcelus, A., Jones, M. H., Goubran, R., & Knoefel, F. (2007). Integration of smart home technologies in a health monitoring system for the elderly. In *21st International Conference on Advanced Information Networking and Applications Workshops (AINAW'07)* (*vol. 2*, pp. 820-825). Niagara Falls, Canada: IEEE. 10.1109/AINAW.2007.209

Arksey, H., & O'Malley, L. (2005). Scoping studies: Towards a methodological framework. *International Journal of Social Research Methodology*, *8*(1), 19–32. doi:10.1080/1364557032000119616

Ashrafuzzaman, M., Huq, M. M., Chakraborty, C. M., Khan, R. M., Tabassum, T., & Hasan, R. (2013). Article. *International Journal of Technology Enhancements and Emerging Engineering Research*, *1*(3), 23–27.

Atzori, L., Iera, A., & Morabito, G. (2010). The Internet of Things: A Survey. *Computer Networks*, *54*(15), 2787–2805. doi:10.1016/j.comnet.2010.05.010

Awad, A., Mohamed, A., & El-Sheriff, A. A. (2013). Energy-efficient cross-layer design for a wireless body area monitoring networks in healthcareapplications. *IEEE 24th International Symposium on Personal, Indoor and Mobile Radio Communication, 6*, 1484-1489.

Axisa, F., Bossuyt, F., Vervust, T., & Vanfleteren, J. (2008). Laser based fast prototyping methodology of producing stretchable and conformable electronic systems. *Proc. 2nd Electronics System-Integration Technology Conference ESTC*, 1387–1390. 10.1109/ESTC.2008.4684558

Azimi, I., Rahmani, A. M., Liljeberg, P., & Tenhunen, H. (2016). Internet of things for remote elderly monitoring: A study from user-centered perspective. *Journal of Ambient Intelligence and Humanized Computing, 8*(2), 273–289. doi:10.100712652-016-0387-y

Bagala, F., Becker, C., Cappello, A., Chiari, L., Aminian, K., Hausdorff, J. M., ... Klenk, J. (2012). Evaluation of accelerometer-based fall detection algorithms on real-world falls. *PLoS One, 7*(5), e37062. doi:10.1371/journal.pone.0037062 PMID:22615890

Balasubramanian, A., Mahajan, R., & Venkataramani, A. (2010). Augmenting mobile 3G using WiFi. In *Proceedings of the 8th international conference on Mobile systems, applications, and services* (pp. 209-222). ACM.

Baldiseera, A. T., & Camarinhamatos, L. (2016). towards a collaborative business ecosystem for elderly care. In Doctral conference on computing, electrical and industrial systems (pp. 24-34). Cham: Springer.

Bandodkar, A. J., Jia, W., Yardimci, C., Wang, X., Ramirez, J., & Wang, J. (2015). Tattoo-based noninvasive glucose monitoring: A proof-of-concept study. *Analytical Chemistry, 87*(1), 394–398. doi:10.1021/ac504300n PMID:25496376

Baoding, Z., & Liu, J. (2010). A kind of design schema of wireless smart water meter reading system based on zigbee technology. *International Conference on E-Product E-Service and E-Entertainment* (pp. 1-4). Henan, China: IEEE.

Basanta, H., Huang, Y.-P., & Lee, T.-T. (2016). Intuitive IoT-based H2U Healthcare System for Elderly People. In *13th International Conference on Networking, Sensing, and Control* (pp. 1-6). Mexico: IEEE. 10.1109/ICNSC.2016.7479018

Bates, M., & Zumla, A. (2015). Rapid infectious diseases diagnostics using Smartphones. *Annals of Translational Medicine, 3*(15). PMID:26488011

Ben Rejab, Nouira, & Trabelsi. (2014). Health Monitoring Systems Using Machine Learning Techniques. *Springer International Journal of Machine Learning, 10*, 234–251.

Ben Said, A., Mohamed, A., Elfouly, T., & Dennis, M. (2018). A Deep learning approach for Vital signs compressions and Energy Efficient delivery in m-health systems. *IEEE Journal of Translational Engineering in Health and Medicine, 6.*

Benaloh, J. (1994, May). Dense probabilistic encryption. In *Proceedings of the workshop on selected areas of cryptography* (pp. 120-128). Academic Press.

Berlin, J. E., Storti, K. L., & Brach, J. S. (2006). Using activity monitors to measure physical activity in free-living conditions. *Journal of American Physical Therapy., 86*, 1137–1145. PMID:16879047

Bernal, Yang, Li, Kumar, Madhvanath, Ramesh, & Bala. (2017). Deep TemporalMultimodal Fusion for Medical Procedure Monitoring using A wearable Sensors. *IEEE Transactions on Multimedia, 10*, 965–982.

Bhatia, G., Lala, A., Chaurasia, A., & Rajpal, R. (2013), Implementation of Cloud computing technology for the improvement of entire healthcare services in India. *IEEE International Conference on Advances in Technology and Engineering (ICATE)*, 1–5. 10.1109/ICAdTE.2013.6524771

Bhattacharyya, A., Pachori, R. B., Upadhyay, A., & Acharya, U. R. (2017). Tunable-Q Wavelet Transform Based Multiscale Entropy Measure for Automated Classification of Epileptic EEG Signals. *Applied Sciences*, *7*(4), 385. doi:10.3390/app7040385

Blinman, P., King, M., Norman, R., Viney, R., & Stockler, M. R. (2012, May). Preferences for cancer treatments: An overview of methods and applications in oncology. *Annals of Oncology: Official Journal of the European Society for Medical Oncology*, *23*(5), 1104–1110. doi:10.1093/annonc/mdr559 PMID:22234737

Bluetooth. (2017). *Bluetooth technology*. Retrieved from https://www.bluetooth.com/

Boi, R., Racca, L., Cavallero, A., Carpaneto, V., Racca, M., Dall' Acqua, F., ... Odetti, P. (2012). Hearing loss and depressive symptoms in elderly patients. *Geriatrics & Gerontology International*, *12*(3), 440–445. doi:10.1111/j.1447-0594.2011.00789.x PMID:22212622

Boneh, D., Goh, E. J., & Nissim, K. (2005, February). Evaluating 2-DNF formulas on ciphertexts. In *Theory of Cryptography Conference* (pp. 325-341). Springer.

Botta, A., de Donato, W., Persico, V., & Pescape, A. (2014). On the Integration of Cloud Computing and Internet of Things. In *2014 International Conference on Future Internet of Things and Cloud* (pp. 23–30). Academic Press. 10.1109/FiCloud.2014.14

Bourke, A. K., O'brien, J. V., & Lyons, G. M. (2007). Evaluation of a threshold-based tri-axial accelerometer fall detection algorithm. *Gait & Posture*, *26*(2), 194–199. doi:10.1016/j.gaitpost.2006.09.012 PMID:17101272

Bourouis, A., Feham, M., & Bouchachia, A. (2011). Ubiquitous mobile health monitoring system for elderly (UMHMSE). *International Journal of Computer Science & Information technology*, *3*(3), 74-82.

Bouslimi, D., & Coatrieux, G. (2016). A crypto-watermarking system for ensuring reliability control and traceability of medical images. *Signal Processing Image Communication*, *47*, 160–169. doi:10.1016/j.image.2016.05.021

Brakerski, Z., & Vaikuntanathan, V. (2011, August). Fully homomorphic encryption from ring-LWE and security for key dependent messages. In *Annual cryptology conference* (pp. 505-524). Springer. 10.1007/978-3-642-22792-9_29

Bravata, D. M., Sundaram, V., & Gienger, A. L. (2007). Using pedometers to increase physical activity and improve health: A systematic review. *Journal of the American Medical Association*, *298*(19), 2296–2304. doi:10.1001/jama.298.19.2296 PMID:18029834

Bray, J., & Sturman, C. F. (2001). *Bluetooth 1.1: connect without cables*. Pearson Education.

Bressler, B. H., Keyes, W. J., Rochon, P. A., & Badley, E. (1999). The prevalence of low back pain in the elderly: A systematic review of the literature. *Spine*, *24*(17), 1813. doi:10.1097/00007632-199909010-00011 PMID:10488512

Brosteaux, D., Axisa, F., Gonzalez, M., & Vanfleteren, J. (2007). Design and Fabrication of Elastic Interconnections for Stretchable Electronic Circuits. *IEEE Electron Device Letters*, *28*(7), 552–554. doi:10.1109/LED.2007.897887

Bruce, J. (2015). *Getting Started with OpenHAB Home Automation on Raspberry Pi*. Academic Press.

Brunelli, Benini, Moser, & Thiele. (2008, March). An efficient solar energy harvester for wireless sensor nodes. *Design, Automation and Test in Europe*, 104-109.

Buratti, C., Conti, A., Dardari, D., & Verdone, R. (2009). An overview on wireless sensor networks technology and evolution. *Sensors (Basel)*, *9*(9), 6869–6896. doi:10.339090906869 PMID:22423202

C, C., B, G., & S.K., G. (2014). Mobile metadata assisted community database of chronic wound. *Int. Journal of Wound MEDICINE, 6*, 34-42.

Calabria, D., Caliceti, C., Zangheri, M., Mirasoli, M., Simoni, P., & Roda, A. (2017). Smartphone-based enzymatic biosensor for oral fluid L-lactate detection in one minute using confined multilayer paper reflectometry. *Biosensors & Bioelectronics, 94*, 124–130. doi:10.1016/j.bios.2017.02.053 PMID:28267667

Callegari, D., Conte, E., Ferreto, T., Fernandes, D., Moraes, F., Burmeister, F., & Severino, R. (2014). EpiCare: A home care platform based on mobile cloud computing to assist epilepsy diagnosis. In *2014 4th International Conference on Wireless Mobile Communication and Healthcare - Transforming Healthcare Through Innovations in Mobile and Wireless Technologies (MOBIHEALTH)* (pp. 148–151). Academic Press. 10.4108/icst.mobihealth.2014.257379

Camarinha-Matos, L. M., Afsarmanesh, H., Ermilova, E., Ferrada, F., Klen, A., & Jarimo, T. (2008). ARCON reference models for collaborative networks. *Collaborative Networks: Reference Modeling*, 83-112.

Cameron, C. (2019). *Cloud computing security risks every company faces*. Retrieved from https://www.skyhighnetworks.com/cloud-security-blog/9-cloud-computing-security-risks-every-company-faces/

Cao, W., Zhou, Y., Philip Chen, C. L., & Xia, L. (2017). Medical image encryption using edge maps. *Signal Processing, 132*, 96–109. doi:10.1016/j.sigpro.2016.10.003

Carrera, A., Pifarré, M., Vilaplana, J., Cuadrado, J., Solsona, S., Mateo, J., & Solsona, F. (2016). BPcontrol: A mobile app to monitor hypertensive patients. *Applied Clinical Informatics, 7*(04), 1120–1134. doi:10.4338/ACI-2015-12-RA-0172 PMID:27924346

Carta, R., Jourand, P., Hermans, B., Thoné, J., Brosteaux, D., Vervust, T., ... Puers, R. (2009). Design and implementation of advanced systems in a flexible-stretchable technology for biomedical applications. *Sensors and Actuators. A, Physical, 156*(1), 79–87. doi:10.1016/j.sna.2009.03.012

Castensøe-Seidenfaden, P., Husted, G. R., Jensen, A. K., Hommel, E., Olsen, B., Pedersen-Bjergaard, U., & Teilmann, G. (2018). Testing a smartphone app (Young with Diabetes) to improve self-management of diabetes over 12 months: Randomized controlled trial. *JMIR mHealth and uHealth, 6*(6), e141. doi:10.2196/mhealth.9487 PMID:29945861

Celik, N., Manivannan, N., & Balachandran, W. (2016). Evaluation of a Behind-the-Ear ECG Device for Smartphone based Integrated Multiple Smart Sensor System in Health Applications. *International Journal of Advanced Computer Science and Applications, 7*(7), 409–418. doi:10.14569/IJACSA.2016.070757

Chakraborty, C. (2011). Mobile Telemedicine Systems for Remote Patient's Chronic Wound Monitoring. In M-Health Innovations for Patient-Centered Care. IGI Global.

Chakraborty, C. B., G., & S.K., G. (2016). Mobile Telemedicine Systems for Remote Patient's Chronic Wound Monitoring. In M-Health Innovations for Patient-Centered Care (pp. 217-243). IGI.

Chakraborty, C., Gupta, B., & Ghosh, S. K. (2014). Tele-wound monitoring through smartphone. In *2014 International Conference on Medical Imaging, m-Health and Emerging Communication Systems (MedCom)* (pp. 197–201). Academic Press. 10.1109/MedCom.2014.7006003

Chakraborty, Gupta, & Ghosh. (2013). A Review on Telemedicine-Based WBAN Framework for Patient Monitoring. *International Journal of Telemedicine and e-Health, 19*(8), 619–626.

Chakraborty, Gupta, & Ghosh. (2016). Mobile Telemedicine Systems for Remote Patient's Chronic Wound Monitoring. In *M-Health Innovations for Patient-Centered Care*, (pp. 217-243). IGI Global.

Chakraborty, T. (2017). EC3: Combining Clustering and Classification for Ensemble Learning. In *Proceedings of IEEE International Conference on Data Mining (ICDM)*. New Orleans, LA: IEEE.

Chakraborty, C. (2013). Review on Telemedicine-Based WBAN Framework for Patient 26Monitoring. *Int. Journal of Telemedicine and e-Health, 19*(8), 619–626.

Chakraborty, C. (2017). Chronic Wound Image Analysis by Particle Swarm Optimization Technique for Tele-Wound Network. *Wireless Personal Communications, 96*(3), 3655–3671. doi:10.100711277-017-4281-5

Chakraborty, C. (2019). Mobile Health (m-Health) for Tele-wound Monitoring. *IGI: Mobile Health Applications for Quality Healthcare Delivery, Ch., 5*, 98–116.

Chakraborty, C. (2019). Mobile health (m-Health) for tele-wound monitoring: Role of m-Health in wound management. In C. Chakraborty (Ed.), *Mobile Health Applications for Quality Healthcare Delivery*. IGI Global. doi:10.4018/978-1-5225-8021-8.ch005

Chakraborty, C. (2019). Performance Analysis of Compression Techniques for Chronic Wound Image Transmission under Smartphone-Enabled Tele-wound Network. *Int. Journal of E-Health and Medical Communications, 10*(2), 1–15.

Chakraborty, C., & Kumari, S. (2016). Bio-metric Identification using Automated Iris Detection Technique. *IEEE: 3rd International Conference on Microelectronics, Circuits, and Systems*, 113-17.

Chakraborty, C., Gupta, B., & Ghosh, S. K. (2014). Mobile metadata assisted community database of chronic wound images. *Wound Medicine, 6*, 34–42. doi:10.1016/j.wndm.2014.09.002

Chakraborty, C., Gupta, B., & Ghosh, S. K. (2016). Mobile telemedicine systems for remote patient's chronic wound monitoring. In A. Moumtzoglou (Ed.), *M-Health Innovations for Patient-Centered Care*. IGI Global. doi:10.4018/978-1-4666-9861-1.ch011

Chakraborty, C., Gupta, B., & Ghosh, S. K. (2016). *Mobile Telemedicine Systems for Remote Patient's Chronic Wound Monitoring. M-Health Innovations for Patient-Centered Care, 11*, 217–243.

Chandel, V., Sinharay, A., Ahmed, N., & Ghose, A. (2016). Exploiting IMU Sensors for IOT Enabled Health Monitoring. In *First Workshop on IoT-enabled Healthcare and Wellness Technologies and Systems* (pp. 21-22). Singapore: ACM. 10.1145/2933566.2933569

Chander & Kumaravelan. (2018). One class outlier detection Using SVM formulations in WSN harsh environments. *International Journal of Recent Technology and Engineering, 7*(4).

Chander. (2018). A Analysis of machine learning in WSN. *International Journal of Engineering & Technology, 7*(4).

Chang, J. D., Chen, B. H., & Tsai, C. S. (2013). LBP-based fragile watermarking scheme for image tamper detection and recovery. *Next-Generation Electronics (ISNE), 2013 IEEE International Symposium on*, 173–176.

Chan, K. L., & Chen, M. (2019). Effects of Social Media and Mobile Health Apps on Pregnancy Care: Meta-Analysis. *JMIR mHealth and uHealth, 7*(1), e11836. doi:10.2196/11836 PMID:30698533

Chatterjee, A., & Sengupta, I. (2018). Translating algorithms to handle fully homomorphic encrypted data on the cloud. *IEEE Transactions on Cloud Computing, 6*(1), 287–300. doi:10.1109/TCC.2015.2481416

Chen, J., Kwong, K., Chang, D., Luk, J., & Bajcsy, R. (2005). Wearable sensors for reliable fall detection. In *IEEE Engineering in Medicine and Biology 27th Annual Conference* (pp. 3551-3554). Shanghai, China: IEEE.

Chen, M., Li, W., Hao, Y., Qian, Y., & Humar, I. (2018). Edge cognitive computing based smart healthcare system. *Future Generation Computer Systems, 86*, 403–411.

Chen, D., Wan, S., Xiang, J., & Bao, F. S. (2017). A high-performance seizure detection algorithm based on Discrete Wavelet Transform (DWT) and EEG. *PLoS One, 12*(3), 1–21. doi:10.1371/journal.pone.0173138 PMID:28278203

Cheng, C., Brown, R. C., Cohen, L. L., Venugopalan, J., Stokes, T. H., & Wang, M. D. (2013). *iACT-An interactive mHealth monitoring system to enhance psychotherapy for adolescents with sickle cell disease.* Paper presented at the Annual International Conference of the IEEE Engineering in Medicine and Biology Society, Osaka, Japan. 10.1109/EMBC.2013.6609992

Chen, M., Gonzalez, S., Vasilakos, A., Cao, H., & Leung, V. C. M. (2011). Body area networks: A survey. *Mobile Networks and Applications, 16*(2), 171–193. doi:10.100711036-010-0260-8

Chen, M., Hao, Y., Hu, L., Hossain, M. S., & Ghoneim, A. (2018). Edge-CoCaCo: Toward Joint Optimization of Computation, Caching, and Communication on Edge Cloud. *IEEE Wireless Communications, 25*(3), 21–27. doi:10.1109/MWC.2018.1700308

Chen, M., Hao, Y., Hwang, K., Wang, L., & Wang, L. (2017). Disease Prediction by Machine Learning Over Big Data From Healthcare Communities. *IEEE Access: Practical Innovations, Open Solutions, 5*, 8869–8879. doi:10.1109/ACCESS.2017.2694446

Chen, M., Herrera, F., & Hwang, K. (2018). Cognitive Computing: Architecture, Technologies and Intelligent Applications. *IEEE Access: Practical Innovations, Open Solutions, 6*, 19774–19783. doi:10.1109/ACCESS.2018.2791469

Chen, M., Wan, J., Gonzalez, S., Liao, X., & Leung, V. C. M. (2014). A Survey of Recent Developments in Home M2M Networks. *IEEE Communications Surveys and Tutorials, 16*(1), 98–114. doi:10.1109/SURV.2013.110113.00249

Chen, X., & Hu, C.-J. (2017). Adaptive medical image encryption algorithm based on multiple chaotic mapping. *Saudi Journal of Biological Sciences, 24*(8), 1821–1827. doi:10.1016/j.sjbs.2017.11.023 PMID:29551931

Cheon, J. H., & Kim, J. (2015). A hybrid scheme of public-key encryption and somewhat homomorphic encryption. *IEEE Transactions on Information Forensics and Security, 10*(5), 1052–1063. doi:10.1109/TIFS.2015.2398359

Chillotti, I., Gama, N., Georgieva, M., & Izabachène, M. (2017). *TFHE: Fast FullyHomomorphicEncryptionLibraryovertheTorus.* Retrieved from https://github.com/tfhe/tfhe

Chin, C. D., Cheung, Y. K., Laksanasopin, T., Modena, M. M., Chin, S. Y., Sridhara, A. A., & Karita, E. (2013). Mobile device for disease diagnosis and data tracking in resource-limited settings. *Clinical Chemistry, 59*(4), 629–640. doi:10.1373/clinchem.2012.199596 PMID:23327782

Chinmay, C. B. G., & Ghosh, S. K. (2013). A Review on Telemedicine-Based WBAN Framework for Patient Monitoring. *Telemedicine Journal and e-Health, 19*(18). PMID:23841489

Chinmay, C., Gupta, B., Ghosh, S. K., Das, D., & Chakraborty, C. (2016). Telemedicine Supported Chronic Wound Tissue Prediction Using Different Classification Approach. *Journal of Medical Systems, 40*(3), 1–12. PMID:26573639

Chipara, O., Lu, C., Bailey, T. C., & Roman, G.-C. (2010), Reliable clinical monitoring using wireless sensor networks: experiences in a step-down hospital unit. *Proceedings of the 8th ACM Conference on Embedded Networked Sensor Systems*, 155–168. 10.1145/1869983.1869999

Chlaihawia, A. A., Narakathua, B. B., Emamiana, S., Bazuina, B. J., & Atashbar, M. Z. (2018). Development of printed and flexible dry ECG electrodes. *Sensing and Bio-Sensing Research, 20*, 9–15. doi:10.1016/j.sbsr.2018.05.001

Choong, C. L., Shim, M. B., Lee, B. S., Jeon, S., Ko, D. S., Kang, T. H., ... Im, J. (2014). Highly stretchable resistive pressure sensors using a conductive elastomeric composite on a micropyramid array. *Advanced Materials*, *26*(21), 3451–3458. doi:10.1002/adma.201305182 PMID:24536023

Chortos, A., & Bao, Z. (2014). Skin-inspired electronic devices. *Materials Today*, *17*(7), 321–331. doi:10.1016/j.mattod.2014.05.006

Chtioui, I., Bossuyt, F., Vanfleteren, J., & Bedoui, M. H. (2017). 2.5/3D dynamically stretchable and permanently shaped electronic circuits. *Microsystem Technologies*, *24*(2), 831–853. doi:10.100700542-017-3582-7

Chung, W.-Y., Lee, Y.-D., & Jung, S.-J. (2008). A wireless sensor network compatible wearable u-healthcare monitoring system using integrated ECG, accelerometer and SpO2. *IEEE 30th Annual International Conference on Engineering in Medicine and Biology Society (EMBS),* 1529–1532.

Clear, M., & McGoldrick, C. (2015, August). Multi-identity and multi-key leveled FHE from learning with errors. In *Annual Cryptology Conference* (pp. 630-656). Springer. 10.1007/978-3-662-48000-7_31

Cook, K. A., Modena, B. D., & Simon, R. A. (2016). Improvement in asthma control using a minimally burdensome and proactive smartphone application. *The Journal of Allergy and Clinical Immunology. In Practice*, *4*(4), 730–737. doi:10.1016/j.jaip.2016.03.005 PMID:27107690

Costa, Â., Castillo, J., Novais, P., Fernández-Caballero, A., & Simoes, R. (2012). Sensor-driven agenda for intelligent home care of the elderly. *Expert Systems with Applications*, *39*(15), 12192–12204. doi:10.1016/j.eswa.2012.04.058

Cover, T., & Hart, P. (2006). Nearest neighbor pattern classification. *IEEE Transactions on Information Theory*, *13*(1), 21–27. doi:10.1109/TIT.1967.1053964

Cunningham, J. P., & Ghahramani, Z. (2015). Linear dimensionality reduction: Survey, insights, and generalizations. *Journal of Machine Learning Research*, *16*(1), 2859–2900.

Cunningham, P., & Delany, S. J. (2007). k-Nearest neighbour classifiers. *Multiple Classifier Systems*, *34*(8), 1–17.

Cushing, A., Manice, M. P., Ting, A., & Parides, M. K. (2016). Feasibility of a novel mHealth management system to capture and improve medication adherence among adolescents with asthma. *Patient Preference and Adherence*, *10*, 2271–2275. doi:10.2147/PPA.S115713 PMID:27853357

Daemen, J. & Rijmen, V. (2002). *The Design of Rijndael*. AES- The Advanced Encryption.

Daemen, J., & Rijmen, V. (2000). The Block Cipher Rijndael. In *Proceedings of International Conference on Smart Cards Research and Applications (CARDS'98), Lecture Notes in Computer Science* (Vol 1820, pp. 247-256). Springer-Verlag. 10.1007/10721064_26

Dahiya, R. S., & Gennaro, S. (2013). Bendable Ultra-Thin Chips on Flexible Foils. *IEEE Sensors Journal*, *13*(10), 4030–4037. doi:10.1109/JSEN.2013.2269028

Dallet, C., Kareem, S., & Kale, I. (2014). *Real time blood image processing application for malaria diagnosis using mobile phones.* Paper presented at the International Symposium on Circuits and Systems, Melbourne, Australia. 10.1109/ISCAS.2014.6865657

Damgård, I., & Jurik, M. (2001, February). A generalisation, a simpli. cation and some applications of paillier's probabilistic public-key system. In *International Workshop on Public Key Cryptography* (pp. 119-136). Springer. 10.1007/3-540-44586-2_9

Dehkordi, A. B., Esfahani, S. N., & Avanaki, A. N. (2011). Robust LSB watermarking optimized for local structural similarity. *2011 19th Iranian Conference on Electrical Engineering*, 1–6.

Demir. (2018). Energy Scavenging Methods for WBAN Applications: A Review. *IEEE Communications*, 1558-1748.

Dennis, C. (2018). A systematic review of chronic disease management interventions in primary care. *BMC Family Practice*, *19*(1). PMID:29316889

Derhamy, H., Eliasson, J., Delsing, J., & Priller, P. (2015). A Survey of Commercial Frameworks for the Internet of Things. *IEEE 20th Conference on Emerging Technologies & Factory Automation (ETFA),* 1-8.

Deshmukh, S., & Shah, R. (2016). Computation offloading frameworks in mobile cloud computing : a survey. In *2016 IEEE International Conference on Current Trends in Advanced Computing (ICCTAC)* (pp. 1–5). IEEE. 10.1109/ICCTAC.2016.7567332

Devanand, D. P.-X., Taylor, S., Gurland, B. J., Wilder, D., Stern, Y., & Mayeux, R. (1996). Depressed mood and the incidence of Alzheimer's disease in the elderly living in the community. *Archives of General Psychiatry*, *53*(2), 175–182. doi:10.1001/archpsyc.1996.01830020093011 PMID:8629893

DeVaul, R., Sung, M., Gips, J., & Pentland, A. (2003). MIThril applications and architecture. *SeventhIEEE International Symposium on Wearable Computers*, 4-11. 10.1109/ISWC.2003.1241386

Diffie, W., & Hellman, M. (1976). New directions in cryptography. *IEEE Transactions on Information Theory*, *22*(6), 644–654. doi:10.1109/TIT.1976.1055638

Dillingham, R., Ingersoll, K., Flickinger, T. E., Waldman, A. L., Grabowski, M., Laurence, C., ... Cohn, W. F. (2018). PositiveLinks: A Mobile health intervention for retention in HIV care and clinical outcomes with 12-month follow-up. *AIDS Patient Care and STDs*, *32*(6), 241–250. doi:10.1089/apc.2017.0303 PMID:29851504

Dobson, R., Carter, K., Cutfield, R., Hulme, A., Hulme, R., McNamara, C., & Whittaker, R. (2015). Diabetes text-message self-management support program (SMS4BG): A pilot study. *JMIR mHealth and uHealth*, *3*(1), e32. doi:10.2196/mhealth.3988 PMID:25830952

Dohler, D., Michael, P., & Binder, W. H. (2017). CuAAC-based click chemistry in self-healing polymers. *Accounts of Chemical Research*, *50*(10), 2610–2620. doi:10.1021/acs.accounts.7b00371 PMID:28891636

Domingos, P., & Pazzani, M. (1997). On the optimality of the simple Bayesian classifier under zero-one loss. *Machine Learning*, *29*(2-3), 103–130. doi:10.1023/A:1007413511361

Dongre, D., & Dongre, E. (2012). *Mobile multi sense disease management platform.* Paper presented at the International Conference on Green Technologies, Trivandrum, India.

Doukas, C., & Maglogiannis, I. (2012). Bringing IoT and Cloud Computing towards Pervasive Healthcare. In *2012 Sixth International Conference on Innovative Mobile and Internet Services in Ubiquitous Computing* (pp. 922–926). Academic Press. 10.1109/IMIS.2012.26

Dowlin, N., Gilad-Bachrach, R., Laine, K., Lauter, K., Naehrig, M., & Wernsing, J. (2017). Manual for homomorphic encryption for bioinformatics. *Proceedings of the IEEE*, *105*(3), 552–567.

Draper, B. M., Poulos, C. J., Cole, A. M., Poulos, R. G., & Ehrlich, F. (1992). A comparison of caregivers for elderly stroke and dementia victims. *Journal of the American Geriatrics Society*, *40*(9), 896–901. doi:10.1111/j.1532-5415.1992.tb01986.x PMID:1512385

Dridi, A., Sassi, S., & Faiz, S. (2017) A Smart IoT platform for personalized healthcare monitoring using semantic technologies. *IEEE International Conference on Tools with Artificial Intelligence (ICTAL)*, 1198-1203. 10.1109/ICTAI.2017.00182

Ducas & Micciancio. (2014). *A Fully Homomorphic Encryption library*. Retrieved from https://github.com/ lducas/FHEW

Ducas, L., & Micciancio, D. (2015, April). FHEW: bootstrapping homomorphic encryption in less than a second. In *Annual International Conference on the Theory and Applications of Cryptographic Techniques* (pp. 617-640). Springer. 10.1007/978-3-662-46800-5_24

Duda, R. O., Stork, D. G., & Hart, P. E. (2001). *Pattern classification* (2nd ed.). Wiley.

Dzaferovic, E., Vrtagic, S., Bandic, L., Kevric, J., Subasi, A., & Qaisar, S. M. (2016). Cloud-based mobile platform for EEG signal analysis. In *2016 5th International Conference on Electronic Devices, Systems and Applications (ICEDSA)* (pp. 1–4). Academic Press. 10.1109/ICEDSA.2016.7818497

Dziak, D., Jachimczyk, B., & Kulesza, W. J. (2017). IoT-Based Information System for Healthcare Application: Design Methodology Approach. *Applied Sciences*, *7*(6), 596. doi:10.3390/app7060596

Easton, C., Philip, N., & Aleksandravicius, A. (2013). Validity of smartphone accelerometers for assessing energy expenditure during fast running. *XIII Mediterranean Conference on Medical and Biological Engineering and Computing*, 1911–1914.

Edwards. (2012). Wireless sensors relay medical insight to patients and caregivers. *IEEE Signal Process. Magzine.*, *29*(3), 8–12.

Ekdahl, P., & Johansson, T. (2002, August). A new version of the stream cipher SNOW. In *International Workshop on Selected Areas in Cryptography* (pp. 47-61). Springer.

ElGamal, T. (1985). A public key cryptosystem and a signature scheme based on discrete logarithms. *IEEE Transactions on Information Theory*, *31*(4), 469–472. doi:10.1109/TIT.1985.1057074

Elola, Aramendi, Irusta, Picon, Alonso, Owens, & Idris. (2019). *Deep Neural Networks for ECG- Based Pulse Detection during Out-of-Hospital Cardiac Arrest*. Academic Press.

Eom, J., Jaisutti, R., Lee, H., Lee, W., Heo, J. S., Lee, J. Y., ... Kim, Y. H. (2017). Highly sensitive textile strain sensors and wireless user-interface devices using all-polymeric conducting fibers. *ACS Applied Materials & Interfaces*, *9*(11), 10190–10197. doi:10.1021/acsami.7b01771 PMID:28251848

Escobar Cruz, N., Solarte, J., & Gonzalez-Vargas, A. (2018). Automated Epileptic Seizure Detection System Based on a Wearable Prototype and Cloud Computing to Assist People with Epilepsy. In J. C. Figueroa-García, J. G. Villegas, J. R. Orozco-Arroyave, & P. A. Maya Duque (Eds.), *Applied Computer Sciences in Engineering* (pp. 204–213). Cham: Springer International Publishing. doi:10.1007/978-3-030-00353-1_18

Escoffery, C., McGee, R., Bidwell, J., Sims, C., Thropp, E. K., Frazier, C., & Mynatt, E. D. (2018). A review of mobile apps for epilepsy self-management. *Epilepsy & Behavior*, *81*, 62–69. doi:10.1016/j.yebeh.2017.12.010 PMID:29494935

Evans, D. (2011). *The Internet of Things - How the Next Evolution of the Internet is Changing Everything*. White Paper. Cisco Internet Business Solutions Group (IBSG).

Fan, K., Wang, P., Hu, Y., & Dou, B. (2017). Fall detection via human posture representation and support vector machine. *International Journal of Distributed Sensor Networks*, *13*(5). doi:10.1177/1550147717707418

Farahani, S. (2011). *ZigBee wireless networks and transceivers*. Newnes.

Fattah, S., Sung, N.-M., Ahn, I.-Y., Ryu, M., & Yun, J. (2017). Building IoT services for aging in place using standard-based IoT platforms and heterogeneous IoT products. *Sensors (Basel), 17*(10), 2311. doi:10.339017102311 PMID:29019964

Faxon, D. P., Schwamm, L. H., Pasternak, R. C., Peterson, E. D., McNeil, B. J., Bufalino, V., & Smaha, L. A. (2004). Improving quality of care through disease management: Principles and recommendations from the American Heart Association's Expert Panel on Disease Management. *Circulation, 109*(21), 2651–2654. doi:10.1161/01.CIR.0000128373.90851.7B PMID:15173048

Fernández, L., Blasco, J.M., & Hernández, J.F. (2009). *Wireless sensor networks in ambient intelligence. Book Wireless Sensor Networks in Ambient Intelligence City*. Univ. Politécnica de Valencia: Technologies for Health and Well-being Institute ITACA.

Finkenzeller, K. (2010). *RFID handbook: fundamentals and applications in contactless smart cards, radio frequency identification and near-field communication*. John Wiley & Sons. doi:10.1002/9780470665121

Foroughi, H., Aski, B. S., & Pourreza, H. (2008). Intelligent video surveillance for monitoring fall detection of elderly in home environments. In *11th international conference on computer and information technology* (pp. 219-224.). Khulna, Bangladesh: IEEE.

Fouchal, H., Herbin, M., & Blanchard, F. (2015, August). Centralized energy monitoring over wireless sensor networks. In *2015 International Wireless Communications and Mobile Computing Conference (IWCMC)* (pp. 788-792). IEEE. 10.1109/IWCMC.2015.7289183

Fox, M. S. (1990). AI and expert system myths, legends, and facts. *IEEE Intelligent Systems, 1*, 8–20.

Fraiwan, L., Ninan, J., & Al-Khodari, M. (2018). Mobile application for ulcer detection. *The Open Biomedical Engineering Journal, 12*(1), 16–26. doi:10.2174/1874120701812010016 PMID:30069252

Frederix, I., Sankaran, S., Coninx, K., & Dendale, P. (2016). *MobileHeart, a mobile smartphone-based application that supports and monitors coronary artery disease patients during rehabilitation*. Paper presented at the 38th Annual International Conference of the IEEE Engineering in Medicine and Biology Society, Lake Buena Vista, FL. 10.1109/EMBC.2016.7590752

Friedl, M. A., & Brodley, C. E. (1997). Decision tree classification of land cover from remotely sensed data. *Remote Sensing of Environment, 61*(3), 399–409. doi:10.1016/S0034-4257(97)00049-7

Friedman, J. H., Bentley, J. L., & Finkel, R. A. (1977). An algorithm for finding best matches in logarithmic expected time. *ACM Transactions on Mathematical Software, 3*(3), 209–226. doi:10.1145/355744.355745

Furht, B., & Escalante, A. (2010). *Handbook of cloud computing* (Vol. 3). New York: Springer. doi:10.1007/978-1-4419-6524-0

G, A., Chakraborty, C., & G, B. (2019). Medical Information Processing Using Smartphone Under IoT Framework. In *Energy Conservation for IoT Devices, Studies in Systems, Decision and Control* (Vol. 206, pp. 283-308). Springer.

Gachet, D., de Buenaga, M., Aparicio, F., & Padron, V. (2012). Integrating Internet of Things and Cloud Computing for Health Services Provisioning: The Virtual Cloud Carer Project. In *2012 Sixth International Conference on Innovative Mobile and Internet Services in Ubiquitous Computing* (pp. 918–921). Academic Press. 10.1109/IMIS.2012.25

Gaddam, A., Mukhopadhyay, S. C., & Gupta, G. S. (2011). Elder care based on cognitive sensor network. *IEEE Sensors Journal, 11*(3), 574–581. doi:10.1109/JSEN.2010.2051425

Galbraith, S. D. (2002). Elliptic curve Paillier schemes. *Journal of Cryptology*, *15*(2), 129–138. doi:10.100700145-001-0015-6

Gall, T., Valkanas, E., Bello, C., Markello, T., Adams, C., Bone, W. P., & Davis, J. (2017). Defining disease, diagnosis, and translational medicine within a homeostatic perturbation paradigm: The national institutes of health undiagnosed diseases program experience. *Frontiers in Medicine*, *4*, 62. doi:10.3389/fmed.2017.00062 PMID:28603714

Gandhi, B., Singh, L., & Gupta, L. (2017). Disease predictor: A disease prediction app. *International Journal for Research in Applied Science and Engineering Technology*, *5*(4), 1509–1512. doi:10.22214/ijraset.2017.4265

Gao, Z.-K., Cai, Q., Yang, Y.-X., Dong, N., & Zhang, S.-S. (2017). Visibility Graph from Adaptive Optimal Kernel Time-Frequency Representation for Classification of Epileptiform EEG. *International Journal of Neural Systems*, *27*(04), 1750005. doi:10.1142/S0129065717500058 PMID:27832712

Garcia, E., Ding, H., Sarela, A., & Karunanithi, M. (2010). *Can a mobile phone be used as a pedometer in an outpatient cardiac rehabilitation program?* Paper presented at the IEEE/ICME International Conference on Complex Medical Engineering, Gold Coast, Australia. 10.1109/ICCME.2010.5558833

Gentry, C., & Boneh, D. (2009). A fully homomorphic encryption scheme: Vol. 20. *No. 09*. Stanford, CA: Stanford University.

Ghadi, M., Laouamer, L., & Moulahi, T. (2015). Enhancing digital image integrity by exploiting JPEG bitstream attributes. *Journal of Innovation in Digital Ecosystems*, *2*(1-2), 20–31. doi:10.1016/j.jides.2015.10.003

Ghayvat, H., Mukhopadhyay, S., Gui, X., & Suryadevara, N. (2015). WSN- and IOT-Based Smart Homes and Their Extension to Smart Buildings. *Sensors (Basel)*, *15*(5), 10350–10379. doi:10.3390150510350 PMID:25946630

Ghose, A., Sinha, P., Bhaumik, C., Sinha, A., Agrawal, A., & Choudhury, A. D. (2013). UbiHeld - Ubiquitous Healthcare Monitoring System for Elderly and Chronic Patients. In *1st Workshop on Human Factors and Activity Recognition in Healthcare, Wellness and Assisted Living* (pp. 1255-1264). Zurich, Switzerland: ACM.

Giannakakis, G., Sakkalis, V., Pediaditis, M., & Tsiknakis, M. (2015). Methods for Seizure Detection and Prediction: An Overview. In V. Sakkalis (Ed.), *Modern Electroencephalographic Assessment Techniques: Theory and Applications* (pp. 131–157). New York, NY: Springer New York. doi:10.1007/7657_2014_68

Goldwasser, S., & Micali, S. (1982, May). Probabilistic encryption & how to play mental poker keeping secret all partial information. In *Proceedings of the fourteenth annual ACM symposium on Theory of computing* (pp. 365-377). ACM. 10.1145/800070.802212

Gomez, J. (2016). Patient Monitoring System Based on Internet of Things: A survey. *Journal of Computer Networks*, *11*, 532–550.

Gonzalez, M., Axisa, F., Bulcke, M. V., Brosteaux, D., Vandevelde, B., & Vanfleteren, J. (2008). Design of metal interconnects for stretchable electronic circuits. *Microelectronics and Reliability*, *48*(6), 825–832. doi:10.1016/j.microrel.2008.03.025

Gould, C., & Edwards, R. (2016). Review on Micro-Energy Harvesting Technologies. *51st International Universities Power Engineering Conference (UPEC)*, 1-5.

Gravina, R., Alinia, P., Ghasemzadeh, H., & Fortino, G. (2017). Multi-Sensor Fusion in Body Sensor Networks: State-of-the-art and research challenges. *Information Fusion*, *35*, 68–80. doi:10.1016/j.inffus.2016.09.005

Grguric A. (2012). *ICT towards elderly independent living*. Research and Development Centre, Ericsson Nikola Tesla.

Gubbi, J., Buyya, R., Marusic, S., & Palaniswami, M. (2013). Internet of Things (IoT) A Vision, Architectural Elements, and Future Directions. *Future Generation Computer Systems*, *29*(7), 1645–1660. doi:10.1016/j.future.2013.01.010

Gutjahr, G., Krishna, C. L, & Nedungadi, P. (2018). Optimal Tour Planning for Measles and Rubella Vaccination in Kochi, South India. *Proceedings of International Conference on Advances in Computing, Communications and Informatics (ICACCI).*

Gwo-Jia, Aripriharta, & Gwo-Jiun. (2017). The PPG Physiological Signal for Heart Rate Variability Analysis. *Wireless Personal Communication, 97*, 5229–5276.

Habib, C., Makhoul, A., Darazi, R., & Salim, C. (2016). Self-adaptive data collection and fusion for health monitoring based on body sensor networks. *IEEE Transactions on Industrial Informatics*, *12*(6), 2342–2352. doi:10.1109/TII.2016.2575800

Haddad, S., Coatrieux, G., Cozic, M., & Bouslimi, D. (2017). Joint watermarking and lossless JPEG-LS compression for medical image security. *Proceedings of the International Conference on Watermarking and Image Processing - ICWIP 2017.* 10.1145/3150978.3150985

Haghi, M., Thurow, K., & Stoll, R. (2017). Wearable Devices in Medical Internet of Things. Scientific Research and Commercially Available Devices: Healthc Inform Res, 4-15.

Halevi & Shoup. (2013). *An Implementation of homomorphic encryption.* Retrieved from https://github.com/ shaih/HElib

Halonen, T., Romero, J., & Melero, J. (2004). *GSM, GPRS and EDGE performance: evolution towards 3G/UMTS.* John Wiley & Sons.

Hamrioui, S., Gonzalez, J. H., Castillo, G., de la Torre-Diez, I., & Lopez-Coronado, M. (2018). *Development and QoE evaluation of an iOS mHealth app for self-controlling and education of patients with heart diseases.* Paper presented at the 13th Iberian Conference on Information Systems and Technologies, Cáceres, Spain. 10.23919/CISTI.2018.8398633

Han, E.-H., Karypis, G., & Kumar, V. (2001). Text Categorization Using Weight Adjusted k-Nearest Neighbor Classification. In *Proceedings of the 5th Pacific-Asia Conference on Knowledge Discovery and Data Mining* (pp. 53-65). Springer-Verlag. 10.1007/3-540-45357-1_9

Hanson, Powell Jr., Barth, & Ringgenberg. (2009). *Body Area Sensor networks: Challenges and opportunities.* IEEE Computer Society.

Hao, J. (2015). Image processing and transmission scheme based on generalized Gaussian mixture with opportunistic networking for a wireless sensor networks. *International Journal of Wireless Communication and Networking*, *21*(1), 226–234. doi:10.118613638-015-0458-3

Harb. (2011). Energy harvesting: State-of-the-art. *Renewable Energy*, *36*, 2641-2654.

Harpale, V., & Bairagi, V. (2018). An adaptive method for feature selection and extraction for classification of epileptic EEG signal in significant states. *Journal of King Saud University - Computer and Information Sciences.*

Hassanalieragh, M., Page, A., Soyata, T., Sharma, G., Aktas, M., Mateos, G., & Andreescu, S. (2015, June). Health monitoring and management using Internet-of-Things (IoT) sensing with cloud-based processing: Opportunities and challenges. In *2015 IEEE International Conference on Services Computing* (pp. 285-292). IEEE. 10.1109/SCC.2015.47

Hayes, B. (2008). Cloud computing. *Communications of the ACM*, *51*(7), 9–11. doi:10.1145/1364782.1364786

He, D., Ye, R., Chan, S., Guizani, M., & Xu, Y. (2018). Privacy in the Internet of Things for Smart Healthcare. *IEEE Communications Magazine*, *56*(4), 38–44. doi:10.1109/MCOM.2018.1700809

Heimerl, K., Menon, A., & Hasan, S. (2015). *Analysis of smartphone adoption and usage in a rural community cellular network.* Paper presented at the Seventh International Conference on Information and Communication Technologies and Development, Singapore, Singapore. 10.1145/2737856.2737880

Hoang, D. C., Tan, Y. K., Chng, H. B., & Panda, S. K. (2009). Thermal energy harvesting from human warmth for wireless body area network in medical healthcare system. In *International Conference on Power Electronics and Drive Systems (PEDS)* (pp.1277-1282). Academic Press. 10.1109/PEDS.2009.5385814

Holtz, B., & Lauckner, C. (2012). Diabetes management via mobile phones: A systematic review. *Telemedicine Journal and e-Health, 18*(3), 175–184. doi:10.1089/tmj.2011.0119 PMID:22356525

Holtz, B., & Whitten, P. (2009). Managing asthma with mobile phones: A feasibility study. *Telemedicine Journal and e-Health, 15*(9), 907–909. doi:10.1089/tmj.2009.0048 PMID:19919198

Honkoop, P. J., Simpson, A., Bonini, M., Snoeck-Stroband, J. B., Meah, S., Chung, K. F., & Sont, J. K. (2017). MyAirCoach: The use of home-monitoring and mHealth systems to predict deterioration in asthma control and the occurrence of asthma exacerbations; study protocol of an observational study. *BMJ Open, 7*(1), e013935. doi:10.1136/bmjopen-2016-013935 PMID:28119390

Hossain, M. M., Fotouhi, M., & Hasan, R. (2015). Towards an analysis of security issues, challenges, and open problems in the internet of things. In *Proc. 2015 IEEE World Congress on Services (SERVICES)*, (pp. 21-28). New York: IEEE. 10.1109/SERVICES.2015.12

Hossain, M. (2016). Patient State Recognition System for Healthcare Using Speech and Facial Expressions. *Journal of Medical Systems, 40*(12), 272. doi:10.100710916-016-0627-x PMID:27757715

Hossain, M. S., Muhammad, G., Song, B., Hassan, M. M., Alelaiwi, A., & Alamri, A. (2015). Audio-Visual Emotion-Aware Cloud Gaming Framework. *IEEE Transactions on Circuits and Systems for Video Technology, 25*(12), 2105–2118. doi:10.1109/TCSVT.2015.2444731

Hossain, M., & Muhammad, G. (2016a). Audio-visual emotion recognition using multi-directional regression and Ridgelet transform. *Journal on Multimodal User Interfaces, 10*(4), 325–333. doi:10.100712193-015-0207-2

Hossain, M., & Muhammad, G. (2016b). Cloud-assisted Industrial Internet of Things (IIoT) – Enabled framework for health monitoring. *Computer Networks, 101*, 192–202. doi:10.1016/j.comnet.2016.01.009

Hosu, O., Ravalli, A., Piccolo, G. M. L., Cristea, C., Sandulescu, R., & Marrazza, G. (2017). Smartphone-based immunosensor for CA125 detection. *Talanta, 166*, 234–240. doi:10.1016/j.talanta.2017.01.073 PMID:28213228

Hou, L., Zhao, S., Xiong, X., Zheng, K., Chatzimisios, P., Hossain, M. S., & Xiang, W. (2016). Internet of Things Cloud: Architecture and Implementation. *IEEE Communications Magazine, 54*(12), 32–39. doi:10.1109/MCOM.2016.1600398CM

Houssein, E. H., Hassanien, A. E., & Ismaeel, A. A. K. (2017). EEG Signals Classification for Epileptic Detection: A Review. In *Proceedings of the Second International Conference on Internet of Things, Data and Cloud Computing* (pp. 70:1--70:9). New York: ACM. 10.1145/3018896.3018970

Hsieh, Y.-Z., & Jeng, Y.-L. (2018). Development of home intelligent fall detection IoT system based on feedback optical flow convolutional neural network. *IEEE Access: Practical Innovations, Open Solutions, 6*, 6048–6057. doi:10.1109/ACCESS.2017.2771389

Hua, Z., Yi, S., & Zhou, Y. (2018). Medical image encryption using high-speed scrambling and pixel adaptive diffusion. *Signal Processing, 144*, 134–144. doi:10.1016/j.sigpro.2017.10.004

Hu, M., Ye, Q., & Tang, Y. (2018). Efficient batch identity-based fully homomorphic encryption scheme in the standard model. *IET Information Security*, *12*(6), 475–483. doi:10.1049/iet-ifs.2017.0567

Humphereys, G. (2012). The health-care challenges posed by population aging. *Bulletin of the World Health Organization, 90.*

Hung, K., Zhang, Y. T., & Tai, B. (2004). Wearable medical devices for tele-home healthcare. *IEEE 26th Annual International Conference on Engineering in Medicine and Biology Society,* 5384–5387.

Hussein, M., Mohamed, A., & Alghoniemy, M. (2015). Scalable real-time energy-efficient EEG compression scheme for a wireless body areasensor network. *Journal of Biomedical Signal Processing Control, 19,* 122–129. doi:10.1016/j.bspc.2015.03.005

Hu, X., Wang, B., & Ji, H. (2013). A a wireless sensor network-based structural health monitoring system for highway bridges. *Computer-Aided Civil and Infrastructure Engineering, 10,* 1623–1637.

Iazzi, A., Rziza, M., & Thami, R. O. (2018). Fall detection based on posture analysis and support vector machine. In *4th International Conference on Advanced Technologies for Signal and Image Processing (ATSIP).* Sousse, Tunisia: IEEE. 10.1109/ATSIP.2018.8364462

Ibarra, E., Antonopoulos, A., Kartsakli, E., Rodrigues, J., & Verikoukis, C. (2016). QoS-aware energy management in body sensor nodes powered by human energy harvesting. *IEEE Sensors Journal, 16*(2), 542–549. doi:10.1109/JSEN.2015.2483064

Ishai, Y., & Paskin, A. (2007, February). Evaluating branching programs on encrypted data. In *Theory of Cryptography Conference* (pp. 575-594). Springer. 10.1007/978-3-540-70936-7_31

Isinkaye, F. O., Awosupin, S. O., & Soyemi, J. (2017). A mobile based expert system for disease diagnosis and medical advice provisioning. *International Journal of Computer Science and Information Security, 15*(1), 568–572.

Islam, M. S., Hasan, M. M., Wang, X., Germack, H. D., & Noor-E-Alam, M. (2018). A Systematic Review on Healthcare Analytics: Application and Theoretical Perspective of Data Mining. *Health Care, 6*(2), 54. PMID:29882866

Istepanian, Jovanov, & Zhang. (2004). Guest editorial introduction to the special section on m-health: Beyond seamless mobility and global wireless health-care connectivity. *IEEE Transactions on Information Technology in Biomedicine,* 405-414.

Istepanian, R. S., & Al-anzi, T. M. (2018). m-Health interventions for diabetes remote monitoring and self management: Clinical and compliance issues. *mHealth, 4*(4), 1–3. PMID:29552566

Iyawa, G. E., & Hamunyela, S. (2019). *mHealth apps and services for maternal healthcare in developing countries.* Paper presented at IST Africa, Nairobi, Kenya.

Iyawa, G. E., Langan-Martin, J., Seville, S., & Masikara, W. (2019). mHealth as tools for development in mental health. In Impacts of Information Technology on Patient Care and Empowerment. In R. W. McHaney, I. Reychev, J. Azuri, M. E. McHaney & R. Moshonov. IGI Global.

Iyawa, G. E., Botha, A., & Herselman, M. (2016). Identifying and defining the terms related to a Digital Health Innovation Ecosystem. In M. Herselman & A. Botha (Eds.), *Strategies, Approaches and Experiences: Towards Building a South African Digital Health Innovation Ecosystem.* Pretoria: CSIR.

Iyawa, G. E., & Coleman, A. (2015). Improving health care delivery in rural communities through the use of mobile phones: A case study in Windhoek. *International Science and Technology Journal of Namibia, 8,* 1–21.

Iyawa, G. E., Herselman, M., & Botha, A. (2016). Digital health innovation ecosystems: From systematic literature to conceptual framework. *Procedia Computer Science*, *100*, 244–252. doi:10.1016/j.procs.2016.09.149

Iyawa, G. E., Velusamy, V., & Palanisamy, P. (2019). Wearable technologies for glucose monitoring: A systematic mapping study of publication trends. In D. Goyal, S. Balamurugan, S. Peng, & D. S. Jat (Eds.), *The IoT and the Next Revolutions Automating the World*. IGI Global. doi:10.4018/978-1-5225-9246-4.ch007

Jain, A. K. (2010). Data clustering: 50 years beyond K-means. *Pattern Recognition Letters*, *31*(8), 651–666. doi:10.1016/j.patrec.2009.09.011

Jalal, A., Kamal, S., & Kim, D. (2014). A depth video sensor-based life-logging human activity recognition system for elderly care in smart indoor environments. *Sensors (Basel)*, *14*(7), 11735–11759. doi:10.3390140711735 PMID:24991942

Jang, S. (2010). Structural health monitoring of a cable-stayed bridge using smart sensor technology: Deployment and evaluation. *Journal of Smart Structural System*, *72*(8), 1156–1173.

Jasper, H. H. (1958). The ten twenty electrode system of the international federation. *Electroencephalography and Clinical Neurophysiology*, *10*, 371–375. Retrieved from https://ci.nii.ac.jp/naid/10020218106/en/

Jimenez, F., & Torres, R. (2015). Building an IoT-aware healthcare monitoring system. In *34th International Conference of the Chilean Computer Science Society (SCCC)* (pp. 1-4). Santiago, Chile: IEEE.

Jingwei Liu, K. S. K. (2010). Hybrid security mechanisms for wireless body area networks. *Second Int. Conf. Ubiquitous Future Networks*, 98–103. 10.1109/ICUFN.2010.5547221

Johnson, R. A., & Wichern, D. W. (2002). *Applied multivariate statistical analysis* (Vol. 5). Upper Saddle River, NJ: Prentice hall.

Jonas, S. M., Deserno, T. M., Buhimschi, C. S., Makin, J., Choma, M. A., & Buhimschi, I. A. (2015). Smartphone-based diagnostic for preeclampsia: An mHealth solution for administering the Congo Red Dot (CRD) test in settings with limited resources. *Journal of the American Medical Informatics Association*, *23*(1), 166–173. doi:10.1093/jamia/ocv015 PMID:26026158

Jose-Luis, B.-M. (2015). *Wearable Sensors Integrated with Internet of Things for Advancing eHealth Care Sensors*. MDPI.

Juen, J., Cheng, Q., & Schatz, B. (2015). A natural walking monitor for pulmonary patients using mobile phones. *IEEE Journal of Biomedical and Health Informatics*, *19*(4), 1399–1405. doi:10.1109/JBHI.2015.2427511 PMID:25935052

Jung, H., Moon, J., Baek, D., Lee, J., Choi, J., Hong, J., & Lee, S. (2012). CNT/PDMS composite flexible dry electrodes for long-term ECG monitoring. *IEEE Transactions on Biomedical Engineering*, *59*(5), 1472–1479. doi:10.1109/TBME.2012.2190288 PMID:22410324

Jutel, A., & Lupton, D. (2015). Digitizing diagnosis: A review of mobile applications in the diagnostic process. *Diagnosis*, *2*(2), 89–96. doi:10.1515/dx-2014-0068 PMID:29540025

Kagen, S., & Garland, A. (2019). Asthma and Allergy Mobile Apps in 2018. *Current Allergy and Asthma Reports*, *19*(1), 6. doi:10.100711882-019-0840-z PMID:30712150

Kale, S., & Khandelwal, C. S. (2013, March). Design and implementation of real time embedded tele-health monitoring system. In *2013 International Conference on Circuits, Power and Computing Technologies (ICCPCT)* (pp. 771-774). IEEE. 10.1109/ICCPCT.2013.6528842

Kamišalić, A., Fister, I., Turkanović, M., & Karakatič, S. (2018). Sensors and functionalities of non-invasive wrist-wearable devices: A review. *Sensors (Basel), 18*(6), 1714–1747. doi:10.339018061714 PMID:29799504

Kamta & Chakraborty. (2019). A Novel Approach Toward Enhancing the Quality of Life in Smart Cities using Clouds and IoT-Based Technologies. Springer: Digital Twin Technologies and Smart Cities, 1-17.

Kanan & Bensalem. (2016). Energy harvesting for wearable wireless healthcare systems. *IEEE Wireless Communications and Networking Conference*.

Kanaparthi, S., & Badhulika, S. (2017). Low cost, flexible and biodegradable touch sensor fabricated by solvent-free processing of graphite on cellulose paper. *Sensors and Actuators. B, Chemical, 242*, 857–864. doi:10.1016/j.snb.2016.09.172

Kanaparthi, S., Sekhar, V. R., & Badhulika, S. (2016). Flexible, eco-friendly and highly sensitive paper antenna based electromechanical sensor for wireless human motion detection and structural health monitoring. *Extreme Mech. Lett, 9*, 324–330. doi:10.1016/j.eml.2016.09.007

Kanso, A., & Ghebleh, M. (2015). An efficient and robust image encryption scheme for medical applications. *Communications in Nonlinear Science and Numerical Simulation, 24*(1-3), 98–116. doi:10.1016/j.cnsns.2014.12.005

Karasz, H. N., Eiden, A., & Bogan, S. (2013). Text messaging to communicate with public health audiences: How the HIPAA Security Rule affects practice. *American Journal of Public Health, 103*(4), 617–622. doi:10.2105/AJPH.2012.300999 PMID:23409902

Kareem, S., Kale, I., & Morling, R. C. (2012). *Automated P. falciparum detection system for post-treatment malaria diagnosis using modified annular ring ratio method.* Paper presented at the UKSim 14th International Conference on Computer Modelling and Simulation, Cambridge, UK.

Karlik, B., & Olgac, A. V. (2011). Performance analysis of various activation functions in generalized MLP architectures of neural networks. *International Journal of Artificial Intelligence and Expert Systems, 1*(4), 111–122.

Kaur, M., Kaur, J., & Kaur, R. (2015). *Low cost cataract detection system using smart phone.* Paper presented at theInternational Conference on Green Computing and Internet of Things, Delhi, India. 10.1109/ICGCIoT.2015.7380724

Kaur, M., & Kaur, R. (2012). Reversible watermarking of medical images: Authentication and recovery- a survey. *J. Inf. Oper. Manag, 3*, 241.

Kavilkrue, M., & Boonma, P. (2015). Dimensionality Reduction Algorithms for Improving Efficiency of PromoRank: A Comparison Study. In H. Unger, P. Meesad, & S. Boonkrong (Eds.), *Recent Advances in Information and Communication Technology 2015. Advances in Intelligent Systems and Computing* (Vol. 361). Springer. doi:10.1007/978-3-319-19024-2_3

Kavis, M. J. (2014). *Architecting the cloud: design decisions for cloud computing service models (SaaS, PaaS, and IaaS).* John Wiley & Sons. doi:10.1002/9781118691779

Kavitha, K. C., & Perumalraja, R. (2014), Smart wireless healthcare monitoring for drivers community. *IEEE International Conference on Communications and Signal Processing (ICCSP)*, 1105–1108 10.1109/ICCSP.2014.6950019

Keller, M. J., Gray, M. R., & Givens, J. A. (1985). A fuzzy k-nearest neighbor algorithm. *IEEE Transactions on Systems, Man, and Cybernetics, SMC-15*(4), 580–585. doi:10.1109/TSMC.1985.6313426

Kelly, T., Suryadevara, N. K., & Mukhopadhyay, S. C. (2013). Towards the implementation of IoT for environmental condition monitoring in homes. *IEEE Sensors Journal, 13*(10), 3846–3853. doi:10.1109/JSEN.2013.2263379

Khambete, N. D., & Murray, A. (2012), National efforts to improve healthcare technology management and medical device safety in India. *7th International Conference on Appropriate Healthcare Technologies for Developing Countries*, 1–5. 10.1049/cp.2012.1474

Khan & Pathan. (2018). The state-of-the-art wireless body area sensor networks: A survey. *International Journal of Distributed Networks*, *14*(4).

Khan, N. S., Muaz, M. H., Kabir, A., & Islam, M. N. (2017). *Diabetes predicting mHealth application using machine learning*. Paper presented at the International WIE Conference on Electrical and Computer Engineering, Dehradun, India. 10.1109/WIECON-ECE.2017.8468885

Khoi, M. N., Saguna, S., Mitra, K., & Åhlund, C. (2015). Irehmo: an efficient iot-based remote health monitoring system for smart regions. In *17th International Conference on E-health Networking, Application & Services (HealthCom)* (pp. 563-568). Boston, MA: IEEE. 10.1109/HealthCom.2015.7454565

Kim, G., Son, J., Park, S., & Kim, W. (2008). Hybrid Process for Fabricating 3D Hierarchical Scaffolds Combining Rapid Prototyping and Electrospinning. *Macromolecular Rapid Communications*, *29*(19), 1577–1581. doi:10.1002/marc.200800277

Kim, H.-S., Seo, J.-S., & Seo, J. (2016). A Daily Activity Monitoring System for Internet of Things-Assisted Livingin Home Area Networks. *Iranian Journal of Electrical and Computer Engineering*, *6*(1), 399–405.

Kittler, J., Hatef, M., Duin, R. P. W., & Matas, J. (1998). On combining classifiers. *IEEE Transactions on Pattern Analysis and Machine Intelligence*, *20*(3), 226–239. doi:10.1109/34.667881

Kleinberger, T., Becker, M., Ras, E., Holzinger, A., & Müller, P. (2007). Ambient intelligence in assisted living: enable elderly people to handle future interfaces. In *International conference on universal access in human-computer interaction* (pp. 103-112). Springer. 10.1007/978-3-540-73281-5_11

Knickerbocker, J. U., Budd, R., Dang, B., Chen, Q., Colgan, E., Hung, L. W., . . . Wen, B. (2018), Heterogeneous Integration Technology Demonstrations for Future Healthcare, IoT, and AI Computing Solutions. *IEEE 68th Conference Electronic Components and Technology (ECTC)*, 1519-1528.

Knowlton, S. M., Sencan, I., Aytar, Y., Khoory, J., Heeney, M. M., Ghiran, I. C., & Tasoglu, S. (2015). Sickle cell detection using a smartphone. *Scientific Reports*, *5*(1), 15022. doi:10.1038rep15022 PMID:26492382

Ko, Lu, Srivastava, & Stankovic. (2010). Wireless sensor networks for healthcare. *Proceedings of the IEEE*, 1947–1960.

Kodali, R. K., Swamy, G., & Lakshmi, B. (2015). *An Implementation of IoT for Healthcare. In IEEE Recent Advances in Intelligent Computational Systems* (pp. 411–416). RAICS.

Koppar, A. R., & Sridhar, V. (2009), A workflow solution for electronic health records to improve healthcare delivery efficiency in rural India. *IEEE International Conference on eHealth, Telemedicine, and Social Medicine*, 227–232. 10.1109/eTELEMED.2009.30

Koppen, M. (2008). The curse of dimensionality. In *Proceedings of the 5th Online World Conference on Soft Computing in Industrial Applications (WSC5)* (pp. 4-8). Academic Press.

Kosse, R. C., Bouvy, M. L., de Vries, T. W., Kaptein, A. A., Geers, H. C., van Dijk, L., & Koster, E. S. (2017). mHealth intervention to support asthma self-management in adolescents: The ADAPT study. *Patient Preference and Adherence*, *11*, 571–577. doi:10.2147/PPA.S124615 PMID:28356720

Kriegel, H.-P., Kröger, P., & Zimek, A. (2009). Clustering high-dimensional data: A survey on subspace clustering, pattern-based clustering, and correlation clustering. ACM Trans. Knowl. Discov. Data., 3(1). doi:10.1145/1497577.1497578

Krishnamurthi, R., & Goyal, M. (2019). Hybrid Neuro-fuzzy Method for Data Analysis of Brain Activity Using EEG Signals. In J. Wang, G. R. M. Reddy, V. K. Prasad, & V. S. Reddy (Eds.), *Soft Computing and Signal Processing* (pp. 165–173). Singapore: Springer Singapore. doi:10.1007/978-981-13-3600-3_16

Laine, K., Chen, H., & Player, R. (2017). *Simple Encrypted Arithmetic Library*. Retrieved from https://sealcrypto.codeplex.com/

Laiphrakpam, D. S., & Khumanthem, M. S. (2017). Medical image encryption based on an improved ElGamal encryption technique. *Optik - International Journal for Light and Electron Optics, 147*, 88–102.

Lakshmi, C., Thenmozhi, K., Rayappan, J. B. B., & Amirtharajan, R. (2018). Encryption and watermark-treated medical image against hacking disease—An immune convention in spatial and frequency domains. *Computer Methods and Programs in Biomedicine, 159*, 11–21. doi:10.1016/j.cmpb.2018.02.021 PMID:29650305

Lakshminarayana, R., Wang, D., Burn, D., Chaudhuri, K. R., Galtrey, C., Guzman, N. V., ... Steiger, M. (2017). Using a smartphone-based self-management platform to support medication adherence and clinical consultation in Parkinson's disease. *MPJ Parkinson's Disease*, *3*(1), 2. doi:10.103841531-016-0003-z PMID:28649602

Landers, R., Hubner, U., Schmelzeisen, R., & Mulhaupt, R. (2002). Rapid prototyping of scaffolds derived from thermoreversible hydrogels and tailored for applications in tissue engineering. *Biomaterials*, *23*(23), 4437–4447. doi:10.1016/S0142-9612(02)00139-4 PMID:12322962

Latre´, B., Braem, B., Moerman, I., Blondia, C., & Demeester, P. (2011). A survey on wireless body area networks. *Wireless Networks*, *17*(1), 1–18. doi:10.100711276-010-0252-4

Lavsky-Shulan, M., Wallace, R. B., Kohout, F. J., Lemke, J. H., Morris, M. C., & Smith, I. M. (1985). Prevalence and functional correlates of low back pain in the elderly: The Iowa 65+ Rural Health Study. *Journal of the American Geriatrics Society*, *33*(1), 23–28. doi:10.1111/j.1532-5415.1985.tb02855.x PMID:3155530

Lee, J.-C., Jeon, J.-H., & Kim, S.-H. (2016), Design and Implementation of Healthcare Resource Model on IoTivity Platform. *IEEE International Conference on Information and Communication Technology Convergence (ICTC)*, 887-891. 10.1109/ICTC.2016.7763322

Lefler, L. L., Rhoads, S. J., Harris, M., Funderburg, A. E., Lubin, S. A., Martel, I. D., ... Beverly, C. J. (2018). Evaluating the use of mobile health technology in older adults with heart failure: Mixed-methods study. *JMIR Aging*, *1*(2), e12178. doi:10.2196/12178

Leidy, N. K., Kimel, M., Ajagbe, L., Kim, K., Hamilton, A., & Becker, K. (2014). Designing trials of behavioral interventions to increase physical activity in patients with COPD: Insights from the chronic disease literature. *Respiratory Medicine*, *108*(3), 472–481. doi:10.1016/j.rmed.2013.11.011 PMID:24315467

LeMoyne, R., Mastroianni, T., Cozza, M., Coroian, C., & Grundfest, W. (2010, August). Implementation of an iPhone for characterizing Parkinson's disease tremor through a wireless accelerometer application. In *2010 Annual International Conference of the IEEE Engineering in Medicine and Biology* (pp. 4954-4958). IEEE. 10.1109/IEMBS.2010.5627240

Lewinski, A. A., Patel, U. D., Diamantidis, C. J., Oakes, M., Baloch, K., Crowley, M. J., ... Bosworth, H. B. (2019). Addressing diabetes and poorly controlled hypertension: Pragmatic mHealth self-management intervention. *Journal of Medical Internet Research*, *21*(4), e12541. doi:10.2196/12541 PMID:30964439

Le, X. H., Khalid, M., Sankar, R., & Lee, S. (2011). An Efficient Mutual Authentication and Access Control Scheme for Wireless Sensor Network in Healthcare. *Journal of Networks*, *27*, 355–364.

Liberale, Dallago, & Barnabei. (2014). Energy harvesting system for wireless body sensor nodes. *IEEE Biomedical Circuits and Systems Conference (BioCAS) Proceedings*, 416-419. 10.1109/BioCAS.2014.6981751

Liew, S. C., & Zain, J. M. (2011). Tamper localization and lossless recovery watermarking scheme. In Software Engineering and Computer Systems. Springer. doi:10.1007/978-3-642-22170-5_48

Li, M., Yu, S., Zheng, Y., Ren, K., & Lou, W. (2013b). Scalable and secure sharing of personal health records in cloud computing using attribute-based encryption. *IEEE Transactions on Parallel and Distributed Systems*, *24*(1), 131–143. doi:10.1109/TPDS.2012.97

Lima, J. B., Madeiro, F., & Sales, F. J. R. (2015). Encryption of medical images based on the cosine number transform. *Signal Processing Image Communication*, *35*, 1–8. doi:10.1016/j.image.2015.03.005

Lin, C., Chiu, M., Hsiao, C., Lee, R., & Tsai, Y. (2006). Wireless health care service system for elderly with dementia. *IEEE Transactions on Information Technology in Biomedicine*, *10*(4), 696–704. doi:10.1109/TITB.2006.874196 PMID:17044403

Li, R. Z., Hu, A., Zhang, T., & Oakes, K. D. (2014). Direct writing on paper of foldable capacitive touch pads with silver nano wire inks. *ACS Applied Materials & Interfaces*, *6*(23), 21721–21729. doi:10.1021/am506987w PMID:25365734

Litt, B., & Echauz, J. (2002). Prediction of epileptic seizures. *Lancet Neurology*, *1*(1), 22–30. doi:10.1016/S1474-4422(02)00003-0 PMID:12849542

Liu, Y., Qu, X., & Xin, G. (2016). An ROI-based reversible data hiding scheme in encrypted medical images. *Journal of Visual Communication and Image Representation*, *39*, 51–57. doi:10.1016/j.jvcir.2016.05.008

Liu, Y., Wang, H., Zhao, W., Zhang, M., Qin, H., & Xie, Y. (2018). Flexible, Stretchable Sensors for Wearable Health Monitoring: Sensing Mechanisms, Materials, Fabrication Strategies and Features. *Sensors (Basel)*, *18*(2), 645. doi:10.339018020645 PMID:29470408

Li, X., Niu, J., Kumari, S., Liao, J., Liang, W., & Khan, M. K. (2016). A new authentication protocol for healthcare applications using wireless medical sensor networks with user anonymity. *Security and Communication Networks*, *9*(15), 2643–2655. doi:10.1002ec.1214

Li, Z., Ma, C., & Wang, D. (2017a). Towards multi-hop homomorphic identity-based proxy re-encryption via branching program. *IEEE Access: Practical Innovations, Open Solutions*, *5*, 16214–16228. doi:10.1109/ACCESS.2017.2740720

Lloyd, S. P. (1982). Least squares quantization in PCM. Information Theory. *IEEE Transactions on Information Theory*, *28*(2), 129–137. doi:10.1109/TIT.1982.1056489

Lokhande, P. P., & Mote, T. S. (2016). *Epilepsy Monitoring and Analysis System using Android Platform*. Academic Press.

Lomotey, R. K., Nilson, J., Mulder, K., Wittmeier, K., Schachter, C., & Deters, R. (2016). Mobile Medical Data Synchronization on Cloud-Powered Middleware Platform. *IEEE Transactions on Services Computing*, *9*(5), 757–770. doi:10.1109/TSC.2016.2555313

Lomotey, R. K., Sofranko, K., & Orji, R. (2018). Enhancing Privacy in Wearable IoT through a Provenance Architecture. *Multimodal Technologies and Interaction*, *2*(2), 18. doi:10.3390/mti2020018

Lopez, B. D. B., Aguirre, J. A. A., Coronado, D. A. R., & Gonzalez, P. A. (2018). *Wearable technology model to control and monitor hypertension during pregnancy*. Paper presented at the 13th Iberian Conference on Information Systems and Technologies, Cáceres, Spain. 10.23919/CISTI.2018.8399200

López-Alt, A., Tromer, E., & Vaikuntanathan, V. (2012, May). On-the-fly multiparty computation on the cloud via multikey fully homomorphic encryption. In *Proceedings of the forty-fourth annual ACM symposium on Theory of computing* (pp. 1219-1234). ACM. 10.1145/2213977.2214086

Lu, C., Raghunathan, V., & Roy, K. (2011). Efficient design of micro-scale energy harvesting systems. *IEEE J. Emerging Sel. Topics Circuits Syst*, *1*(3), 254–266. doi:10.1109/JETCAS.2011.2162161

Lv, Y., Zhao, H., Liang, Z., Dong, H., Liu, L., Zhang, D., & Cai, S. (2012). A mobile phone short message service improves perceived control of asthma: A randomized controlled trial. *Telemedicine Journal and e-Health*, *18*(6), 420–426. doi:10.1089/tmj.2011.0218 PMID:22667695

Lynch, J. P., & Loh, K. J. (2006). A summary review of a wireless sensors and sensor networks for structural health monitoring. *Journal of Shock and Vibration*, *4*, 2354–2362.

MacQueen, J. (1967). Some methods for classification and analysis of multivariate observations. In *Proceedings of the Fifth Berkeley Symposium on Mathematical Statistics and Probability. Volume 1: Statistics* (pp. 281-297), University of California Press.

Mahbub, Wang, Islam, Pullano, & Fiorillo. (2016). A low power wireless breathing monitoring system using piezo electric transducer, *IEEE International Symposium on Medical Measurements and Applications. (MeMeA)*, 1-5.

Mahmoodian, N., Boese, A., Friebe, M., & Haddadnia, J. (2019). Epileptic seizure detection using cross-bispectrum of electroencephalogram signal. *Seizure*, *66*, 4–11. doi:10.1016/j.seizure.2019.02.001 PMID:30769009

Mainetti, L., Patrono, L., Secco, A., & Sergi, I. (2017). An IoT-aware AAL System to Capture Behavioral Changes of Elderly People. *Journal of Communications Software and Systems*, *13*(2), 68-76.

Mainetti, L., Patrono, L., Secco, A., & Sergi, I. (2016). An IoT-aware AAL system for elderly people. In *2016 International Multidisciplinary Conference on Computer and Energy Science (SpliTech)* (pp. 1-6). Split, Croatia: IEEE. 10.1109/SpliTech.2016.7555929

Majumdar, A., Gogna, A., & Ward, R. (2014). A low-rank matrix recovery approach for energy-efficient EEG acquisition for a wireless body area network. *Journal of Sensors*, *14*(9), 15729–15748. doi:10.3390140915729 PMID:25157551

Malhi, S. C., Mukhopadhyay, S. C., Schnepper, J., Haefke, M., & Ewald, H. (2012). A Zigbee-based wearable physiological parameters monitoring system. *IEEE Sensors Journal*, *12*(3), 423–430. doi:10.1109/JSEN.2010.2091719

Malik, D. S., Mordeson, J. N., & Sen, M. K. (2007). *MTH 581-582 Introduction to Abstract Algebra*. Academic Press.

Manadhata, P. K., & Wing, J. M. (2011). An Attack Surface Metric. *IEEE Transactions on Software Engineering*, *37*(3), 371–386. doi:10.1109/TSE.2010.60

Manikandan, S., & Kulkarni, A. S. (2019). IoT based Low Power Wearable ECG Monitoring System. *Current Signal Transduction Therapy*, *14*(1), 68–74. doi:10.2174/1574362413666180622105447

Manisha, N. D. (2015). Fault detection in wireless sensor networks. *International Journal of Computer Science*, *3*(3), 6-10.

Marschollek, M., Goevercin, M., & Wolf, K. H. (2008). A performance comparison of accelerometry-based step detection algorithms on a large, non-laboratory sample of healthy and mobility-impaired persons. *Conference Proceedings; ... Annual International Conference of the IEEE Engineering in Medicine and Biology Society. IEEE Engineering in Medicine and Biology Society. Conference*, *2008*, 1319–1322. PMID:19162910

Martin, A., Osswald, C., Dezert, J., & Smarandache, F. (2008). *General combination rules for qualitative and quantitative beliefs*. Infinite Study.

Martin, C. K., Gilmore, L. A., Apolzan, J. W., Myers, C. A., Thomas, D. M., & Redman, L. M. (2016). Smartloss: A personalized mobile health intervention for weight management and health promotion. *JMIR mHealth and uHealth*, *4*(1), e18. PMID:26983937

Mazzeo, A. D., Kalb, W. B., Chan, L., Killian, M. G., Bloch, J. F., Mazzeo, B. A., & Whitesides, G. M. (2012). Paper-based, capacitive touch pads. *Advanced Materials*, *24*(21), 2850–2856. doi:10.1002/adma.201200137 PMID:22539155

McEvedy, C., & Jones, R. (1978). Atlas of world population history. Harmondsworth, UK: Penguin Books Ltd.

Megalingam, R. K., Veliyara, P. S., Prabhu, R., Krishna, R. R., & Katoch, R. (2014), Wheeled Patient Monitoring System. In L.C. Jain, S. Patnaik, & N. Ichalkaranje (Ed.), *Intelligent Computing, Communication and Devices: Proceedings of ICCD* (vol. 1, pp. 779-786). New Delhi: Academic Press.

Megiddo, I., Colson, A., Chisholm, D., Dua, T., Nandi, A., & Laxminarayan, R. (2016). Health and economic benefits of public financing of epilepsy treatment in India: An agent-based simulation model. *Epilepsia*, *57*(3), 464–474. doi:10.1111/epi.13294 PMID:26765291

Mell, P., & Grance, T. (2011). *The NIST definition of cloud computing*. Academic Press.

Memon, N. A., Chaudhry, A., Ahmad, M., & Keerio, Z. A. (2011). Hybrid watermarking of medical images for ROI authentication and recovery. *International Journal of Computer Mathematics*, *88*(10), 2057–2071. doi:10.1080/00207160.2010.543677

Meneilly, S. G., & Tessier, D. (2001). Diabetes in elderly adults. *The Journals of Gerontology. Series A, Biological Sciences and Medical Sciences*, *56*(1), M5–M13. doi:10.1093/gerona/56.1.M5 PMID:11193234

Meskó, B., Drobni, Z., Bényei, É., Gergely, B., & Győrffy, Z. (2017). Digital health is a cultural transformation of traditional healthcare. *mHealth*, *3*(38), 1–8. PMID:29184890

Metcalfe, R. M., & Boggs, D. R. (1976). Ethernet: Distributed packet switching for local computer networks. *Communications of the ACM*, *19*(7), 395–404. doi:10.1145/360248.360253

Michielli, N., Acharya, U. R., & Molinari, F. (2019). Cascaded LSTM recurrent neural network for automated sleep stage classification using single-channel EEG signals. *Computers in Biology and Medicine*, *106*, 71–81. doi:10.1016/j.compbiomed.2019.01.013 PMID:30685634

Mineraud Julien, O. (2016). A gap analysis of Internet-of-Things Platforms. *Computer Communications*, *89-90*, 5–16. doi:10.1016/j.comcom.2016.03.015

Miori, V., & Russo, D. (2017). *Improving life quality for the elderly through the Social Internet of Things (SIoT). In 2017 Global Internet of Things Summit (GIoTS)* (pp. 1–6). Geneva, Switzerland: IEEE.

Mishra, N., Lin, C.-C., & Chang, H.-T. (2014). Cognitive Inference Device for Activity Supervision in the Elderly. *The Scientific World Journal*, 1–12. PMID:25405211

Mohammadzadeh, N., & Safdari, R. (2014). Patient monitoring in mobile health: Opportunities and challenges. *Medicinski Arhiv*, *68*(1), 57. doi:10.5455/medarh.2014.68.57-60 PMID:24783916

Moosavi, S. R., Gia, T. N., Nigussie, E., Rahmani, A. M., Virtanen, S., Tenhunen, H., & Isoaho, J. (2016). End-to-end security scheme for mobility enabled healthcare Internet of Things. *Future Generation Computer Systems*, *64*, 108–124. doi:10.1016/j.future.2016.02.020

Mora, H., Gil, D., Terol, R. M., Azorín, J., & Szymanski, J. (2017). An IoT-Based Computational Framework for Healthcare Monitoring in Mobile Environments. *MDPI Sensors*, *17*(10), 2302. doi:10.339017102302 PMID:28994743

Mubashir, M., Shao, L., & Seed, L. (2013). A survey on fall detection: Principles and approaches. *Neurocomputing*, *100*, 144–152. doi:10.1016/j.neucom.2011.09.037

Muhtaroglu. (2017). Micro-scale energy harvesting for battery less information technologies in Energy Harvesting and Energy Efficiency: Technology. *Methods and Applications*, *37*, 63-85.

Muller, N., Emmrich, P. M. F., Rajemison, E. N., De Neve, J. W., Bärnighausen, T., Knauss, S., & Emmrich, J. V. (2019). A Mobile Health Wallet for Pregnancy-Related Health Care in Madagascar: Mixed-Methods Study on Opportunities and Challenges. *JMIR mHealth and uHealth*, *7*(3), e11420. doi:10.2196/11420 PMID:30457972

Munn, Z., Peters, M. D., Stern, C., Tufanaru, C., McArthur, A., & Aromataris, E. (2018). Systematic review or scoping review? Guidance for authors when choosing between a systematic or scoping review approach. *BMC Medical Research Methodology*, *18*(1), 143. doi:10.118612874-018-0611-x PMID:30453902

Munos, B., Baker, P. C., Bot, B. M., Crouthamel, M., de Vries, G., Ferguson, I., & Ozcan, A. (2016). Mobile health: The power of wearables, sensors, and apps to transform clinical trials. *Annals of the New York Academy of Sciences*, *1375*(1), 3–18. doi:10.1111/nyas.13117 PMID:27384501

Murphy, K. P. (2013). *Machine Learning: a Probabilistic Perspective*. MIT Press.

Murphy, S. L. (2009). Review of physical activity measurement using accelerometers in older adults: Considerations for research design and conduct. *Preventive Medicine*, *48*(2), 108–114. doi:10.1016/j.ypmed.2008.12.001 PMID:19111780

Naccache, D., & Stern, J. (1998, November). A new public key cryptosystem based on higher residues. In *Proceedings of the 5th ACM conference on Computer and communications security* (pp. 59-66). ACM. 10.1145/288090.288106

Najafi, B., Aminian, K., Loew, F., Blanc, Y., & Robert, P. A. (2002). Measurement of stand-sit and sit-stand transitions using a miniature gyroscope and its application in fall risk evaluation in the elderly. *IEEE Transactions on Biomedical Engineering*, *49*(8), 843–851. doi:10.1109/TBME.2002.800763 PMID:12148823

Nangalia, V., Prytherch, D., & Smith, G. (2010). Health technology assessment review: Remote monitoring of vital signs current status and future challenges. *Journal of Critical Care*, *14*(5), 552–565. PMID:20875149

Nanthini, B., & Santhi, B. (2017). Electroencephalogram signal classification for automated epileptic seizure detection using genetic algorithm. *Journal of Natural Science, Biology, and Medicine*, *8*(2), 159–166. doi:10.4103/jnsbm.JNSBM_285_16 PMID:28781480

Nasution, H. A., & Emmanuel, S. (2007). Intelligent video surveillance for monitoring elderly in home environments. In *9th Workshop on Multimedia Signal Processing* (pp. 203-206). IEEE. 10.1109/MMSP.2007.4412853

Nedungadi, P., Iyer, A., Gutjahr, G., Bhaskar, J., & Pillai, A. B. (2018). Data-Driven Methods for Advancing Precision Oncology. *Current Pharmacology Reports*, *4*(2), 145–156. doi:10.100740495-018-0127-4

Negra, R., Jemili, I., & Belghith, A. (2016). Wireless body area networks: Applications and technologies. *Procedia Computer Science*, *83*, 1274–1281. doi:10.1016/j.procs.2016.04.266

Nematzadeh, H., Enayatifar, R., Motameni, H., Guimarães, F. G., & Coelho, V. N. (2018). Medical image encryption using a hybrid model of modified genetic algorithm and coupled map lattices. *Optics and Lasers in Engineering*, *110*, 24–32. doi:10.1016/j.optlaseng.2018.05.009

Nguyen, H. H., Mirza, F., Naeem, M. A., & Nguyen, M. (2017). A review on iot healthcare monitoring applications and a vision for transforming sensor data into real-time clinical feedback. In *21st International Conference on Computer Supported Cooperative Work in Design (CSCWD)* (pp. 257-262). Wellington, New Zealand: IEEE. 10.1109/CSCWD.2017.8066704

Nie, P., & Li, B. (2011, July). A cluster-based data aggregation architecture in WSN for structural health monitoring. In *2011 7th International Wireless Communications and Mobile Computing Conference* (pp. 546-552). IEEE. 10.1109/IWCMC.2011.5982592

Nie, P. (2006). *An open standard for instant messaging: eXtensible Messaging and Presence Protocol (XMPP). In TKK T-110.5190 Seminar on Internetworking* (pp. 1–6). Helsinki University of Technology.

Niu, K., Zhao, F., & Zhang, S. (2013). A Fast Classification Algorithm for Big Data based on KNN. *Journal of Applied Sciences (Faisalabad)*, *13*(12), 2208–2212. doi:10.3923/jas.2013.2208.2212

Ni, Z., Shi, Y. Q., Ansari, N., & Su, W. (2006). Reversible data hiding. *IEEE Transactions on Circuits and Systems for Video Technology*, *16*(3), 354–362. doi:10.1109/TCSVT.2006.869964

Nkosi, M. T., & Mekuria, F. (2010). Cloud Computing for Enhanced Mobile Health Applications. In *2010 IEEE Second International Conference on Cloud Computing Technology and Science* (pp. 629–633). IEEE. 10.1109/CloudCom.2010.31

Noel & Abdaoui. (2017). Structural Health monitoring using A Wireless Sensor Networks. *IEEE Journal of Communication*, *19*(3), 1924–1936.

Nordin, A. N., & Ramli, N. (2019). Flexible and Stretchable Circuits for Smart Wearables. *Journal of Telecommunication*, *9*(3-8), 117–122.

Noury, N., Fleury, A., Rumeau, P., Bourke, A., Laighin, G., & Rialle, V. (2007). Fall detection-principles and methods. In *29th Annual International Conference of the IEEE Engineering in Medicine and Biology Society* (pp. 1663-1666). Lyon, France: IEEE.

Odunmbaku, A., Rahmani, A. M., Liljeberg, P., & Tenhunen, H. (2015). *Elderly monitoring system with sleep and fall detector. In International Internet of Things Summit* (pp. 473–480). Cham: Springer.

Oh, H., Rizo, C., Enkin, M., & Jadad, A. (2005). What is eHealth (3): A systematic review of published definitions. *Journal of Medical Internet Research*, *7*(1), e1. doi:10.2196/jmir.7.1.e1 PMID:15829471

Okamoto, T., & Uchiyama, S. (1998, May). A new public-key cryptosystem as secure as factoring. In *International conference on the theory and applications of cryptographic techniques* (pp. 308-318). Springer. 10.1007/BFb0054135

Olivero, M., Tosi, D., & Perrone, G. (2018). *Low-cost fiber Bragg Grating vibroacoustic sensor for voice and heartbeat detection.* Academic Press.

Otto, C., & Milenković, A. (2006). System Architecture of a Wireless Body Area Sensor network for Ubiquitous Health Monitoring. *Journal OF Mobile Multimedia*, *1*(4), 307–326.

Ougiaroglou, S., & Nanopoulos, A. (2007). Adaptive k-Nearest-Neighbor Classification Using a Dynamic Number of Nearest Neighbors. In Y. Ioannidis, B. Novikov, & B. Rachev (Eds.), *Advances in Databases and Information Systems* (pp. 66–82). Springer Berlin Heidelberg. doi:10.1007/978-3-540-75185-4_7

Ou, J., & Li, H. (2010). Structural health monitoring in mainland China: Review and future trends. *Journal of Structural Health Monitoring*, *3*(1), 874–890.

Oyelami, O. M. (2012). A Mobile Phone-Based Expert System for Disease Diagnosis. In E-Healthcare Systems and Wireless Communications: Current and Future Challenges. IGI Global. doi:10.4018/978-1-61350-123-8.ch011

Pacheco, J., Tunc, C., & Hariri, S. (2018). Security Framework for IoT Cloud Services. *Proc. IEEE/ACS 15th International Conference on Computer Systems and Applications (AICCSA)*.

Page, R., Shankar, R., McLean, B. N., Hanna, J., & Newman, C. (2018). Digital Care in Epilepsy: A Conceptual Framework for Technological Therapies. *Frontiers in Neurology*, *9*, 99. doi:10.3389/fneur.2018.00099 PMID:29551988

Paillier, P. (1999, May). Public-key cryptosystems based on composite degree residuosity classes. In *International Conference on the Theory and Applications of Cryptographic Techniques* (pp. 223-238). Springer. 10.1007/3-540-48910-X_16

Pang, Z., Zheng, L., Tian, J., Kao-Walter, S., Dubrova, E., & Chen, Q. (2015). Design of a terminal solution for integration of in-home health care devices and services towards the Internet-of-Things. *Enterprise Information Systems*, *9*(1), 86–116. doi:10.1080/17517575.2013.776118

Pan, J., & Tompkins, W. (1985). A real-time QRS detection algorithm. *IEEE Transactions on Biomedical Engineering*, *32*(3), 230–236. doi:10.1109/TBME.1985.325532 PMID:3997178

Panyasoponlert, N., Piboonudompornkul, P., Rudahl, K. T., & Goldin, S. E. (2012). *Flu incident reporting on mobile phone*. Paper presented at the International Conference on Communication, Networks and Satellite, Bali, Indonesia.

Park, S.J., Subramaniyam, M., Kim, S.E., Hong, S., Lee, J.H., & Jo, C.M. (2017). Development of the elderly healthcare monitoring system with IoT. *Advances in Human Factors and Ergonomics in Healthcare*, 309-315.

Park, S., Kim, J. Y., Lee, J. C., Kim, H. R., Song, S., Kwon, H., ... Choi, C. M. (2019). Mobile phone app–based pulmonary rehabilitation for chemotherapy-treated patients with advanced lung cancer: Pilot study. *JMIR mHealth and uHealth*, *7*(2), e11094. doi:10.2196/11094 PMID:30714943

Park, Y. T. (2016). Emerging new era of mobile health technologies. *Healthcare Informatics Research*, *22*(4), 253–254. doi:10.4258/hir.2016.22.4.253 PMID:27895955

Parzen, E. (1962). On estimation of a probability density function and mode. *Annals of Mathematical Statistics*, *33*(3), 1065–1076. doi:10.1214/aoms/1177704472

Patel, S., Park, H., Bonato, P., Chan, L., & Rodgers, M. (2012). A review of wearable sensors and systems with application in rehabilitation. *Journal of Neuroengineering and Rehabilitation*, *9*(1), 21. doi:10.1186/1743-0003-9-21 PMID:22520559

Peters, D. H., Garg, A., Bloom, G., Walker, D. G., Brieger, W. R., & Hafizur Rahman, M. (2008). Poverty and access to health care in developing countries. *Annals of the New York Academy of Sciences*, *1136*(1), 161–171. doi:10.1196/annals.1425.011 PMID:17954679

Petersen, C. L., Wechsler, E. V., Halter, R. J., Boateng, G. G., Proctor, P. O., Kotz, D. F., & Batsis, J. A. (2018). *Detection and monitoring of repetitions using an mHealth-enabled resistance band*. Paper presented at the IEEE/ACM International Conference on Connected Health: Applications, Systems and Engineering Technologies, Washington, DC.

Petersen, R. C., Smith, G. E., Waring, S. C., Ivnik, R. J., Tangalos, E. G., & Kokmen, E. (1999). Mild cognitive impairment: Clinical characterization and outcome. *Archives of Neurology*, *5*(3), 303–308. doi:10.1001/archneur.56.3.303 PMID:10190820

Peterson, J., Pearce, P. F., Ferguson, L. A., & Langford, C. A. (2017). Understanding scoping reviews: Definition, purpose, and process. *Journal of the American Association of Nurse Practitioners*, *29*(1), 12–16. doi:10.1002/2327-6924.12380 PMID:27245885

Petrie, K. J., Perry, K., Broadbent, E., & Weinman, J. (2012). A text message programme designed to modify patients' illness and treatment beliefs improves self-reported adherence to asthma preventer medication. *British Journal of Health Psychology*, *17*(1), 74–84. doi:10.1111/j.2044-8287.2011.02033.x PMID:22107110

Piette, J. D., Blaya, J. A., Lange, I., & Sanchis, J. B. B. (2011). *Experiences in mHealth for chronic disease management in 4 countries*. Paper presented at the 4th International Symposium on Applied Sciences in Biomedical and Communication Technologies, Barcelona, Spain. 10.1145/2093698.2093868

Piller, L. B., Ford, C. E., Davis, B. R., Nwachuku, C., Black, H. R., Oparil, S., ... Probstfield, J. L. (2006). Incidence and predictors of angioedema in elderly hypertensive patients at high risk for cardiovascular disease: A report from the Antihypertensive and Lipid-Lowering Treatment to Prevent Heart Attack Trial (ALLHAT). *Journal of Clinical Hypertension*, *8*(9), 649–658. doi:10.1111/j.1524-6175.2006.05689.x PMID:16957427

Pinto, S., Cabral, J., & Gomes, T. (2017). We-care: An IoT-based health care system for elderly people. In *IEEE International Conference on Industrial Technology (ICIT)* (pp. 1378-1383). Toronto, Canada: IEEE. 10.1109/ICIT.2017.7915565

Prince, S. A., Adamo, K. B., Hamel, M. E., Hardt, J., Gorber, S. C., & Tremblay, M. (2008). A comparison of direct versus self-report measures for assessing physical activity in adults: A systematic review. *The International Journal of Behavioral Nutrition and Physical Activity*, 5. PMID:18990237

Punit, Agrawal, Chhabra, & Dhir. (2016). IoT based smart healthcare kit. *IEEE International Conference on Computational Techniques in Information and Communication Technologies (ICCTICT)*, 237-242.

Qadir, Q. M., Rashid, T. A., Al-Salihi, N. K., Ismael, B., Kist, A. A., & Zhang, Z. (2018). Low Power Wide Area Networks: A Survey of Enabling Technologies, Applications and Interoperability Needs. *IEEE Access: Practical Innovations, Open Solutions*, *6*, 77454–77473. doi:10.1109/ACCESS.2018.2883151

Qasim, A. F., Meziane, F., & Aspin, R. (2018). Digital watermarking: Applicability for developing trust in medical imaging workflows state of the art review. *Computer Science Review*, *27*, 45–60. doi:10.1016/j.cosrev.2017.11.003

Quintiliani, L. M., Mann, D. M., Puputti, M., Quinn, E., & Bowen, D. J. (2016). Pilot and feasibility test of a mobile health-supported behavioral counseling intervention for weight management among breast cancer survivors. *JMIR Cancer, 2*(1), e4.

Qureshi, F. U., Muhtaroğlu, A., & Tuncay, K. (2017). Near-optimal design of scalable energy harvester for underwater pipeline monitoring applications with consideration of impact to pipeline performance. *IEEE Sensors Journal*, *17*(7), 1981–1991. doi:10.1109/JSEN.2017.2661199

Rahman, M. M., Bhuiyan, M. I. H., & Das, A. B. (2019). Classification of focal and non-focal EEG signals in VMD-DWT domain using ensemble stacking. *Biomedical Signal Processing and Control*, *50*, 72–82. doi:10.1016/j.bspc.2019.01.012

Rajagopal, M. K., & Rodriguez-Villegas, E. (2013). Towards wearable sleep diagnostic systems for point-of-care applications. *Proceedings of the 2013 IEEE point-of-care healthcare technologies (PHT)*. 10.1109/PHT.2013.6461276

Rajaraman & Ullman. (2011). *Mining of Massive Datasets*. New York: Cambridge University Press.

Ramgopal, S., Thome-Souza, S., Jackson, M., Kadish, N. E., Fernández, I. S., Klehm, J., … Loddenkemper, T. (2014). Seizure detection, seizure prediction, and closed-loop warning systems in epilepsy. *Epilepsy & Behavior, 37*, 291–307.

Ranganathan, L. N., Aadhimoolam Chinnadurai, S., Samivel, B., Kesavamurthy, B., & Mehndiratta, M. M. (2015). Application of mobile phones in epilepsy care. *International Journal of Epilepsy*, *02*(01), 28–37. doi:10.1016/j.ijep.2015.02.002

Rashid, F. Y. (2017). Top cloud security controls you should be using. *InfoWorld*. Retrieved from https://www.csoonline.com/article/3208905/top-cloud-security-controls-you-should-be-using.html

Rashid, T.A., &Abdulla, S. A. (2018). A Hybrid of Artificial Bee Colony, Genetic Algorithm, and Neural Network for Diabetic Mellitus Diagnosing, *ARO-The Scientific Journal of Koya University, 6*(1), 55-64.

Rashidi, P., & Mihailidis., A. (2013). A survey on ambient-assisted living tools for older adults. *IEEE Journal of Biomedical and Health Informatics*, *17*(3), 579-590.

Rashid, T. A., & Abdullah, S. M. (2018). A Hybrid of Artificial Bee Colony, Genetic Algorithm, and Neural Network for Diabetic Mellitus Diagnosing. *ARO-The Scientific Journal of Koya University.*, *6*(1), 55–64. doi:10.14500/aro.10368

Rashid, T. A., Abdullah, S. M., & Abdullah, R. M. (2016). An Intelligent Approach for Diabetes Classification, Prediction, and Description. In V. Snášel, A. Abraham, P. Krömer, M. Pant, & A. Muda (Eds.), *Innovations in Bio-Inspired Computing and Applications* (Vol. 424, pp. 323–335). Cham: Springer. doi:10.1007/978-3-319-28031-8_28

Rashid, T. A., Abdulla, S. M., & Abdulla, R. M. (2016). Decision Support System for Diabetes Mellitus through Machine Learning Techniques. *International Journal of Advanced Computer Science and Applications*, *7*(7), 170–178.

Rashid, T. A., Fattah, P., & Awlaa, D. K. (2018). Using Accuracy Measure for Improving the Training of LSTM with Metaheuristic Algorithms. *Procedia Computer Science*, *140*, 324–333. doi:10.1016/j.procs.2018.10.307

Rashid, T. A., Hassan, M. K., Mohammadi, M., & Fraser, K. (2019). Improvement of variant adaptable LSTM trained with metaheuristic algorithms for healthcare analysis. In C. Chakraborty (Ed.), *Advanced Classification Techniques for Healthcare Analysis*. IGI Global. doi:10.4018/978-1-5225-7796-6.ch006

Rashidzadeh, H., Kasargod, P. S., Supon, T. M., Rashidzadeh, R., & Ahmadi, M. (2016). Energy harvesting for IoT sensors utilizing MEMS technology. *2016 IEEE Canadian Conference on Electrical and Computer Engineering (CCECE 2016)*. 10.1109/CCECE.2016.7726622

Ray, & P, P. (2014). Home Health Hub Internet of Things (H 3 IoT): An architectural framework for monitoring health of elderly people. In *International Conference on Science Engineering and Management Research (ICSEMR)* (pp. 1-3). Chennai, India: IEEE.

Ren, Jin, Chen, Ghayvat, & Chen. (2018). A Novel cardiac Auscultation monitoring system based a wireless sensing for healthcare. *IEEE Journal of Translational Engineering in Health and Medicine, 6*, 1324-1331.

Reyes, B., Olvera-Montes, N., Charleston-Villalobos, S., González-Camarena, R., Mejía-Ávila, M., & Aljama-Corrales, T. (2018). A Smartphone-Based System for Automated Bedside Detection of Crackle Sounds in Diffuse Interstitial Pneumonia Patients. *Sensors (Basel)*, *18*(11), 3813. doi:10.339018113813 PMID:30405036

Reyes-Ortiz, J. L., Oneto, L., Sama, A., Parra, X., & Anguita, D. (2016). Transition-aware human activity recognition using smartphones. *Neurocomputing*, *171*, 754–767. doi:10.1016/j.neucom.2015.07.085

Riazul Islam, S. M., Daehan Kwak, M. D., Humaun Kabir, M., Hossain, M., & Kyung-Sup Kwak. (2015). The Internet of Things for Health Care: A Comprehensive Survey. *IEEE Access: Practical Innovations, Open Solutions*, *3*, 678–708. doi:10.1109/ACCESS.2015.2437951

Riazul Islam, S. M., Kwak, D., Humaun Kabir, M., Hossain, M., & Kwak, K. S. (2015). The Internet of Things for health care: A comprehensive survey. *IEEE Journal of Translational Engineering in Health and Medicine*, *3*, 678–708.

Richardson, M. L., Frank, M. S., & Stern, E. J. (1995). Digital image manipulation: What constitutes an acceptable alteration of a radiologic image? *AJR. American Journal of Roentgenology*, *164*(1), 228–229. doi:10.2214/ajr.164.1.7998545 PMID:7998545

Rivest, R. L., Adleman, L., & Dertouzos, M. L. (1978a). On data banks and privacy homomorphisms. *Foundations of Secure Computation, 4*(11), 169-180.

Rivest, R. L., Shamir, A., & Adleman, L. (1978b). A method for obtaining digital signatures and public-key cryptosystems. *Communications of the ACM*, *21*(2), 120–126. doi:10.1145/359340.359342

Rodrigues, J. J., Pedro, L. M., Vardasca, T., de la Torre-Díez, I., & Martins, H. M. (2013). Mobile health platform for pressure ulcer monitoring with electronic health record integration. *Health Informatics Journal*, *19*(4), 300–311. doi:10.1177/1460458212474909 PMID:24255053

Rohokale, V. M., Prasad, N. R., & Prasad, R. (2011), A cooperative internet of things (IoT) for rural healthcare monitoring and control. *IEEE 2nd International Conference on Wireless Communication, Vehicular Technology, Information Theory and Aerospace & Electronic Systems Technology (Wireless VITAE),* 1–6.

Saeb, S., Lattie, E. G., Kording, K. P., & Mohr, D. C. (2017). Mobile phone detection of semantic location and its relationship to depression and anxiety. *JMIR mHealth and uHealth*, *5*(8), e112. doi:10.2196/mhealth.7297 PMID:28798010

Saleh, E., Błaszczyński, J., Moreno, A., Valls, A., Romero-Aroca, P., de la Riva-Fernández, S., & Słowiński, R. (2017). Learning ensemble classifiers for diabetic retinopathy assessment. *Artificial Intelligence in Medicine*, *85*, 50–63. doi:10.1016/j.artmed.2017.09.006 PMID:28993124

Salih & Abraham. (2015). *Intelligent Decision Support for Real-time Health CareMonitoring System.* Afro-European Conference for Industrial Advancement.

Salimien, N., Ehteshami, A., & Talouki, M. A. (2019). Developing Ghasedek: A mobile application to improve the quality of cancer palliative care. *Acta Medica Informatica*, *27*(1), 19–22. doi:10.5455/aim.2019.27.19-22

Sander, T., Young, A., & Yung, M. (1999). Non-interactive cryptocomputing for NC/SUP 1. In *Foundations of Computer Science, 1999. 40th Annual Symposium on* (pp. 554-566). IEEE.

Sareen, S., Sood, S. K., & Gupta, S. K. (2016). An Automatic Prediction of Epileptic Seizures Using Cloud Computing and Wireless Sensor Networks. *Journal of Medical Systems*, *40*(11), 226. doi:10.100710916-016-0579-1 PMID:27628727

Sathya, S., Joshi, S., & Padmavathi, S. (2017). Classification of breast cancer dataset by different classification algorithms. *Proceedings of 4th International Conference on Advanced Computing and Communication Systems.* 10.1109/ICACCS.2017.8014573

Satija, U., Barathram, R., & Manikandan, M. S. (2016). Real-Time Signal Quality-Aware ECG Telemetry System for IoT-Based Health Care Monitoring. *IEEE Internet of Things*, 1-9.

Saxena, A., & Saad, A. (2017). Evolving an artificial neural network classifier for condition monitoring of rotating mechanical systems. *Journal of Applied Soft Computing*, *7*(1), 135–154.

Sebbak, F., & Benhammadi, F. (2017). Majority-consensus fusion approach for elderly IoT-based healthcare applications. *Annales des Télécommunications*, *72*(3-4), 157–171. doi:10.100712243-016-0550-7

Seelam, Vasavi Sai Viswanada Prabhu Deva Kumar, & Akashe, S. (2017). Implementation of GSM Based Security System with IOT Applications. *International Journal of Computer Network and Information Security*, *6*, 13–20.

Seppala, J., De Vita, I., Jamsa, T., Miettunen, J., Isohanni, M., Rubinstein, K., … Bulgheroni, M. (2019). Mobile phone and wearable sensor-based mHealth approaches for psychiatric disorders and symptoms: systematic review. *JMIR Mental Health, 6*(2), 1-14.

Shabut, A. M., Tania, M. H., Lwin, K. T., Evans, B. A., Yusof, N. A., Abu-Hassan, K. J., & Hossain, M. A. (2018). An intelligent mobile-enabled expert system for tuberculosis disease diagnosis in real time. *Expert Systems with Applications*, *114*, 65–77. doi:10.1016/j.eswa.2018.07.014

Shaladi, R., Alatshan, F., & Yang, C. (2015). An overview on the applications of structural health monitoring using a wireless sensor networks in bridge engineering. *International Conference in Advanced Science and Engineering Technology National Resources*, 19(3), 1542-1553.

Sharma, M., Shah, S., & Achuth, P. V. (2019). A Novel Approach for Epilepsy Detection Using Time–Frequency Localized Bi-orthogonal Wavelet Filter. *Journal of Mechanics in Medicine and Biology*, *19*(01), 1940007. doi:10.1142/S0219519419400074

Sharma, R. R., & Pachori, R. B. (2017). Time–frequency representation using IEVDHM–HT with application to classification of epileptic EEG signals. *IET Science, Measurement & Technology*. doi:10.1049/iet-smt.2017.0058

Shehab, A., Ismail, A., Osman, L., Elhoseny, M., & El-Henawy, I. (2017). Quantified self using IoT wearable devices. In *International Conference on Advanced Intelligent Systems and Informatics* (pp. 820-831). Cham: Springer.

Shelhamer, E., Long, J., & Darrell, T. (2017). Fully convolutional networks for semantic segmentation. *IEEE Transactions on Pattern Analysis and Machine Intelligence*, *39*(4), 1753–1768. doi:10.1109/TPAMI.2016.2572683 PMID:27244717

Shesternikova, O. P., Agafonov, M. A., Vinokurova, L. V., Pankratova, E. S., & Finn, V. K. (2016). Intelligent system for diabetes prediction in patients with chronic pancreatitis. *Scientific and Technical Information Processing*, *43*(5-6), 315–345. doi:10.3103/S0147688216050051

Shirane, Ito, Ishihara, & Masu. (2015). An RF energy harvesting power management circuit for appropriate duty-cycled operation. *Japanese Journal of Applied Physics*, *54*(4S), 04DE11.1-04DE11.6. March.

Simpson, A. J., Honkoop, P. J., Kennington, E., Snoeck-Stroband, J. B., Smith, I., East, J., & Usmani, O. (2017). Perspectives of patients and healthcare professionals on mHealth for asthma self-management. *The European Respiratory Journal*, *49*(5), 1601966. doi:10.1183/13993003.01966-2016 PMID:28461291

Singh, P., & Panjwani, M. (2016). mHealth: Meaning, purpose and outcome. *International Journal of Computer Science and Information Technologies*, *7*(5), 2216–2221.

Sirikham, A. (2011). *Abnormal heart rate detection device warning via mobile phone network.* Paper presented at the International Conference on Multimedia Computing and Systems, Ouarzazate, Morocco. 10.1109/ICMCS.2011.5945590

Skeppstedt, E. A. T. F. M., & Kvist, M. (2014), Medical text simplification using synonym replacement: Adapting assessment of word difficulty to a compounding language. *Proceedings of the 3rd Workshop on Predicting and Improving Text Readability for Target Reader Populations*, 57–65.

Skulic, J., & Leung, K. K. (2015). Application of network coding in a wireless sensor networks for bridge monitoring. *Proceedings of IEEE 23rd International Symposium on Personal, Indoor and Mobile Radio Communication, 10*(1), 789–795.

Sonderman, K. A., Nkurunziza, T., Kateera, F., Gruendl, M., Koch, R., Gaju, E., ... Riviello, R. (2018). Using mobile health technology and community health workers to identify and refer cesarean-related surgical site infections in rural Rwanda: A randomised controlled trial protocol. *BMJ Open*, *8*(5), e022214. PMID:29739786

Song, Y., Huang, J., Zhou, D., Zha, H., & Giles, C. L. (2007). IKNN: Informative K-Nearest Neighbor Pattern Classification. In *Proceedings of the 11th European conference on Principles and Practice of Knowledge Discovery in Databases* (pp. 248-264), Springer Berlin Heidelberg.

Sonune, S., Kalbande, D., Yeole, A., & Oak, S. (2017), Issues in IoT Healthcare Platforms: A Critical Study and Review. *IEEE International Conference on Intelligent Computing and Control (I2C2)*, 1-5. 10.1109/I2C2.2017.8321898

Sopic, D., Aminifar, A., & Atienza, D. (2018). e-Glass: A Wearable System for Real-Time Detection of Epileptic Seizures. In *2018 IEEE International Symposium on Circuits and Systems (ISCAS)* (pp. 1–5). IEEE. 10.1109/ISCAS.2018.8351728

Sourav, Chakraborty, & Paul. (2019). Programming Paradigm and Internet of Things. In A Handbook of Internet of Things & Big Data. CRC.

Sourav, Chakraborty, & Sumit. (2018). A Survey on IoT based Traffic Control and Prediction Mechanism. In *Internet of Things and Big data Analytics for Smart Generation, Intelligent Systems Reference Library*. Springer.

Springer, D. B., Zuhike, L. J., Mayosi, B. M., Tarassenko, L., & Clifford, G. D. (2014). *Mobile phone-based rheumatic heart disease diagnosis*. Paper presented at the Appropriate Healthcare Technologies for Low Resource Settings, London, UK. 10.1049/cp.2014.0761

Sravanth, C. C., & Anudeep, B. G. (2019). Classification Algorithms for EEG-based Brain-Computer Interface: A Review. IGI Global.

Stamate, D., Katrinecz, A., Alghamdi, W., Stahl, D., Delespaul, P., van Os, J., & Guloksuz, S. (2017). *Predicting Psychosis Using the Experience Sampling Method with Mobile Apps*. Paper presented at the IEEE International Conference on Machine Learning and Applications, Cancun, Mexico. 10.1109/ICMLA.2017.00-84

Standard. Information Security and Cryptography. (2002). New York, NY: Springer.

Stankevich, E., Paramonov, I., & Timofeev, I. (2012). *Mobile phone sensors in health applications*. Paper presented at the 12th Conference of Open Innovations Association, Oulu, Finland.

Stauffer, C., & Grimson, W. (1999). Adaptive Background Mixture Models for Real-time Tracking. In *IEEE Computer Society Conference on Computer Vision and Pattern Recognition* (Vol. 2, pp. 246-252). Fort Collins, CO: IEEE. 10.1109/CVPR.1999.784637

Sterken, T., Vanfleteren, J., Torfs, T., de Beeck, M. O., Bossuyt, F., & Van Hoof, C. (2011). Ultra-Thin Chip Package (UTCP) and Stretchable Circuit Technologies for Wearable ECG System. *Proc. Annual International Conference of the IEEE Engineering in Medicine and Biology Society*. 10.1109/IEMBS.2011.6091734

Subasi, A., Radhwan, M., Kurdi, R., & Khateeb, K. (2018). IoT based Mobile Healthcare System for Human Activity Recognition. *IEEE 15th Learning and Technology Conference (L&T)*, 29-34.

Sufi, F., Khalil, I., & Tari, Z. (2010). *A cardiod based technique to identify cardiovascular diseases using mobile phones and body sensors.* Paper presented at theIEEE Engineering in Medicine and Biology, Buenos Aires, Argentina. 10.1109/IEMBS.2010.5626578

Sun, B., Chen, W., & Zheng, X. (2012). The System Design for the Extraction and Pre-processing of Surface EMG. *Proc. World Congress on Medical Physics and Biomedical Engineering*, 33, 8 – 13. 10.1016/j.phpro.2012.05.023

Sun, Y., Lo, F. P.-W., & Lo, B. (2019). EEG-based user identification system using 1D-convolutional long short-term memory neural networks. *Expert Systems with Applications*, *125*, 259–267. doi:10.1016/j.eswa.2019.01.080

Suo, H., Wan, J., Zou, C., & Liu, J. (2012). Security in the internet of things: a review. In *Proc. 2012 IEEE International Conference on Computer Science and Electronics Engineering (ICCSEE)*, (Vol. 3, pp. 648-665). Hangzhou, China: IEEE. 10.1109/ICCSEE.2012.373

Suresh, S., Omkar, S. N., & Mani, V. (2005). Parallel implementation of back-propagation algorithm in networks of workstations. *IEEE Transactions on Parallel and Distributed Systems*, *16*(1), 24–34. doi:10.1109/TPDS.2005.11

Sur, S., Crotty, T. B., Kephart, G. M., Hyma, B. A., Colby, T. V., Reed, C. E., ... Gleich, G. J. (1993). Sudden-onset fatal asthma: A distinct entity with few eosinophils and relatively more neutrophils in the airway submucosa? *The American Review of Respiratory Disease*, *148*(3), 713–719. doi:10.1164/ajrccm/148.3.713 PMID:8368644

Tang, S., Ghose, B., Hoque, M. R., Hao, G., & Yaya, S. (2019). Women Using Mobile Phones for Health Communication Are More Likely to Use Prenatal and Postnatal Services in Bangladesh: Cross-Sectional Study. *JMIR mHealth and uHealth*, *7*(2), e10645. doi:10.2196/10645 PMID:30816850

Taniar, D. (2008). *Data Mining and Knowledge Discovery Technologies*. Hershey, PA: IGI Global. doi:10.4018/978-1-59904-960-1

Teng, M. H., Hou, Y. M., Chang, S. H., & Cheng, H. J. (2019). Home-delivered attention bias modification training via smartphone to improve attention control in sub-clinical generalized anxiety disorder: A randomized, controlled multi-session experiment. *Journal of Affective Disorders*, *246*, 444–451. doi:10.1016/j.jad.2018.12.118 PMID:30599367

Thap, T., Yoon, K. H., & Lee, J. (2016). Graphite based electrode for ecg monitoring: Evaluation under freshwater and saltwater conditions. *Sensors (Basel)*, *16*(4), 542. doi:10.339016040542 PMID:27092502

Toh, W. Y., Tan, Y. K., Koh, W. S., & Siek, L. (2014). Autonomous wearable sensor nodes with flexible energy harvesting. *IEEE Sensors Journal*, *14*(7), 2299–2306. doi:10.1109/JSEN.2014.2309900

Tsiouris, K. M., Gatsios, D., Rigas, G., Miljkovic, D., Seljak, B. K., Bohanec, M., & Fotiadis, D. I. (2017). PD_Manager: an mHealth platform for Parkinson's disease patient management. *Healthcare Technology Letters, 4*(3), 102-108.

Tsoutsos, N. G., & Maniatakos, M. (2018). Efficient Detection for Malicious and Random Errors in Additive Encrypted Computation. *IEEE Transactions on Computers*, *67*(1), 16–31. doi:10.1109/TC.2017.2722440

Tzanis, G. (2018). Healthcare data analysis in the Internet of things era. In D. B. A. Khosrow-Pour (Ed.), *Encyclopedia of information science and technology* (4th ed.; pp. 1984–1994). Hershey, PA: IGI Global. doi:10.4018/978-1-5225-2255-3.ch172

Tzimourta, K. D., Tzallas, A. T., Giannakeas, N., Astrakas, L. G., Tsalikakis, D. G., Angelidis, P., & Tsipouras, M. G. (2019). A robust methodology for classification of epileptic seizures in EEG signals. *Health and Technology*, *9*(2), 135–142. doi:10.100712553-018-0265-z

Ullah, S., Higgins, H., & Braem, B. (2012). A comprehensive survey of wireless body area networks. *Journal of Med Systems, 36*(3), 1065–1094.

Ullah, K., Shah, M. A., & Zhang, S. (2016). Effective ways to use Internet of Things in the field of medical and smart health care. *IEEE International Conference on Intelligent Systems Engineering (ICISE)*, 372-379. 10.1109/INTELSE.2016.7475151

USEFIL. (2013). *USEFIL project.* Available at: http://www.usefil.eu/

Vagg, T., Tan, Y. Y., Shortt, C., Hickey, C., Plant, B. J., & Tabirca, S. (2018). *MHealth and serious game analytics for cystic fibrosis adults.* Paper presented at the 31st International Symposium on Computer-Based Medical Systems, Karlstad, Sweden. 10.1109/CBMS.2018.00025

Van Dijk, M., Gentry, C., Halevi, S., & Vaikuntanathan, V. (2010, May). Fully homomorphic encryption over the integers. In *Annual International Conference on the Theory and Applications of Cryptographic Techniques* (pp. 24-43). Springer.

Vergara, M., de la Cal, E., Villar, J. R., González, V. M., & Sedano, J. (2017). An IoT Platform for Epilepsy Monitoring and Supervising. *Journal of Sensors*, *2017*, 1–18. doi:10.1155/2017/6043069

Vicnesh, J., & Hagiwara, Y. (2019). Accurate Detection of Seizure using Nonlinear Parameters Extracted from EEG Signals. *Journal of Mechanics in Medicine and Biology*, *19*(01), 1940004. doi:10.1142/S0219519419400049

Vippalapalli, V., & Ananthula, S. (2016, October). Internet of things (IoT) based smart health care system. In *2016 International Conference on Signal Processing, Communication, Power and Embedded System (SCOPES)* (pp. 1229-1233). IEEE. 10.1109/SCOPES.2016.7955637

Wagenmakers, E.-J., Steyvers, M., Raaijmakers, J. G. W., Shiffrin, R. M., van Rijn, H., & Zeelenberg, R. (2004). A model for evidence accumulation in the lexical decision task. *Cognitive Psychology*, *48*(3), 332–367. doi:10.1016/j.cogpsych.2003.08.001 PMID:15020215

Waher, P. (2014). Securing the Life Cycle of Things. *Internet of Things using Thing Registries.*

Wang, J. (2014). An enhanced fall detection system for elderly person monitoring using consumer home networks. *IEEE Transactions on Consumer Electronics*, *60*(1), 23–29. doi:10.1109/TCE.2014.6780921

Wang, L. F., Liu, J. Q., Yan, X. X., Yang, B., & Yang, C. S. (2013). A MEMS-based pyramid micro-needle electrode for long-term EEG measurement. *Microsystem Technologies*, *19*(2), 269–276. doi:10.100700542-012-1638-2

Wang, S.-W., Im, J.-P., & Cho, G.-H. (2011). Dual-input dual-output energy harvesting DC-DC boost converter for wireless body area network. In *IEEE Biomedical Circuits and Systems Conference (BioCAS)* (pp.217-220). IEEE. 10.1109/BioCAS.2011.6107766

Wang, Y., Wu, K., & Ni, L. M. (2017). Wifall: Device-free fall detection by wireless networks. *IEEE Transactions on Mobile Computing*, *16*(2), 581–594. doi:10.1109/TMC.2016.2557792

Weinstein, E. B., Spitzer, J. B., & Ventry, I. M. (1986). Test-retest reliability of the Hearing Handicap Inventory for the Elderly. *Ear and Hearing*, *7*(5), 295–299. doi:10.1097/00003446-198610000-00002 PMID:3770324

Wenyin, Z., & Shih, F. Y. (2011). Semi-fragile spatial watermarking based on local binary pattern operators. *Optics Communications*, *284*(16-17), 3904–3912. doi:10.1016/j.optcom.2011.04.004

Wilson, S., & Liang, R. (2018). *Wearable technology: Present and future*. Paper presented at the 91st World Conference of the textile institute, Leeds, UK

Wood, C. S., Thomas, M. R., Budd, J., Mashamba-Thompson, T. P., Herbst, K., Pillay, D., ... Stevens, M. M. (2019). Taking connected mobile-health diagnostics of infectious diseases to the field. *Nature*, *566*(7745), 467–474. doi:10.103841586-019-0956-2 PMID:30814711

World Health Organisation. (2011). mHealth: New horizons for health through mobile technologies. WHO Press.

World Health Organization. (2012). *Health Topics Ageing*. Available at: http://www.who.int/topics/ageing/en/

World Health Organization. (2013). *Physical Activity and Older Adults*. Available at: http://www.who.int/ dietphysicalactivity/factsheet_olderadults

Wu, D. N., Gan, Q. Q., & Wang, X. M. (2018). Verifiable Public Key Encryption With Keyword Search Based on Homomorphic Encryption in Multi-User Setting. *IEEE Access: Practical Innovations, Open Solutions*, *6*, 42445–42453. doi:10.1109/ACCESS.2018.2861424

Wu, J., Cai, Z., & Gao, Z. (2010). Dynamic K-Nearest-Neighbor with Distance and Attribute Weighted for Classification. In *Proceedings of the International Conference on Electronics and Information Engineering* (vol. 1, pp. 356-360). Kyoto. 10.1109/ICEIE.2010.5559858

Wu, X., & Vipin Kumar, J. (2007). Top 10 algorithms in data mining. *Knowledge and Information Systems*, *14*(1), 1–37. doi:10.100710115-007-0114-2

Xia, H., Asif, I., & Zhao, X. (2013). Cloud-ECG for real time ECG monitoring and analysis. *Computer Methods and Programs in Biomedicine*, *110*(3), 253–259. doi:10.1016/j.cmpb.2012.11.008 PMID:23261079

Xie, Liu, & Xue. (2017). *A survey of dimensionality reduction techniques based on random projection*. CoRR abs/1706.04371.

Xna, S., & Lee, H.K. (2013). Neural network approach for damaged area location prediction of a composite plate using Electromechanical impedance technique. *Journal of Composite Science and Technology*, *56*, 794–804.

Yang, X., Yi, X., Nepal, S., Kelarev, A., & Han, F. (2018). A Secure Verifiable Ranked Choice Online Voting System Based on Homomorphic Encryption. *IEEE Access: Practical Innovations, Open Solutions*, *6*, 20506–20519. doi:10.1109/ACCESS.2018.2817518

Yang, Z., Zhou, Q., Lei, L., Zheng, K., & Xiang, W. (2016). An IoT-cloud Based Wearable ECG Monitoring System for Smart Healthcare. *Journal of Medical Systems*, *40*(286), 1–11. PMID:27796840

Yao, A. C. (1982, November). Protocols for secure computations. In *Foundations of Computer Science, 1982. SFCS'08. 23rd Annual Symposium on* (pp. 160-164). IEEE. 10.1109/SFCS.1982.38

Yasuda, M. (2017). Secure Hamming distance computation for biometrics using ideal-lattice and ring-LWE homomorphic encryption. *Information Security Journal: A Global Perspective, 26*(2), 85-103.

Ying, H., Schnitzer, A., Leonhardt, S., & Schiek, M. (2007). *Automatic step detection in the accelerometer signal.* Body Sensor Networks BSN2007, Aachen, Germany.

Yu, D. X., Parmanto, B., Dicianno, B. E., Watzlaf, V. J., & Seelman, K. D. (2014). *Accessible mHealth for patients with dexterity impairments*. Paper presented at the 16th International ACM SIGACCESS Conference on Computers & Accessibility, Rochester, NY. 10.1145/2661334.2661402

Zanella, A., Bui, N., Castellani, A., Vangelista, L., & Zorzi, M. (2014). Internet of Things for Smart Cities. *IEEE Internet of Things Journal*, *1*(1), 22–32. doi:10.1109/JIOT.2014.2306328

Zennifa, F., Filtrilina, H. &Iramina, K. (2014). *Prototype early warning system for heart disease detection using android application*. Paper presented at the Annual International Conference of the IEEE Engineering in Medicine and Biology Society, Chicago, IL. 10.1109/EMBC.2014.6944369

Zhang, E., Peng, J., & Li, M. (2017). Outsourcing secret sharing scheme based on homomorphism encryption. *IET Information Security*, *12*(1), 94–99. doi:10.1049/iet-ifs.2017.0026

Zhang, Q., Cheng, L., & Boutaba, R. (2010). Cloud computing: State-of-the-art and research challenges. *Journal of Internet Services and Applications*, *1*(1), 7–18. doi:10.100713174-010-0007-6

Zhang, S.-L., Zhang, B., Su, Y.-L., & Song, J.-L. (2019). A novel EEG-complexity-based feature and its application on the epileptic seizure detection. *International Journal of Machine Learning and Cybernetics*. doi:10.100713042-019-00921-w

Zhou, J., Leppanen, T., Harjula, E., Ylianttila, M., Ojala, T., & Yu, C., … Yang, L. T. (2013). CloudThings: A common architecture for integrating the Internet of Things with Cloud Computing. In *Proceedings of the 2013 IEEE 17th International Conference on Computer Supported Cooperative Work in Design (CSCWD)* (pp. 651–657). IEEE. 10.1109/CSCWD.2013.6581037

Zhou, T., Yang, X., Liu, L., Zhang, W., & Li, N. (2018). Faster bootstrapping with multiple addends. *IEEE Access: Practical Innovations, Open Solutions*, *6*, 49868–49876. doi:10.1109/ACCESS.2018.2867655

Zhou, Y., Ding, X., Zhang, J., Duan, Y., Hu, J., & Yang, X. (2014). Fabrication of conductive fabric as textile electrode for ECG monitoring. *Fibers and Polymers*, *15*(11), 2260–2264. doi:10.100712221-014-2260-y

Zhu, Bojian, Li, Gu, & Yang. (2018). On the development of security monitoring system via a wireless sensing network. *Journal of a Wireless Communication Networking, 16*(6), 1685-1697.

About the Contributors

Chinmay Chakraborty is a Senior Assistant Professor in the Dept. of Electronics and Communication Engineering, BIT Mesra, Jharkhand, India. His primary areas of research include WBAN, Internet of Medical Things, Medical Imaging and Telemedicine. Prior to BIT, he worked at the Faculty of Science and Technology, ICFAI University, Agartala, India as a Sr. Lecturer. He worked as a Research Consultant in the Coal India project at Industrial Engineering & Management, IIT Kharagpur. He worked as a project coordinator of Telecom Convergence Switch project under the Indo-US joint initiative. He also worked as a Network Engineer in System Administration at MISPL under Global Teleservice Ltd., India. He is the author of "PSTN-IP Telephony Gateway for Ensuring QoS in Heterogeneous Networks" (2014) and "Advanced Classification Techniques for Healthcare Analysis" (2019). He is an Editorial Board Member in the Journal of Wireless Communication Technology, Int. Journal of Telecomm. Engg. etc. and also a member of the International Advisory Board for Malaysia Technical Scientist Congress and the MIR Labs. He has been also editing four books on IGI, IET, CRC, and Pan Standford Publishing. He is a guest editor of Future Internet journal special issue (Internet of Healthcare Things (IoHT): Methods, Advances, and Applications) and SoCTA-19 Int. Conf., Patna on Computational Intelligence and Bioinformatics for Smart Healthcare Technology. He received a young research excellence award, Global Peer Review Award, Young Faculty Award, and Outstanding Researcher Award. He was the speakers for AICTE, DST sponsored FDP and CEP Short Term Courses.

* * *

Shyam Akashe was born in Achalpur, a city in Maharashtra, India on 22nd May 1976. He did M.Tech in Electronics & Communication Engineering from Rajiv Gandhi Proudyogiki Vishwavidyalaya (RGPV), Bhopal in 2006 and Ph.D Thapar University, Patiala (previously Thapar Institute of Engineering and Technology), Punjab in 2013. Dr. Akashe worked as Assistant Professor at Institute of Technology & Management (ITM) Gwalior. Currently, he is working as Professor and Post-graduation Coordinator, Electronics & Communication Engineering department at ITM University Gwalior. Dr. Akashe is authored/co-authored more than 200 research papers in peer reviewed international/national journals and conferences. He has also published 5 patent, 2 copyright, 2 books and 1 chapter.His biography published in Marquis's Who's Who in Engineering Field, USA awarded by Marquis, 2015. His areas of research are Low Power VLSI Design, Modeling, FinFET based memory design, Circuits for future VLSI Technology, Digital Design and FPGA implementation. He is life member of the Institution of Engineers (IE), Life Member of the Indian Society for Technical Education (IETE), Life Member of the Indian Society for Technical Education (ISTE) and Life Member of the Instrumentation Society of India (ISOI), also he is member of VLSI Society of India (VSI). Dr. Akashe is editorial board member of the IEEE African Journal of Computing & ICTS (IEEE Nigeria). He is also a reviewer for IEEE Transaction on VLSI Systems, IEEE Transactions on Nanotechnology, International Journal of Electronics (Taylor and Francis), Microelectronics Journal (Elsevier).

Arunadevi B. is presently Associate Professor, Department of Electronics and Communication Engineering, Dr. N.G.P Institute of Technology, Coimbatore. She has 13 years of teaching and research experience in the fields of Digital Image Processing, Medical Image Analysis, Pattern Recognition, Soft Computing, Multi-dimensional System and Knowledge-based System and Robotics. She has published 12 papers in International and National Journals to her credit.

Pradeep Reddy CH is currently working as Associate Professor in VIT-AP University, Amaravati, India. He has a total of thirteen years experience in both teaching and research. He received his B.Tech in Computer Science and Engineering from PBR VITS, JNTU Andhra Pradesh, India and M.Tech in Computer Science and Engineering from VIT University, Vellore, India. He did his PhD in Computer Science and Engineering from VIT University, Vellore. He has published various journals and served as reviewer and editor for reputed journals. His research interests include Wireless Networks, IoT, Security systems and Cloud computing.

Bhanu Chander received B.Tech Degree in Computer science and Engineering from Acharya Nagarjuna University in 2013, Received M.Tech degree form Computer science and Engineering From Central university of Rajasthan in 2016 and Presntly am Full time Research Scholar in Department of computer science and Engineering form Pondicherry University. my research interest areas are Wireless sensor networks, Internet of Things, Cryptography, Image processing.

Jeyamala Chandrasekaran is working currently as Assistant Professor in the Department of Information Technology, Thiagarajar College of Engineering. Her Academic qualifications include Post graduate of Computer Science and Engineering from Anna University, Chennai. She has completed her research in the domain of Multimedia Security. She has been part of the teaching fraternity since 2005 guiding Under graduate and Post graduate Information Technology Students. Her teaching interests include Cryptography, Artificial intelligence, Network security and Information Systems. Her research publications include 5 international journals and 10 international conferences. She has undergone various pedagogical training programmes and has a keen interest in using different teaching learning methodologies. She has been an active reviewer in various international journals like Multidimensional Systems and Signal processing, 3D Research and in various international conferences.

Mahendra Kumar Das received his BSc degree from V. B. U. Hazaribag and MSc degree from Ranchi University, Ranchi, Jharkhand, India. Currently, he is working in Birla Institute of Technology, Deoghar Campus, Jharkhand, India. He has two years research experience in B. I. T. Mesra, Ranchi from March 2006 to July 2008 and ten years teaching experience. His area of research interest is sensors and transducers.

Akash Gupta received his Bachelor's degree in Electronics and Communication Engineering from SVITS, Indore and Master's degree in Electrconics and Communication Engineering from Birla Institute of technology, Mesra, Ranchi. He is pursuing PhD from National Institute of Technology, Patna. Presently, he is working as an Assistant Professor in Birla Institute of Technology, Mesra, Deoghar campus, Jharkhand. His area of interest is bio-medical signal processing and Brain-Computer Interface.

Bharat Gupta attached to the field of education and research for last fifteen years. He is a senior member of IEEE (USA). He did his graduation in (honors) 2000 and post-graduation in 2003. He did his doctorate from University of Rome, Tor Vergata, Italy. Presently, He is working as an Assistant Professor in Department of Electronics & Communication Engineering, National Institute of Technology Patna, Bihar. He is the Professor In-Charge of Incubation Centre, NIT Patna and Nodal officer for Bihar startup at NIT Patna. Dr. Gupta is the Chief Investigator for the project "Scheme for Financial Assistance for setting up of Electronics and ICT Academies" at NIT Patna sponsored by Ministry of Electronics and Information Technology (MeitY), Govt. of India. Dr. Gupta is also Co-Chief Investigator for the project "Remote Detection of Humans Trapped under Debris in Disaster Affected Areas Using RF Sensing of Cardiopulmonary Motion" under SMDP Project. He has delivered many lectures in International & National conferences and workshops. He has published more than 60 paper in International and National Journals and conferences. He has acted as reviewer of many international conferences & journals. He was in Advisory Committee in National Conference on "Emerging Trends in Electronics and Telecommunication Engineering" and has also chaired many sessions in conferences. He has organized the workshops at national and international level. His research area covers mainly Wireless Body Area Network, Routing and MAC protocol for Medical Wireless Communication, ICT for Health care, Internet of Thing (IoT), Medical IoT (MioT), FM-UWB communication technology, etc.

Sandhya Harikumar received her B.E in Computer Engineering from Birla VishwaKarma Mahavidyalaya, Gujarat, India and M.Tech in Computer Science & Engineering from Indian Institute of Technology, Delhi. She is pursuing her Ph.D in the area of machine learning. She is an academician and has more than 15 years of teaching experience. Her areas of interest include DBMS, Machine Learning, and Distributed computing.

Gloria Ejehiohen Iyawa is a Senior Lecturer in the Department of Informatics, Namibia University of Science and Technology. Her research interests include Digital Health and Health Informatics.

Ambika Nagaraj Nagaraj has completed her MCA in the year 2001 and M.Phil in the year 2008. She has completed her Ph.D. from Bharathiar University, Coimbatore. She has 12 years of teaching experience. She has published a significant amount of papers in chapters in books, national/ International conference papers and Journals. Presently she is working as a faculty in the computer science department at SSMRV degree college.

Ibtihel Nouira received the B.Eng. degree in industrial electronics in 2008 from NATIONAL Engineering School of Sousse, Tunisia. In 2010, she received the M. Eng. Degree in intelligent and communicating systems from the same School. In 2015, she obtained her PhD in Electrical Engineering from the National School of Engineers of Sfax, Tunisia. Currently, she is a member of the Medical Imaging and Technology Laboratory at the Faculty of Medecine of Monastir, Tunisia and both she is an assistant professor at the Higher Institute of Computer Science and Mathematics of Monastir, Tunisia. Her research interests are on the treatment and analysis of physiological signals, acceleration on GPU and IOT system.

Collins Oduor is an assistant professor Information systems at the School of Science and Technology, United States International University and he has good teaching and research experience at university level. He also have a vast experience in the fields of ICT Consultancies and Teaching, lifelong learning, and ICT integration in Education Programs, Collins has done vast experience in ICT integration in education through training for teacher trainees in Primary Teacher Training Colleges in Kenya. Collins has also participated in the Accelerated 21st Century Education (ACE) ICT integration in Education Pilot Project for Ministry of Education, Teacher Education Professional Development Programme 2009-2012 as a consultant and as a master trainer. Collins has also participated in the Inter University Council of East Africa (IUCEA) Staff mobility programme as external examiner 2015 & 2018 and Third United Nations Environmental Assembly (UNEA) general assembly as delegate and recently he was a speaker at the world summit on information systems (WSIS) held in Geneva Switzerland and, he has supervised twelve masters students thesis/projects, participated in various curricula development for so many universities in the region. In addition to the membership in professional bodies, Dr Oduor have also done three book chapter publications and presented at least ten papers in referred journals plus additional international conferences on ICT.Collins is also a review editor of papers in the International Journal of research publications. Collins is now keen on research areas covering more on ICT integration in Education, Citizen Science, Community services and linkages.

Jude Osakwe is a Senior Lecturer, Department of Informatics, Faculty of Computing and Informatics, Namibia University of Science and Technology, Windhoek.

S. Preethi received the B.E. and M.E. Degrees in Electronics & Communication Engineering in 2011, 2016 respectively. Initially, she have been associated with Nokia Solutions & Networks Ltd as Network Planning & Optimization Engineer for 2.4 years and have worked with various operators globally (Tele2-Russia, MTS-Russia, TMobile-Germany, Airtel-Kenya, Claro Colombia) for planning and optimization of Core elements such as MSS, MGW & HLR in real time networks. Currently she is associated with Dr.N.G.P. Institute of Technology as Assistant Professor in the Department of Electronics & Communication. She has published several papers and book chapters in National and International Conferences and Journals. She is a fellow of ISRD and IAENG. Her research interests are Medical Image & Signal Processing, Machine Learning, Optimization techniques, and Mobile Communication Networks.

Mohamed Hadj Said was born in Monastir, Tunisia in 1987. He received the B.Sc.'10 and M.Sc'12 degrees both from the Higher Institute of informatics and Mathematics of Monastir (ISIMM, Tunisia). His Master is done in collaboration with the laboratory of Sensors, Microsystems and Actuators of Louvain-la-Neuve (SMALL), Belgium. He received the PhD student from the National Engineering

School of Monastir (ENIM) in collaboration with TIMA Laboratory France and Indian Institute of Technology in Mumbai. Actually he working on the design, modeling and simulation of a novel MEMS microphone based in magnetic detection in CMOS Technology. Furthermore, he interests in magnetic sensors, surface acoustic wave modeling sensors, acoustic sensors, MEMS and NEMS, microfabrication, IOT, Instrumentation and Analog devices.

Pavithra V. is currently pursuing masters degree in the Department of Computer Science and Information Security at Thiagarajar College of Engineering, Madurai. She completed her Bachelor's degree in the stream of Information Technology at Velammal College of Engineering and Technology. Her areas of interest are Security and Ethical Hacking. Her current research project is in the area of Medical Image Security.

Prasannadevi V. is Assistant Professor at the Department of Electronics and Communication Engineering, Dr. NGP Institute of Technology. She obtained a bachelor degree in Electronics and Communication Engineering in Government College of Engineering Tirunelveli under Manonmaniam Sundaranar University and Masters degree in VLSI Design in Arulmigu Kalasalingam Engineering College under Anna University. Worked in Teknoturf Info Service since 2006 as tutor on various technologies and programming languages as C, C++, Java, Linux till 2013. Following which she joined Dr. NGP Institute of Technology as Assistant professor since 2014, supported Placement department while being integral part of Electronics and Communication Engineering Department.

Desam Vamsi is studying PhD in VIT-AP University, Amaravati, India. She received her B.Tech in Computer Science and Engineering from NIET, JNTUK Andhra Pradesh, India and M.Tech in Computer Science and Engineering from NIT, JNTUK, Andhra Pradesh. Her research area is Information Security.

Seelam Vasavi Sai Viswanada Prabhu Deva Kumar born at Chintalapudi, a city in Andhra Pradesh, India on 15th June 1996. He is a Certified Chartered Engineer (CEng) in the division of Electronics and Telecommunication from the Institution of Engineers, India (IEI), Master's Degree from Electrical & Computer Engineering (Majoring in Electrical Engineering) and currently working as a Graduate Researcher in Laser & Sensor Application Laboratory from Pusan National University, Busan, South Korea in 2018-2020 and completed B.Tech in Electronics & Communication Engineering from Institute of Technology & Management University (ITM U), Gwalior, India in 2014-2018 and his area of research are Energy Storage Systems (ESS), High Frequency DC-DC Converters, Control Systems, LED Fabrication and Designing, Real Time Embedded Systems (Atmel, ARM), IoT (Internet of Things), Low Power VLSI Design, Modeling, CMOS based memory design, Memristor based circuit design, Circuits for future VLSI Technology, Digital Design & FPGA Implementation. He worked as an Intern in Fuzinix Infotech Pvt. Ltd. and SION Semiconductors Pvt. Ltd. Seelam Vasavi Sai Viswanada Prabhu Deva Kumar is authored few research papers in peer reviewed international journals, conferences and magazines. He is an Editorial Member in International Journal of Information Technology and Computer Science (IJOIT). Associate Member of the Institution of Engineers, India (IEI), Life Member of the Solar Energy Society of India (SESI), Member of the International Association of Engineers (IAENG) (Hong Kong), Member of Institute of Electrical and Electronics Engineers (IEEE) (Seoul) and The Institute of Engineering and Technology (IET) (UK).

Index

P

R

S

T

W

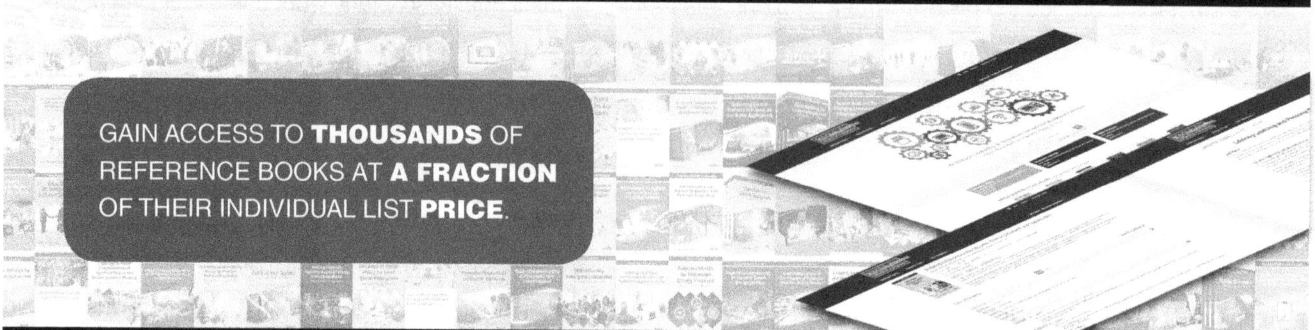
GAIN ACCESS TO **THOUSANDS** OF REFERENCE BOOKS AT **A FRACTION** OF THEIR INDIVIDUAL LIST **PRICE**.

www.ingramcontent.com/pod-product-compliance
Lightning Source LLC
LaVergne TN
LVHW062152300926
849161LV00010B/2646